Life Balance

Multidisciplinary Theories and Research

Life Balance

MULTIDISCIPLINARY THEORIES AND RESEARCH

EDITORS:

KATHLEEN MATUSKA
ST. CATHERINE UNIVERSITY
ST. PAUL, MN

CHARLES H. CHRISTIANSEN
THE AMERICAN OCCUPATIONAL THERAPY FOUNDATION
BETHESDA, MD

ASSOCIATE EDITORS:

HELENE J. POLATAJKO
UNIVERSITY OF TORONTO
TORONTO, ONTARIO, CANADA

JANE A. DAVIS
UNIVERSITY OF TORONTO
TORONTO, ONTARIO, CANADA

FOREWORD BY BRIAN R. LITTLE

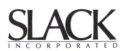

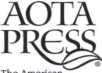

The American
Occupational Therapy
Association, Inc.

www.slackbooks.com • www.aota.org

ISBN: 978-1-55642-906-4

The procedures and practices described in this book should be implemented in a manner consistent with the professional standards set for the circumstances that apply in each specific situation. Every effort has been made to confirm the accuracy of the information presented and to correctly relate generally accepted practices. The authors, editor, and publishers cannot accept responsibility for errors or exclusions or for the outcome of the material presented herein. There is no expressed or implied warranty of this book or information imparted by it. Care has been taken to ensure that drug selection and dosages are in accordance with currently accepted/recommended practice. Due to continuing research, changes in government policy and regulations, and various effects of drug reactions and interactions, it is recommended that the reader carefully review all materials and literature provided for each drug, especially those that are new or not frequently used. Any review or mention of specific companies or products is not intended as an endorsement by the authors or publishers.

SLACK Incorporated and AOTA Press use a review process to evaluate submitted material. Prior to publication, educators or clinicians provide important feedback on the content that we publish. We welcome feedback on this work.

Published by: SLACK Incorporated   AOTA Press
                 6900 Grove Road   4720 Montgomery Lane
                 Thorofare, NJ 08086 USA   Bethesda, MD 20824-1220 USA
                 Telephone: 856-848-1000   Telephone: 301-652-6611
                 Fax: 856-848-6091   Fax: 301-652-7711
                 www.slackbooks.com   www.aota.org
                                                  To order: 877-404-AOTA or store.aota.org

Contact SLACK Incorporated or AOTA Press for more information about other books in this field or about the availability of our books from distributors outside the United States.

Library of Congress Cataloging-in-Publication Data

Life balance : multidisciplinary theories and research / editors, Kathleen Matuska, Charles H. Christiansen ; associate editors, Helene Polatajko, Jane A. Davis.
    p. ; cm.
  Includes bibliographical references and index.
  ISBN 978-1-55642-906-4 (hardcover)
  1. Lifestyles--Congresses. 2. Quality of life--Congresses. 3. Health behavior--Congresses. 4. Health--Congresses. I. Matuska, Kathleen M. II. Christiansen, Charles.
  [DNLM: 1. Life Style--Congresses. 2. Quality of Life--Congresses. 3. Health Behavior--Congresses. WA 30 L722 2009]
  HQ2042.L53 2009
  646.7001--dc22
                        2009023938

Printed in the United States of America.

Last digit is print number: 10 9 8 7 6 5 4 3 2 1

DEDICATIONS

To Charles, for opening doors.
—Kathleen Matuska

To Carrie, Erik, and Kalle, who constantly remind me of the blessings of parenthood.
—Charles H. Christiansen

To my parents and my students and my clients, for teaching me about work and life.
—Helene J. Polatajko

To my parents, Caroline and Norman Davis, for their continued support
in helping me pursue my goals.
—Jane A. Davis

CONTENTS

Contents

ABOUT THE EDITORS

Kathleen Matuska is the Master of Arts in Occupational Therapy Program Director in the School of Health at St. Catherine University. She has contributed to the life balance scholarly discussion through published journal articles and presentations at national and international conferences. Her research and scholarly interests are primarily about understanding or clarifying the construct of life balance and determining ways to measure life balance for ongoing research and clinical application.

Dr. Charles Christiansen is Executive Director of The American Occupational Therapy Foundation. Previously, he spent three decades in academic roles at various universities, including the University of Minnesota, The University of Texas Medical Branch, and The University of British Columbia. Dr. Christiansen holds degrees in educational administration, counseling psychology, and occupational therapy. His scholarly and scientific interests inhabit the domain of lifestyle and health, with a particular focus on individual patterns of activity over the life course and how these influence well-being. He is particularly interested in how the interconnections of social, psychological, and neurophysiological mechanism explain adaptation to stressful circumstances.

Dr. Helene J. Polatajko is an internationally acclaimed researcher, educator, and clinician with extensive experience in assessment and intervention research. Dr. Polatajko is extremely well-published with over 200 publications, including books, chapters, and peer-reviewed articles. She has given over 400 presentations in over 20 countries. Dr. Polatajko is one of the authors of the well-known *Canadian Occupational Performance Measure*, now published in over 20 languages. She is also a primary author of *Enabling Occupation II: Advancing an Occupational Therapy Vision for Health, Well-Being, & Justice Through Occupation*. She has received numerous honors and awards, including the Muriel Driver Lectureship and induction into the American Occupational Therapy Foundation Academy of Research.

Jane A. Davis is a lecturer in the Department of Occupational Science and Occupational Therapy at the University of Toronto. Jane's current research is focused on examining the causal mechanisms that have lead to the production and reproduction of the current work–life balance discourse. She has presented her work at numerous conferences, published in occupation-based journals, and is a co-author of numerous book chapters related to enabling occupation, occupational development, and methods of inquiry. She serves as a board member for the Canadian Society of Occupational Scientists and co-edits a column entitled "Sense of Doing," on behalf of CSOS, in the Canadian Association of Occupational Therapists *OT Now* journal.

CONTRIBUTING AUTHORS

Beatriz C. Abreu, PhD
University of Texas Medical Branch at
Galveston
Transitional Learning Center at Galveston
Galveston, Texas

Dana Anaby, Doctoral Candidate
Rehabilitation Sciences
University of British Columbia
Vancouver, British Columbia, Canada

Catherine Backman, PhD, OT(C), FCAOT
Division of Occupational Therapy
University of British Columbia
Vancouver, British Columbia, Canada

Jerome Bickenbach, PhD
Department of Philosophy
Queens University
Kingston, Ontario, Canada

Joan C. Borod, PhD
Neuropsychology Subprogram
Queens College, New York

Robert A. Cummins, PhD
Department of Psychology
Deakin University
Melbourne, Australia

Janet Dunn, PhD
Department of Behavioral Sciences
University of Michigan–Dearborn
Dearborn, Michigan

Thomas Glass, PhD
Department of Epidemiology
Johns Hopkins University
Baltimore, Maryland

Andrew S. Harvey, PhD
Department of Economics
St. Mary's University
Halifax, Nova Scotia, Canada

Lena-Karin Erlandsson, PhD
Division of Occupational Therapy
Lund University
Lund, Sweden

Carita Håkansson, PhD
School of Health Sciences
Jönköping Universty
Jönköping, Sweden

Amy Heinz, MA
Department of Occupational Science and
Occupational Therapy
College of St. Catherine
St. Paul, Minnesota

Sandra Hofferth, PhD
Department of Family Studies
University of Maryland
College Park, Maryland

Hans Jonsson, PhD
Karolinska Institutet
Division of Occupational Therapy
Huddinge, Sweden

David A. Kinney, PhD
Department of Sociology, Anthropology, and
Social Work
Central Michigan University
Mount Pleasant, Michigan

Stephen Marks, PhD
Department of Sociology
University of Maine
Orono, Maine

Mary Ann McColl, PhD
School of Rehabilitation Therapy
Queens University
Kingston, Ontario, Canada

Contributing Authors

Glenn V. Ostir, PhD
University of Texas Medical Branch at Galveston
Galveston, Texas

Kenneth J. Ottenbacher, PhD, OTR, FAOTA
University of Texas Medical Branch at Galveston
Galveston, Texas

Wendy Pentland, PhD
School of Rehabilitation Therapy
Queens University
Kingston, Ontario, Canada

Dennis Persson, PhD
Division of Occupational Therapy
Lund University
Lund, Sweden

Gary Seale, MS
Transitional Learning Center at Galveston
Galveston, Texas

Kennon Sheldon, PhD
Department of Psychology
University of Missouri–Columbia
Columbia, Missouri

Jerome Singleton, PhD
School of Health and Human Performance
Dalhousie University
Halifax, Nova Scotia, Canada

Richard O. Temple, PhD
University of Texas Medical Branch at Galveston
Transitional Learning Center at Galveston
Galveston, Texas

Ruut Veenhoven, PhD
Department of Social Sciences
Erasmus University Rotterdam
The Netherlands

Gail Whiteford, PhD
Macquarie University
Sydney, Australia

Dennis Zgaljardic, PhD
University of Texas Medical Branch at Galveston
Transitional Learning Center at Galveston
Galveston, Texas

Jiri Zuzanek, PhD
Department of Recreation and Leisure Studies
University of Waterloo
Waterloo, Ontario, Canada

PREFACE

The best and safest thing is to keep a balance in your life, acknowledge the great powers around us and in us. If you can do that, and live that way, you are really a wise man.
—*Euripides, Greek tragic dramatist (484 BC–406 BC)*

The early Greeks alerted us to the importance of life balance some 2,500 years ago, yet humankind has still not divined the secrets of achieving it. As the contents of this book will reveal, at the beginning of the third millennium of the common era, our understanding of the concept remains in its infancy. Indeed, as some people struggle to define and quantify the concept, others question its very existence, or at least its desirability, while still others provide formulas for its achievement.

This book, which offers a unique compilation of the diversity of modern thought on the concept of life balance, began as an idea that owes its origin to early thinking about treating mental illness in the late years of the 19th century in the United States. Those early years were characterized by significant cultural change associated with immigration and industrialization. The reform of medical education and the creation of medical schools at universities led to an emphasis on science and research. Psychology and psychiatry emerged as disciplines interested in the mind and behavior.

Adolph Meyer, known as the father of American psychiatry and an early proponent of systematic study, was intent on showing that people could best be understood by studying their lives. Meyer believed that the regular patterns of life were a key to normalizing behavior and helping mental patients recover. His early writings suggested that balanced lives were necessary for mental health.

Sadly, Meyer's writings were as difficult to understand as his lectures, delivered with a thick German accent. Before Meyer's ideas could have much lasting impact, Sigmund Freud burst on the scene with his psychodynamic theories based, in part, on unconscious motives.

In the present era, also characterized by the profound changes of Meyer's time, it is perhaps understandable that thoughts about life characteristics and how they influence well-being would raise interest in the idea of life balance, inviting us to reconsider some of Meyer's original concepts.

Although there has been widespread interest among the public about how to balance lives, the community of scholars has been slow to take up the idea seriously. It was the need to begin thinking more critically about life balance that led to the idea of an invitational conference that would bring together scholars from around the world whose work had touched on this issue in one way or another. In the spring of 2007, a cadre of international scholars convened in the lakeside city of Kingston, Ontario, Canada, to share insights and debate ideas. This book is a compendium of the papers that emerged as a consequence of that scholarly exchange.

This conference was realized thanks to the fine work of the members of the core planning committee: Jane Davis, Betty Abreu, Wendy Pentland, Kathleen Matuska, Catherine Backman, Helene Polatajko and Charles Christiansen and the administrative and financial support of the University of Texas Medical Branch, the American Occupational Therapy Association, the Social Sciences and Humanities Research Council of Canada, the Department of Occupational Science and Occupational Therapy at the University of Toronto, the publishing division of SLACK Incorporated, represented by John Bond and Brien Cummings, and AOTA Press, represented by Chris Davis.

Obviously, a conference cannot succeed without the active participation of scholars. This conference had participants from many disciplines. Despite differences in terminology, they were able to communicate their ideas effectively. Brian Little was masterful in getting things started with a superb keynote address. He then accepted an invitation to write the foreword for the volume, for which we are deeply grateful. Our hope is that the contributions here will help advance thinking about the ways people can organize their lives in a manner that will lead to greater health, happiness, and general well-being.

Charles H. Christiansen
Rockville, Maryland, USA

Kathleen Matuska
St. Paul, Minnesota, USA

Helene J. Polatajko
Toronto, Ontario, Canada

Jane A. Davis
Toronto, Ontario, Canada

June, 2009

FOREWORD

At the risk of losing my balance, I wish to glance backward as I write the foreword to this land-mark volume. I was honored to give the opening address at the conference upon which this book is based, and I wish to revisit parts of the rather personal message about the quality of lives and the subtleties of balance that I presented on that occasion.

But I wish to glance back even farther than that. I must confess to a four-decade–long affair with occupational therapy. Just one week before I began lecturing on psychology at Oxford University in the late 1960s, a colleague was invited to give a course on human personality at the nearby Dorset House School of Occupational Therapy. Fortunately for me, he was unable to do it, and I agreed to take it on for a little extra pocket money.

Although I knew virtually nothing about their field, my very first experience as a lecturer was with occupational therapy students. Once a week, I would bicycle up to Dorset House. There, after tea and scones, I would instruct the "young ladies" on the complexities of human personality and, rather presumptuously, how such knowledge might inform their eventual practice. In turn, the staff and students patiently taught me about human occupation and its relationship to health and well-being. Four decades later, I realize how lucky I was to get early exposure to occupational therapy, particularly its openness to multidisciplinary influences and its focus on the quality of lives. It was to have an enduring effect on my research career and some of my students and col-leagues. The tea and scones were salutary as well.

The influence of Dorset House took a few years to seep through. My early work on "personal projects" (Little, 1972, 1983), though designed to advance the field of personality and developmental psychology, had a clear family resemblance to occupational therapy and the emerging field of occupational science.

But it was not until many years later that I was able to dig deeper into the link between occupational therapy and personal projects by collaborating with Charles Christiansen and his colleagues. Those who know Chuck will realize how fortuitous this was: Among his many other accomplishments he became a leading researcher with personal projects analysis and a dissemina-tor *nonpareil* of the methodology and its applied implications. We were intrigued by the possible role of balanced project pursuit in enhancing the quality of life. The result of these explorations led to some unanticipated conclusions, some of which I will mention in a moment.

But first I need to say a few words about what personal projects are and how they provide a perspective not only on the diverse topics presented in this book but also about the presenters themselves. Consistent with one of the key assumptions of project analytic theory, our conceptual framework should be reflexive; that is, it should equally apply to ourselves and those other selves about whom we explicitly theorize.

Details on the conceptual development, methodology, and applications of personal projects analysis appear in a recent volume and a short online overview is also available.[1] For present purposes I want to summarize where our theorizing and research has taken us when we adopt a personal-projects perspective on human well-being.

Personal projects are extended sets of personally salient action in context. They can range from seemingly trivial tasks like "putting out the cat" to the passionate pursuits of one's life such as "taking care of my daughter." Although personal, they are not restrictively individualistic. Although some are self-focused, many others are utterly selfless or merge with community con-cerns. Although we may be completely absorbed in a single project at any given point in time, we typically live out our days engaged in multiple projects. I believe that these form project systems and their systemic nature entails tradeoffs, conflicts, mutual facilitation, and a variety of other

---

[1]See Little, B. R., Salmela-Aro, & S. D. Phillips (2007). *Personal project pursuit: Goals, action and human flourishing.* Mahwah, NJ: Lawrence Erlbaum and Little, B. R. (2008). Personal projects and free traits: Personality and motivation reconsidered. *Social and Personality Psychology Compass, 2(3),* 1235–1254.

dynamic features. This, of course, takes us to the very heart of this book—the question of balance. Two questions can be posed: *What kind of balancing acts are personal projects,* and *how does such balancing relate to human well-being?*

PERSONAL PROJECTS AS BALANCING ACTS

There are several different ways in which personal project pursuit can be out of balance. First, project pursuit entails the risk of a *meaning–manageability tradeoff.* Those projects that bring us the greatest sense of meaning in our lives may be the least manageable and most chaotic. Therefore, individuals may tilt in the direction of pursuing highly accomplishable projects that are essentially pointless or passionately meaningful projects that can't get off the ground. Similarly, personal projects are pursued at the precise point at which internal aspirations and propensities (e.g., goals, traits) meet external constraints and affordances (e.g., behavior settings, socioeconomic contexts). Individuals therefore require skills of self-regulation and insight into values as well as skills in negotiating the social ecology within which projects are embedded. For example, a person may have an elegantly articulated set of personal projects that are hierarchically linked so as to serve her needs and core values. But that same individual may simply not know how to proceed through the contextual thickets that constrain us when a project moves from inception to the action stage. Again, in contrast one might have strength and subtlety to negotiate the micropolitics of project pursuit yet feel challenged in articulating precisely what one is getting out of these pursuits.

Second, irrespective of their manageability and meaning, projects may interfere with each other in ways that cause imbalance in the project system as a whole. That is, if one considers all of the projects one is doing at a given time (i.e., the *project system*), some projects may compete with others for time, attention, or other reasons. Although the research literature on this topic is complex, I believe that interference is particularly problematic when core projects are involved. A *core project* is one that, were it to be removed from the system (for whatever reason), would directly compromise the rest of one's personal projects. The loss of a core project and the inability to conceive of constructive alternatives can have devastating consequences. Conversely, to create or discover a core project, even late in one's life, can be transformational.

Third, we live in a world of other *project pursuers* and the interference and facilitation of personal projects is not simply an intra-individual balancing act. One of the key adaptive challenges in marriage and in work life is balancing the claims of oneself and other selves. This means that living a balanced life often involves more than just finding ways to manage one's own projects. It also requires accommodating the projects of others. At the very least, such accommodation, or balancing, involves taking turns with others at having one's projects gain ascendency or go unfulfilled.

Fourth, imbalance may arise from having an overload of projects in one domain of human occupation. We have found that having too many *intrapersonal* projects (e.g., projects focused on the inner self such as "become more extraverted") is inversely associated with well-being and directly related to depressed mood. The fact that such projects are also associated with creativity, however, shows some of the complexities of postulating a simple direct link between project balance and well-being.

PROJECT BALANCE AND WELL-BEING

In reviewing the conceptual development and empirical research on personal projects, the following captures the most general proposition about how projects relate to human well-being or, in its fullest reach, flourishing: *Human flourishing is contingent upon the sustainable pursuit of core projects.*

Our findings about personal projects indicate that the concept of sustainability is directly related to the various types of balance we have briefly noted. For example, a core project that has lost its meaning is not sustainable. *Why* go on? A core project that has become unmanageable is not sustainable. *How* do I go on? The inability to create a reasonably coherent set of project priorities is not sustainable. *Which* do I do? Or assume that you have been able to generate meaningful, manageable projects but they are systematically undermining the projects of people you love. How sustainable are they? With unusual forbearance from others you might muddle through, but the more that your core projects have a negative impact on those you love or are seen to be in defiance of normal standards, the less likely they are to be sustainable. In such instances, others may be saying, "What do you think you're doing?" At a still more general level, in our earliest work in the 1970s on the social ecology of personal projects, we postulated that project pursuits, however balanced they may be within and among individuals, will ultimately be unsustainable if they collectively destroy the ecosystem that sustains life. At the time it was posited, this rather greenish proposition was greeted with loud yawns. Now we are more likely to ask, "What on earth are we all doing?"

I mentioned earlier that the conclusions that we were to draw about project balance and well-being were rather different than anticipated. In looking at some of the sources of project balance discussed above it became apparent that these various ways of viewing life balance using projects had, at best, moderate relationships with traditional measures of subjective well-being, health, and quality of life. Sometimes the relationship was simply not discernible at all. Other times, pursuing sets of projects that were balanced provided a sense of meaning but compromised the person's physical health.

One of the possible reasons for these various findings about project balance is that they needed to be viewed within a longer time frame. When one analyzes life balance based on a person's personal projects, it becomes clear that at various points and moments in our lives we may appear to be radically unbalanced, but if we examine what is happening over time, something approaching a stable equilibrium might be observed. I also mentioned earlier that my opening comments were personal and that they were reflexive; they applied to my colleagues in the audience who were either professors like me or practitioners in diverse areas. My challenge to them was to consider that much of the richness of our lives is achieved by choosing to be strategically unbalanced in at least some of our project pursuits. For a conference on life balance this may have seemed somewhat perverse, so an explanation is in order.

There are three vital sources of human conduct that we call *biogenic, sociogenic,* and *idiogenic* influences. The first two refer to our traditional notions of *biological factors* (i.e., genetic, evolutionary) and *environmental factors* (i.e., cultural scripts, social roles), respectively. Idiogenic influences comprise the intentional acts that can override both biogenic and sociogenic influences. Commitment to a core project is the prototypic example of idiogenic action. When we consider this tripartite approach to human natures, one of the derivative analytic units that emerges is what we call "free traits."

Free traits are socially expected patterns of action that we enact in order to advance our core personal projects, irrespective of our biogenic traits. An example is an introvert (I happen to be one) who has a biogenic disposition toward introversion but who frequently acts as a "pseudo-extravert" in order to advance a core project. As professors, many of us have found ourselves engaged in free-traited behavior. I happen to adore my students and my field of study. They are both core projects, so that I feel the need to stand and deliver my lectures with gusto (or as one student put it, with great "pesto"!). We can view such conduct as acting "out of character"—in the sense that the behavior required by the project is not really typical of a person's biogenic tendencies. But at the same time the project can also reflect the person's "character"—in the sense that it expresses one's core values. There are many other examples of free traits that can be spotted in our daily lives, such as essentially agreeable people who need to act in a disagreeable manner in order to advance a core project. Note that such behavior is strategic. It is consciously chosen to advance our projects—to help us attain our goals. In one fundamental sense it is unbalanced; our idiogenic commitments and projects are in conflict with our biogenic needs and dispositions. The critical question is whether we can do this with impunity, or whether we pay a cost for "free-traited" behavior? Other words, what price do we pay when social expectations influence us to act in ways that are contrary to our natural instincts?

I suggest that, while we may advance our well-being by acting out of character in the short term, in the long term we run the risk of burning out. However, we can mitigate the costs of acting out of character by having available restorative resources such as states, places, or niches in which we can regain the conditions most consistent with our biogenic natures. As a self-professed introvert I have confessed to my students that during the break in a three-hour lecture, I will disappear to the men's room in order to avoid the stimulation that increases neocortical arousal, which is already at too high a level. And just to avoid having to carry out conversations with some of the more extraverted students who walk into the restroom I have developed another strategy in the stall: I lift my feet up so they can't be seen.

In short, when we consider the question of balance in lives from a personal projects perspective a number of key issues come into view, including intentional action, environmental affordances and constraints, values, behavior settings, roles, conflict, time horizons, niches, and restorative resources. We also regard the question of life quality and balance as concepts that are complex, nuanced, and contestable.

It should now be apparent why I was not only honored to address the attendees at the symposium on which this book is based but utterly absorbed by the findings, insights, and cautions about assessing the quality of lives that appear in chapters written by colleagues from a diversity of disciplines. Each of the aforementioned concepts is discussed in different chapters amid many other compelling topics. Several chapters deal head-on with the value questions that the study of life balance and well-being inevitably raise.

That professors and practitioners of occupational science and therapy largely stimulated the conference was of particular significance for me. Just as my *first* lecture had been given to occupational therapy students, by sheer coincidence my address to this conference occurred a few hours after my *last* lecture, given as a visiting professor in the Department of Psychology at McGill University.

As one for whom professing was a passion, I realized that I was in transition to a new stage of life. And frankly, I felt a little wobbly. When we give up a core project, or in my case move away from its daily enactment, we need to create alternative projects that reflect the same deep convictions and engender the same sense of self-definition. As I was wrapping up my opening presentation something wonderful happened to me. I realized that I was still professing with passion but that my students were just a little older and wiser. They had experienced some of the perplexities of life in the immortal profession, and I shared some thoughts with the duly gathered about how we sometimes, in the very act of being strategically out of balance, become most fully ourselves. I felt less wobbly.

Recently, I told a Portuguese colleague that I was retiring. She sternly informed me that in Portugal professors do *not* retire—rather, they *jubilate!* I found this a wonderful way of capturing the new stage of life that I was entering. So I am now planning some jubilant projects, such as transforming groups of unsuspecting folks into students and lecturing to any gathering of people (and some pets) for the sheer love of it. This afternoon I am pursuing a project that is simultaneously provocative, entertaining, and enlightening—a third reading of the chapters in this superb book. I am also enjoying a symbolic serving of tea and scones.

REFERENCES

Little, B. R. (1972). Psychological man as a scientist, humanist, and specialist. *Journal of Experimental Research in Personality, 6,* 95–118.

Little, B. R. (1983). Personal projects: A rationale and method for investigation. *Environment and Behavior, 112,* 273–309.

Brian R. Little
Distinguished Research Professor Emeritus
Department of Psychology
Carleton University, Ottawa, Ontario, Canada
Adjunct Professor
Department of Psychology
McGill University, Montreal, Quebec, Canada

SECTION I

Life Balance
in Perspective

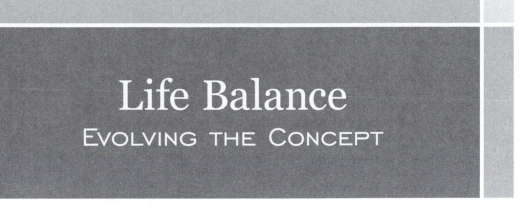

Life Balance
EVOLVING THE CONCEPT

CHARLES H. CHRISTIANSEN, KATHLEEN MATUSKA,
HELENE J. POLATAJKO, AND JANE A. DAVIS

INTRODUCTION

Every day it seems, there is talk about the stress of managing time in modern living and how difficult it has become to cope with the demands of this age. Undeniably, in this first decade of the 21st century, life has changed significantly for many people. The early years of the new millennium have witnessed several events of historical significance, ranging from dramatic terrorist attacks on the symbols of Western capitalism to devastating storms, armed conflict in the Middle East and elsewhere, and the avian influenza scare.

In addition, emerging shortages of natural resources (including oil and water); the rapid modernization of China, India, and other countries; and famine and disease (e.g., HIV/AIDS) on the continent of Africa have resulted in an array of issues that, in a world with instant communication made possible by cell phones and the Internet, would have seemed distant only a generation ago but are now deemed worthy of local concern.

Emerging technologies made possible in the digital age are enabling not only rapid communication but also an unprecedented and accelerated explosion of knowledge. This, in turn, has created changes in the ways people live; how they think about work and play; how they spend their time; what activities they value; and how they contemplate, interpret, and make meaning in their lives.

Because these changes have been rapid and profound, they have challenged the abilities of most people to cope with them. This has created a widespread urge to slow down the pace of life or, at the very least, find ways of living that enable one to catch up with the burden of having too much to do with too little time to do it. This perceived imbalance between the demands of current lives and people's abilities to adequately cope with them results in an experience of stress. Little wonder then that people want to find ways to avoid these stressful conditions and learn better ways of coping with them. Often, coping strategies include finding leisure and recreational outlets that promote relaxation, spending more time with family and friends, seeking more satisfactory working conditions, getting life coaching, moving to the country, or simply retiring early. Of course, not everyone has the resources or opportunity to cope, and their stories may include circumstances that are tabulated in statistical reports of burnout, depression, insomnia, self-inflicted injury, substance abuse, and suicide.

K. Matuska & C. Christiansen (Eds.)
Life balance: Multidisciplinary theories and research (pp 3–12)
© 2009 SLACK Incorporated and AOTA Press

At the same time that the popular press has been discussing the issues of work–life balance and reporting the consequences of time stress, it has also been reported that some governments are describing these problems of living as lifestyles out of balance. For example, the government of Canada has funded initiatives aimed at measuring the extent that family life is jeopardized by economic demands requiring people to work longer hours. The spillover of work into family time is seen as a particular source of stress and also as a threat to the workforce. This stress translates into higher turnover, absenteeism, and lowered productivity, making it a socioeconomic issue worthy of government attention.

Yet, despite the temptation to view life balance as a 21st century concern, it is worth noting that the association between living a balanced life and enjoying health and well-being is an ancient idea. The notion has roots in Chinese, Native American, and ayurvedic medicine. Examples of this are noted in some of the chapters in this volume. More recent support for living balanced lives is found in the contemporary literature from diverse perspectives, such as the economic, social, and behavioral sciences (Christiansen & Matuska, 2006; Sternberg, 1997). Nowhere, however, does the concept enjoy more widespread support than in the popular press. One can hardly pass a magazine rack without seeing tips for achieving some form of a better life—be it health, love, money, or beauty—all in *balance*. This obsession surely emanates from the complexities of modern living, where balance seems unobtainable.

The demands of modern life in developed nations have led to perceptions that stressful circumstances are increasing, and the time available to participate in activities viewed as fundamental to well-being is declining (Bachmann, 2000; Bond, Galinsky, & Swanberg, 1998). Government reports in the United States clearly show that perceived stress is increasing. Not surprisingly, epidemiologists predict that stress-related diseases will be among the leading and most costly health conditions in the next two decades (Murray & Lopaz, 1996). In fact, researchers have linked nearly all of the top ten conditions projected to place demands on world health resources over the coming decades to circumstances perceived to be psychologically stressful, whether those conditions involve cardiopulmonary systems or psychological perceptions of well-being.

At the heart of this discussion is how people allocate time, because human time use reflects the what, when, where, how, and why (and with whom) that describes human lives. A central influence in the lives of most adults involves how they make a living, and thus, changing practices associated with paid work, such as longer hours and increased shift work, are key topics in discussions of time use and time stress.

Within the workforce of many developed nations, it is commonly believed that modern work has been encroaching on nonwork occupations to create an undesirable and unhealthy imbalance between what gives people relaxation, enjoyment, and personal fulfillment or meaning and that which provides them with the economic means to sustain their lives—make a living. Over time, growing concern with this perceived imbalance of how time is used to personal advantage has given rise to such concepts as *quality time, workaholism,* and *burnout* (Hochschild, 1997; Perlow, 1999; Robinson & Godbey, 1997).

Although it is widely accepted that certain daily activities or occupations are more beneficial to health and quality of life than others, little theoretical and empirical work has been done to identify patterns of time use that are an optimal balance between meeting the practical necessities of life and engaging in fulfilling activities that meet psychological needs and create a satisfactory sense of self (Christiansen, 1999). Some studies seem to provide objective evidence that a failure to allocate time (and activities) to address certain fundamental needs related to well-being may lead to perceptions of increased stress, dissatisfaction, and unhappiness (Matuska & Christiansen, 2008). Over time, this failure can lead to objectively measured levels of physiological stress (now called *allostasis*) leading to chronic diseases (McEwen, 2004).

For example, investigators in management sciences, sociology, and family studies have reported research regarding the negative consequences of work requirements spilling over into nonwork domains (Frone, Russell, & Cooper, 1992; Greenhaus, Collins, & Shaw, 2002; Marks &

MacDermid, 1996). Meanwhile, scholars in psychology, leisure studies, nursing, public health, and occupational therapy have studied patterns of human occupation in an attempt to identify characteristics that contribute to higher levels of life satisfaction, health, and general well-being (Camporese, Freguja, & Sabbadini, 1998; Marino-Schorn, 1986; Walker, Sechrist, & Pender, 1987; Zuzanek, 1998). An implicit assumption underlying these studies is that some lifestyle configurations are more likely than others to promote health and well-being by meeting essential needs and reducing stressful circumstances over time.

If the assumption of relationships between lifestyle patterns and well-being is reasonable, then an understanding of the lifestyle activities that reduce stress and promote health should be of interest to social scientists. Yet surprisingly little attention has been paid to patterns of life activities (and their relationship to health) within the biomedical and social sciences literature. Instead, the biomedical sciences (particularly public health) are more likely to focus on the links between particular aspects of life activity or behavior (e.g., smoking, unsafe sex, nutritional habits, sleep, exercise) and how these are associated with illness or disease. This lack of attention to the overall pattern of life activities may be due to the breadth and complexity of the topic, or it may be explained by the tendency of scientists to focus their work in narrow (and therefore more manageable) specialized areas. Given this dearth of research, it is hardly surprising that there exists no universally accepted definition of *life balance*, even though the concept appears regularly in the popular press under the rubric of *work–life balance* and seems to be implicitly (even if simplistically) understood by the public.

DETERMINING THE STATE OF THE SCIENCE

However, it is not as though scientists have been ignoring the issue entirely. The literature across disparate disciplines clearly reveals an interest in the concept of how humans live their lives and how this influences their well-being. Not surprisingly, the particular approaches used to define and study the concepts in the various disciplines tend to reflect the traditions and methods of the particular discipline. For example, sociologists approaching the idea of *balance* define and measure it within the context of theories of social roles, while behavioral scientists describe the concept from the standpoint of motivations, need fulfillment, or discrepancies between perceived and actual life characteristics. Time-use scientists, in turn, are more interested in particular patterns of activities that reflect allocations of time within days and throughout particular life periods.

We have been interested in life balance from the standpoint of *occupational science*, an emerging interdisciplinary field dedicated to understanding humans as doers, as occupational beings whose activities influence their health and well-being. A review of the related literature (Christiansen & Matuska, 2006) conducted several years ago made it clear that researchers from many disciplines had something valuable to contribute to the dialogue about balanced lives. Scientists from different disciplines were found to describe the phenomenon differently but shared a common interest—a presumed relationship between various states (e.g., happiness, well-being, work satisfaction, job performance, marital harmony) and how time was allocated to various activities. This early appraisal of the state of the science in work–life balance suggested the need for an approach that would acknowledge the growing interest in the topic and promote efforts to link scientists from the disparate disciplines who were interested in the topic but approached it from largely different definitions, terminology, and conceptual approaches. An invitational conference on the topic was deemed a useful and timely way to begin an interdisciplinary dialogue and link the disparate perspectives.

AN INTERDISCIPLINARY CONFERENCE

In an effort to initiate an interdisciplinary dialogue, we organized an international, multidisciplinary conference in the spring of 2007 to bring scientists together for a thoughtful discussion about work–life balance as viewed from the standpoint of their various disciplinary perspectives. A conference committee of colleagues from occupational science who were interested in or doing research related to the topic was organized to plan the event. The committee consisted of Charles Christiansen (American Occupational Therapy Foundation), Kathleen Matuska (St. Catherine University), Helene J. Polatajko (University of Toronto), Jane Davis (University of Toronto), Catherine Backman (University of British Columbia), Wendy Pentland (Queen's University), and Beatriz C. Abreu (Transitional Learning Center at Galveston, University of Texas Medical Branch). A grant from the Canadian Social Science and Health Research Council (SSHRC) was instrumental to the effort, as was support from the publishers at SLACK Incorporated (Thorofare, NJ) and AOTA Press (Bethesda, MD). Substantial support was also provided by the University of Texas Medical Branch at Galveston from the George T. Bryan Distinguished Professorship Endowment.

The conference was held in April 2007, in Kingston, Ontario, Canada, with the following aims:

◘ To share current theory and research in life balance, lifestyle patterns, and health across the lifespan

◘ To identify conceptual commonalities, links, and divergences across this research

◘ To determine if life balance is a legitimate construct, worthy of study, and of benefit to people in all societies

◘ To foster opportunities for networking and collaboration

◘ To develop a research agenda based on identified weaknesses and gaps in research.

Another aim was to document the discussion and the presentations of the conference in an edited volume, as represented by this publication—the ultimate purpose being to stimulate further interest, discourse, and collaboration around the topic.

The scientists who attended the conference represented the disciplines of philosophy, psychology, sociology, occupational science, occupational therapy, leisure sciences, family studies, public health, business management, and economics. The challenges of clarifying a concept of life balance soon became evident in the discussions among the gathered scientists. Major questions emerged about whether the topic was even worth studying; if it could be defined or conceptualized; if it could be measured; and if it was an important, distinct component of health and well-being. Other questions arose concerning its applicability to people regardless of their age, culture, background, or living situation. For example, Does the concept of life balance pertain to infants and children? Is the concept relevant to people who are incarcerated or who have physical or mental limitations that interfere with or limit their choices and participation in the usual life activities and experiences of people without such limitations? Does the concept reflect a decidedly Western view of the world? In addressing these and related questions, the scientists at the conference discussed and debated their perspectives over three days. The chapters in this volume document their ideas, as they have been revised and extended since the conference.

THE CONFERENCE AS REFLECTED IN THIS VOLUME

Section 1: Life Balance in Perspective

The first section of this book consists of a compilation of research and theory from philosophical and sociological traditions that consider the concept of a balanced life from a broader, societal perspective. Appropriately, a discussion of whether or not balance is even worth studying begins this book. In Chapter 2, Jerome E. Bickenbach and Thomas A. Glass combine both philosophical and public health viewpoints to explore basic questions such as Why, and in what manner, is a balanced life good? What does it mean to be balanced? Is life balance an effort to "medicalize" life patterns and identify deviance or pathology when none really exists? These questions are approached by reviewing the historical and philosophical teachings of balance and drawing connections to modern times. Birckenbach and Glass challenge us to question our ideas about a balanced life and assert that what some may view as imbalance may not be a problem for others.

In Chapter 3, Gail Elizabeth Whiteford expands on the question about whether life balance is worth studying and asks if a balanced life is important to people of all ages and from all backgrounds. She adopts a global view of human occupation by exploring the impact of the social, economic, political, and cultural context on peoples' opportunities to engage in patterns of meaningful and health-promoting occupations. She asserts that lifestyle balance is shaped and understood in a Eurocentric discursive tradition and the labor-market issues associated with late Western capitalism. In her chapter, Whiteford questions whether life balance is a universal, cross-cultural value and whether life balance is attainable or even relevant in the face of significant forces that militate against it. She supports her assertions with in-depth narratives of South African women faced with daily struggles against poverty and poor health.

Notwithstanding the importance of the fundamental questions raised in Chapters 2 and 3 regarding the essential relevance of balanced living, the volume continues with a discussion of several basic questions.

In Chapter 4, Ruut Veenhoven uses a sociological perspective to advocate for critical analysis of the concept and challenges scientists interested in the topic to be specific about what is meant when the term life balance is used. He describes three potential ways to assess balanced lives and argues that, depending on which approach is chosen, the results will be quite different. For example, should balance be a subjective sense of how balanced people *think* their lives are? Should it be based on a preconceived idea of what balance should be (such as so much time devoted to certain types of activities)? Or is balance best defined as the lifestyle mix that yields the most happiness? Veenhoven provides readers with useful schemata for understanding the relationships among the many variables related to living a balanced life, including ways to conceptualize how happiness and quality of life contribute to the concept.

An important acknowledgement among the researchers at the conference was the fact that life balance is still a very embryonic concept, lacking consensus about its definition. Although several participants have spent significant portions of their life's work addressing questions related to concepts of life balance, these efforts constitute largely isolated work because of the penchant of scientists working in different disciplines to use terms differently—either using different terms to describe similar concepts or similar terms to describe different phenomena. Given these circumstances, it is understandable that consensus or unified agreement about the construct remains a distant aspiration.

In Chapter 5, Stephen Marks takes us through a retrospective of his personal 30-year journey studying balance, showing us how his work was influenced by traditional sociological theorists, the Protestant ethic, and the counterculture of the 1960s. Marks narrates the story of his own personal interest in living a balanced life and shares his professional interest in understanding how that would be represented. His narrative includes an account of how his interests and personal experiences led to the development of a theory of role balance that explains his nonhierarchical approach of studying peoples' entire role systems in a holistic framework. Marks explains how role balance, viewed from the perspective of role systems, can influence how lives are experienced, which he demonstrates in different approaches to measurement.

Section 2: Measuring Life Balance

The second section of the book reflects the intense discussion of the conference participants regarding the idea of life balance and how it can be distinguished from other positive-state constructs such as *life satisfaction* or *subjective well-being*. For example, if people who report living balanced lives also report more life satisfaction or happiness (or any other positive state), then, is life balance a unique characteristic or is it simply another name (or proxy) for the same concept? One requirement for elaborating or clarifying a concept rests on how it is measured in ways that show it is unique or distinct from existing constructs. For a concept to be distinct and worthy of study its own right, it should add new information to our understanding of phenomena.

Appropriately, during the conference, a vigorous discussion arose about how to measure or determine if a life is balanced. Two psychologists, Kennon M. Sheldon (Chapter 6) and Robert A. Cummins (Chapter 7) believed that it is the *balance* idea that needs to be clarified for the concept of life balance to be differentiated from other concepts describing positive psychological states. They agreed that if balance is to be viewed as a unique characteristic of lives, distinct from other concepts, the key challenge will be to identify and define exactly what balance is through measurement of some specific properties.

Sheldon and Cummins each argue that time use constitutes an excellent framework with which to define and measure the construct and that the time spent by an individual engaging in a particular pursuit can be compared with the amount of time a person wants or needs to be engaging in that pursuit. In other words, in a 24-hour time span, are people actually doing what they want or need to do? The match between actual and desired time use can thus be used to represent, along a continuum, the degree of concordance, or balance, within a given life.

According to such a framework, if life balance is a unique construct, then a discrepancy between desired and actual time use in daily activities would relate to stress, life satisfaction, and other psychological constructs in predictable ways. Sheldon argues that current definitions and measures are inadequate to encompass the true potential richness of the life–balance concept, and, as a result, he proposes a new assessment approach and two complementary measures of life balance.

Cummins, for his part, also discusses the measurement challenges associated with isolating the construct of life balance and describes an approach using discrepancy analysis to conceptualize *subjective well-being*, a more established psychological construct. In his schema, the ultimate measure of a balanced life is whether or not it results in a sense of well-being within a given lifestyle.

Andrew S. Harvey and Jerome Singleton (Chapter 8) extend the discussion of time use by examining the relationship between perceived balance and imbalance based on the allocation of time. Using data from Canadian time-use studies, they explore the allocation of time from a daily and life-course perspective in terms of actual time allocation in relation to perceived time balance, stress, and happiness. By comparing time allocation to activities, social space (locations), and social circle (contacts) in the light of self-reported satisfaction with work–life balance, they provide insights into how people feel regarding their time use and perceptions of balance from a framework dichotomizing work and other life activities.

One of the complexities associated with measuring what people do with their time (and whether or not there is a mismatch between actual and desired time use) is that they often do more than one thing at a time, such as cooking dinner and helping a child with homework or driving while talking on the phone. To complicate things further, people also ascribe different meanings to what they are doing at different times. For example, reading might be considered work in one context and leisure in another.

In Chapter 9, Lena-Karin Erlandsson and Carita Håkansson describe a time-geography approach to visually illustrating people's activities in time by showing the patterns of activity in a given day. They report use of this method to categorize Swedish women's everyday patterns of activity (occupations). Using a 24-hour diary, direct observations, video documentation, and an experience sampling method, the researchers were able to graph time and activity logs to describe what activities were performed and at what time of day. Using the graphs, the researchers visually analyzed similarities and differences among actual patterns of daily activities, seeking insights into what patterns might constitute more or less balance by relating the different patterns to measures of the women's health and well-being.

Section 3: Conceptualizing Life Balance

As noted by the participants, given the complexities associated with definitions, measurement, and competing constructs, developing a rigorous and practical model or theory of life balance is clearly fraught with difficulties. Given this reality, is it worthwhile to pursue the concept? The organizers, sponsors, and participants associated with the conference clearly believe it is. This viewpoint is shaped considerably by public interest in the concept. The concept has also been embraced by people in government and business influenced by what they perceive to be the quality of life and economic consequences associated with lives that are out of balance. All these groups—the general public, government, and business—are not too concerned about how balance is defined or measured from a scientific perspective.

The third section of this book offers three models or theories of life balance. In each case, the authors propose frameworks that attempt to identify dimensions of daily life that contribute to balance according to the respective definitions of their models.

Swedish scientists Dennis Persson and Hans Jonsson (Chapter 10) describe an experiential model within which they propose a balanced mix of everyday experiences as important for health and well-being. The experiences necessary for this balanced mix are derived from Csikszentmihalyi's theory of *flow* (1975, 1990, 1997). Persson and Jonsson's model defines three key dimensions: (1) highly or moderately challenging experiences that are matched with high skills, (2) highly challenging experiences that cannot be matched with high skills, and (3) low to moderately challenging experiences. They theorize that all three experience types and their relationships are important for achieving balance in life, meaning that none of them is intrinsically positive or negative.

The three experience types have different relationships to each other, and Persson and Jonsson hypothesize that all three are needed within the context of everyday experience. If any of these three experiences is too dominating, an imbalance arises that in the long-term might risk developing into a destructive process; one that would lead to occupational deprivation or overload with negative consequences on health and well-being. Persson and Jonsson illustrate their experiential balance model with case studies, offer empirical support, and describe its applicability within a global perspective.

Chapter 11 provides an overview of a proposed model of lifestyle balance by Kathleen Matuska and Charles Christiansen, where balance is congruence between desired and actual patterns of activity across five proposed need-based activity dimensions necessary for well-being. Matuska and Christiansen (2008) assert that balance is based on how patterns of daily activities meet important needs and are congruent with a person's values and expectations. Five need-based dimensions are identified as essential to a life with greater balance: (1) having daily activities enabling people to meet needs related to biological health and physical safety, (2) having rewarding relationships with others, (3) feeling engaged and competent, (4) creating self-relevant meaning, and (5) satisfactorily recruiting personal resources necessary for goal attainment. In this model, the level of congruence between individual values and expectations across activities that represent the need dimensions should be predictive of positive state and measures of health.

Wendy Pentland and Mary Ann McColl (Chapter 12) offer an alternative perspective on life balance, one they believe is missing from the current discourse. They propose that the extent to which people perceive their lives to be in balance derives from the extent to which they are living lives that are congruent with their personal values and strengths. They define this congruence as *occupational integrity*. Pentland and McColl assert that the metaphor of balance, as used in every-day conversation, focuses on an idealistic and dualistic outcome that obscures the fundamental characteristics and nature of this sought-after state.

The three models of a balanced life presented in this section each identify different, but related aspects of daily activity patterns seen as essential for life balance. Depending on one's lens for viewing the phenomenon, life balance could be viewed as a balance among (a) types of activity experiences, (b) activities that meet essential needs, or (c) activities that are congruent with one's values and strengths.

Section 4: Approaches for Achieving Life Balance

The fourth section of this book brings together research from specific populations—adolescents, children, and people with acquired brain injury—and concludes with a chapter devoted to life coaching.

In Chapter 13, Sandra L. Hofferth, David A. Kinney, and Janet S. Dunn present important research about activity levels for various social classes of American children. They approach the concept of balance from the standpoint of time use and how parents influence the lifestyles of their children through planned activities. They ask if children are overscheduled and experience unnecessary psychological stress as a result. Given the common Western perception that family schedules in general are out of control, the issue of overscheduled children may be a topic that is both timely and important to parents who worry about how much activity is too much or too little. Their studies show differences in children's activity levels based on family income and maternal education and indicate that high levels of activity are not associated with more symptoms of stress. Instead, their data indicate that children who are uninvolved (i.e., participate in few activities) tend to be more withdrawn, socially immature, and have lower self-esteem. Hofferth, Kinney, and Dunn conclude that the common perception that most children are overscheduled and experience stress as a result may be erroneous and that a certain level of scheduled activity appears to be beneficial.

In Chapter 14, Jiri Zuzanek uses data from the 1998 Canadian General Social Survey and the Ontario Survey of Adolescent Time Use, conducted in 2002–2003 by the Research Group on Leisure and Cultural Development of the University of Waterloo, to explore adolescent time arrangements that best correspond with desirable well-being and health outcomes. His concept of life balance for adolescents is a time-use configuration that best suits their developmental, emotional, and health needs. Zuzanek examined multiple configurations, such as time in paid work, time doing homework, and time socializing with friends. A breakdown of adolescents' access to free time showed that students had higher life satisfaction and perceived happiness when they had moderate amounts of free time. Conversely, too much free time and too little free time resulted in poorer outcomes.

In Chapter 15, Beatriz C. Abreu and her colleagues from the rehabilitation sciences examine how a person's appraisal of life balance, as an emotional judgment influenced by culture, may be compromised in people with acquired brain injury (ABI) because of difficulties with emotional regulation and cognitive processing. This examination is important to rehabilitation specialists who work with individuals with ABI, because ultimately, the goal of rehabilitation is to help those clients attain the highest quality of life possible, and a balanced life is viewed as an enabling factor toward that outcome. Aside from its obvious value to those in rehabilitation, it also adds an important contribution to this volume by examining how notions of life balance are considered within populations who have limitations in their ability to move, sense, think, or feel. Abreu and colleagues provide a thorough description of the neurological influences on these life appraisals after a brain injury. They also suggest that these are important considerations for assisting clients following brain injury to adapt to or compensate for their emotional and cognitive limitations.

In Chapter 16, Amy Heinz and Wendy Pentland discuss *life coaching*, an emerging type of personal and family intervention that focuses on helping people live their lives with greater satisfaction. Instead of theory, the authors provide a practical application of the concept of lifestyle balance viewed from the perspective of an emerging industry comprised of life coach professionals. In this chapter, Heinz and Pentland describe the profession's aim to promote optimal living, healthy habits, and personal life enrichment. They then provide an account of the historical and philosophical roots of the profession, current uses of life coaching, and some methods and techniques used by life coaches.

They note that even if the construct of lifestyle balance remains theoretically vague from the vantage point of science, this is not a limitation for life coaches. Heinz and Pentland argue that rather than concern themselves with definitions of constructs, life coaches focus their efforts on helping their clients achieve a unique view of a good life.

Section 5: Future Research on Life Balance

One of the aims of the conference was to develop a research agenda based on identified weaknesses and gaps in research. In the concluding chapter, Catherine Backman and Dana Anaby offer their synthesis of the questions and concerns raised by the participating scholars, emphasizing potential research directions. They share a structure for organizing hypotheses for further study and suggest that life balance defies a single, universal definition and requires careful consideration of specific elements when operationalized for research purposes. Their conclusion resounds wholeheartedly that life balance is indeed a construct worthy of further study.

The summary of the contents of this volume should convey that the various offerings provide a comprehensive view of a very complex construct. One goal for the conference was to foster continued research and create networks of scholars interested in the topic of life balance. That this has already occurred is evident in the shared contributions to this volume as well as in other forms. Several of the participants have started collaborative research or made plans for their next projects. Others have been inspired to test some of the propositions contained in the various models presented here.

We hope that the ideas presented here will stimulate additional thought and research to further advance the construct of life balance in ways that can be helpful to people who may not be able to define or measure life balance but who feel a compelling need to live their lives in ways that enable them to experience it, however it may be defined.

REFERENCES

Bachmann, K. D. (2000). *Work–life balance: Measuring what matters.* Ottawa: Conference Board of Canada.

Bond, J., Galinsky, E., & Swanberg, J. (1998). *The national study of the changing workforce.* New York: Families and Work Institute.

Camporese, R., Freguja, C., & Sabbadini, L. L. (1998). Time use by gender and quality of life. *Social Indicators Research, 44,* 119–144.

Christiansen, C. (1999). Defining lives: Occupation as identity: An essay on competence, coherence, and the creation of meaning [Eleanor Clarke Slagle Lecture]. *American Journal of Occupational Therapy, 53,* 547–558.

Christiansen, C., & Matuska, K. (2006). Lifestyle balance: A review of concepts and research. *Journal of Occupational Science, 13,* 49–61.

Csikszentmihalyi, M. (1975). *Beyond boredom and anxiety: The experience of play in work and games.* San Francisco: Jossey-Bass.

Csikszentmihalyi, M. (1990). *Flow: The psychology of optimal experience.* New York: Harper & Row.

Csikszentmihalyi, M. (1997). *Finding flow.* New York: HarperCollins.

Frone, M., Russell, M., & Cooper, M. (1992). Antecedents and outcomes of work family conflict: Testing a model of the work-family interface. *Journal of Applied Psychology, 77,* 65–78.

Greenhaus, J., Collins, K., & Shaw, J. (2002). The relation between work–family balance and quality of life. *Journal of Vocational Behavior, 63,* 510–531.

Hochschild, A. R. (1997). *The time bind: When work becomes home and home becomes work.* New York: Metropolitan.

Marks, S. R., & MacDermid, S. M. (1996). Multiple roles and the self: A theory of role balance. *Journal of Marriage and the Family, 58,* 417–432.

Marino-Schorn, J. A. (1986). Morale, work, and leisure in retirement. *Physical and Occupational Therapy in Geriatrics, 4,* 49–59.

Matuska, K., & Christiansen, C. (2008). A proposed model of lifestyle balance. *Journal of Occupational Science. 15,* 1, 9–19.

McEwen, B. S. (2004). Protection and damage from acute and chronic stress: Allostasis and allostatic overload and relevance to the pathophysiology of psychiatric disorders. *Annals of the New York Academy of Sciences. 1032,* 1–7.

Murray, C. J. L., & Lopaz, A. D. (Eds.). (1996). *The global burden of disease: A comprehensive assessment of mortality and disability from diseases, injuries, and risk factors in 1990 and projected to 2020* (Vol. 1). Cambridge, MA: Harvard School of Public Health.

Perlow, L. A. (1999). The time famine: Toward a sociology of work time. *Administrative Science Quarterly, 44,* 57–81.

Robinson, J. P., & Godbey, G. (1997). *Time for life: The surprising ways Americans use their time.* University Park: Pennsylvania University Press.

Sternberg, E. (1997). Emotions and disease: From balance of humors to balance of molecules. *Natural Medicine, 3,* 264–267.

Walker, S., Sechrist, K., & Pender, N. (1987). The health-promoting lifestyle profile: Development and psychometric characteristics. *Nursing Research, 36,* 76–81.

Zuzanek, J. (1998). Time use, time pressure, personal stress, mental health, and life satisfaction from a life cycle perspective. *Journal of Occupational Science, 5,* 26–39.

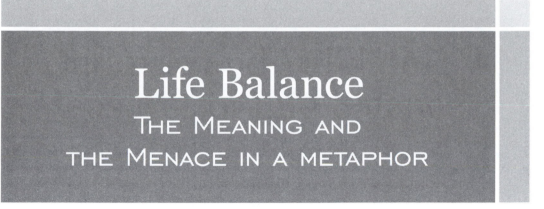

Life Balance
THE MEANING AND
THE MENACE IN A METAPHOR

JEROME E. BICKENBACH AND THOMAS A. GLASS

INTRODUCTION

Although it draws on many professions and disciplines, methodologies, and sources of evidence, the life balance literature is fundamentally grounded in the assumption that *balance* in spheres of life activity is an essential human good, something that should be valued and achieved. In a recent review piece, for example, Roberts (2007) assembled evidence about hours of work and time use, attitudes toward overwork, and complaints about work stress and lack of time for family life. Then he immediately moved to controversies about how this sad state of affairs came about and what might be done about it. The fundamentally problematic nature of the concept of balance itself is neither acknowledged nor addressed. Its historical and philosophical roots are never explored. As is the case with almost all of the life balance literature, it is simply taken for granted that balance is a good thing. There is no mention of why balance ought to be the solution or even an improvement on people's lives. Even discussions that are highly critical of the life balance literature and argue for wholesale reconceptualization of the relationship between work and life (e.g., Eikhof, Warhurst, & Haunschild, 2007) appear to be unconcerned about the prevailing assumption that balance in life is something that needs be achieved.

This essay is an attempt to call this assumption into question and to shine a systematic and historical light on it. We argue that before scholarship on life balance can proceed productively, some very simple but fundamental questions, rarely asked, must be directly confronted:

- Why is the life in balance better than a life not so?

- In what manner, precisely, is the life in balance better?

- What is being balanced in the balanced life?

Are the answers to these questions self-evident (as the total absence of consideration of them would suggest)? We believe that even if well-reasoned and evidence-based answers to these questions can be provided, they are not, in any straightforward sense, self-evident. There are countless examples in literature and in real life where singular individuals have lead astonishingly "imbalanced lives but are nonetheless immensely creative, productive, and socially valuable. Genius, eccentric or otherwise; great artistic ability; or obsessiveness and boundless industry may drive someone to shift all of their energy to their work—or their family—to the exclusion of all other areas of life. These people may be happier that way, but even if they are miserable, why should we

K. Matuska & C. Christiansen (Eds.)
Life-balance: Multidisciplinary theories and research (pp 13–22)
© 2009 SLACK Incorporated and AOTA Press

immediately think that they (or the rest of us) would be better off if they were persuaded to spend more time at home or engage in other nonwork activities?

The main thesis of this chapter is that scientific progress in life balance research requires careful examination of fundamental assumptions. While the topic of life balance has attracted researchers across several disciplines, the concept itself begs several fundamental questions—to which philosophers and ethicists are well positioned to contribute. The failure to engage in careful and systematic consideration of the ethical implications of these issues contributes to the essential hollowness and absence of depth seen in the life balance discourse. The concept of life balance (and the implied epidemic of people living an unbalanced life) risks the implication of culpability for individuals for failing to manage their lives in a society in which balance is increasingly difficult to achieve. Said differently, it is important to guard against the risk that the concept of life balance does not become one more example that serves only to medicalize personal troubles that are reflections of broader social and cultural tensions.

After a quick review of some recent life balance literature, we will offer some conceptual and ethical context to the notion of life balance, with the aim of elucidating the unexamined assumptions that undergird it. In particular, we wish to draw attention to the potential contribution of Aristotle's moral psychology to life balance discourse. For Aristotle does have an account of what it means for a life to be "in balance" but it is very different from our own default account that is rooted in our Judeo-Christian heritage. For Aristotle, balance is primarily an aesthetic ideal, indeed one only achieved when the individual ultimately removed him or herself (although, sadly, Aristotle would never imagine this to be a possibility for a woman) from family and public entirely and inhabited the world of ideas alone. In the more dominant Judeo-Christian tradition, balance is entirely a matter of fulfilling ones duties. What this means for the life balance debate, we leave for later.

CRITICAL EXAMINATION OF LIFE BALANCE LITERATURE

At the heart of the balance literature is the assumption, plausible enough on its face, that work–life balance is important because everyone wants, and derives satisfaction from, balancing work and life. In one working definition, *imbalance* is said to be an "occupational stressor" characterized by "lost resources of time and energy" leading to a failure of goal accomplishment and resulting strain and stress (Aziz & Zickar, 2006, p. 63; O'Driscoll et al., 2003). The assumption here is that working too much is a problem because the individual cannot satisfactorily attend to other goals—some in the work sphere, others in spheres outside of work—that compete for scarce time and energy resources. While this kind of goal imbalance might be a cause of considerable stress and strain, is the problem truly one of imbalance, or is it something else? Surely, the stress comes from being frustrated that there is not enough time to do what one wants to do. An eccentric and utterly imbalanced artist may face precisely these stresses because she cannot finish all the art she wants to. Her problem is not balancing art and life—she consciously abandoned that goal—but meeting the goals of one sphere.

The persistence of the assumption that people demand a balance between work and life is everywhere in the literature—once you look for it. It is an essential component of the standard argument for balancing (e.g., Frone, 2001; Quick, Henley, & Quick, 2004). It is the central argument in the literature on "occupational balance" (Bryden & McColl, 2003). It underwrites recent strategies to solve the problem, such as telecommuting, by making it possible for parents to work from home (Golden, Veiga, & Simsek, 2006). And it is an unstated assumption in the management literature that deals with sources of employee stress and loss of productivity—namely, that employees want to spend more time at home (Kenny & Cooper, 2003; O'Drisoll et al., 2003; Worrall & Cooper, 2001).

These are assumptions about the importance of balance, not arguments that demonstrate that balance is important. If people truly want balance, then denying them that will cause stress. But what if they do not? Why should a balanced life always be preferable? Rarely in the literature have researchers investigated whether employees actively sought balance or asked them if imbalance made working stressful. Interestingly, when studies are focused not on the work–balance issue but on sources of work satisfaction or its absence, imbalance is not as important as level of control and involvement in decision making, recognition for accomplishments, and the potential for growth and development (Grawitch, Gottschalk, & Munz, 2006; Grawitch, Trares, & Kohler, 2007).

Because fundamental questions about the balanced life are not directly confronted, insufficient attention is given to linking the idea of balance to a larger discussion of the good life. This becomes clearer when we ask how we turn the idea of life balance into an operational and measurable phenomenon. Arguably, these discussions cannot be sufficiently well developed using the tools of positivist science alone, and that leaves the normative underpinnings of the issue unexamined.

CULTURAL TRENDS AS MEDICAL ISSUES

We are also concerned that, in the absence of careful attention to the normative assumptions underlying this debate, we will end up with a crass medicalization of the life balance problem. This risk is well illustrated by the putative disorder of *workaholism* (Aziz & Zickar, 2006), defined as the psychological problem of—perhaps willingly —rejecting the need for a work–life balance. It is merely assumed that this is a problem, indeed a medical one. This is an example of *medicalization*, a term first described by the medical sociologist Irving Zola, referring to the turning over of some facet of life to the jurisdiction of medical supervision and treatment (Zola, 1972). It is at the core of objections to the overly broad 1948 definition of health by the World Health Organization (Callahan, 1982). When applied to conditions of life that spring from broader social forces outside of the control of individuals, medicalization risks blaming the victims of those conditions (Mills, 1959).

While medicalization creates an air of legitimacy for intervention by medical specialties, it does nothing to solve fundamental questions that are nonmedical in nature, such as how best to live one's life. Further, the risk we run is to pathologize a problem that is deeply rooted in cultural and normative structures for which medical solutions are insufficient and potentially punitive. If we accept that workaholism is a problem, are we at risk of turning deviation from a cultural norm into a medical problem? Is being out of balance with regard to work and nonwork obligations really a matter of a deficiency of collective character or judgment? A casual look at basic economic data suggests otherwise. Americans and other Westerners, explains psychiatrist Peter Whybrow in his book *American Mania* (Whybrow, 2005), have entered a period of pervasive stress, overwork, and dissatisfaction, not in pursuit of any personal ideal, but due to pressures largely beyond their control or understanding. The past 30 years has seen the unparalleled expansion of U.S. productivity, which has become the envy of the world. Yet, at what cost? Figure 2-1 shows change over time in average hours worked in the United States.

What this figure shows is a general pattern visible in many sources of data. Americans are working harder and longer and getting further behind in the quest for adequate compensation. The figure shows dramatic escalation in average hours worked. This is the miracle of American productivity. It also shows an increase in income inequality in lockstep with that pattern. Americans are working harder than ever, but reaping a smaller fraction of the rewards from their efforts. We have seen a substantial shrinkage of the middle class, as unionization has declined and middle-class jobs have been exported to lower-wage countries like China. We have entered a period where workers are increasingly under-rewarded as the profits of managers and owners escalate. To the extent that life imbalance is a product of a exploitation, the focus of investigation belongs on that

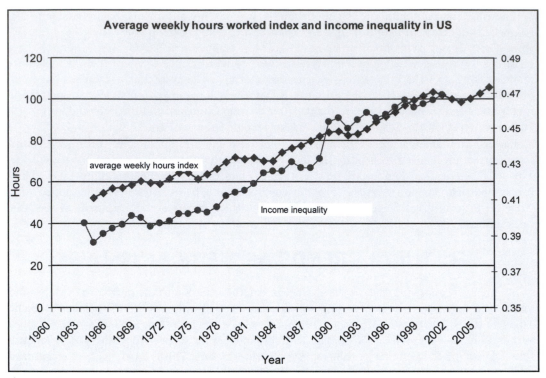

Figure 2-1. Time trends of average hours worked and income inequality in the United States.

exploitation, not on the bind in which individual workers find themselves. In this sense, to the extent the life balance discourse is constructed as an account of individual values and desires, we risk blaming individuals for being stuck in a situation that is not of their own making.

Absent a closer scrutiny of the implicit value of balancing, there is a danger, not merely of transforming character traits into syndromes that require intervention, but engaging in debates that are academic in the worst sense, namely, debates spun out of disagreements over misunderstanding and assumptions that are never pinned down or made sense of. If we are not clear what about a balanced makes it a better life, how can we, ethically, recommend such a life, or alter our public policy to further it?

BALANCE AS HEALTH: THE SOURCE OF THE METAPHOR IN THE ANCIENT WORLD

The preoccupation with balance as an essential feature of the good life stems from a deep-seated idea, but its origins and implications remain largely unexamined. This is where philosophy, we argue, has an indispensable role to play. Philosophers engage in the systematic evaluation of the origins, implications, and complexities underlying precisely this kind of concept. Indeed, the history of philosophy, from the ancient Greeks (at least) onward is an attempt to critically and systematically evaluate competing claims about what we mean by "the good life." Philosophers of ethics and values have been at the forefront of this discussion.

For that reason, the need for careful and systematic philosophical consideration of this question seems to us of considerable importance. As in discussions of health care rationing, economic justice, or quality of life, science and its methods are insufficient to deal with the full dimension of the issue. The issue of life balance hangs essentially on philosophical considerations closely related to theories of what constitutes the good, moral, just, and desired life. Those questions, as history teaches, cannot be answered solely through application of the scientific method. We suggest then, at least for a start, that we look at the roots, conceptual and historical, of the metaphor of the balanced life using the lens of philosophy.

The beginnings of what can properly be called *medical knowledge* arose when the practical, naturalistic healing craft was organized and systematized to explain the behavior of the body in health and illness (Wulff, 1999). In the Western world, this was first attempted by Hippocrates (c. 460–380 BCE). Rejecting superstitious accounts of diseases as sacred or as punishment for evil deeds—suggested by the legendary 12th-century Asclepius who was thought to be a demigod—his approach was empirical and practical. He asked What do we see in the body, and what role do they play in times of health and illness? Knowing nothing of anatomy or physiology, Hippocrates and his school observed what the body ingested, exuded, and processed. From this came the theory of the four *humors:* black bile, yellow bile, phlegm, and blood—the basic body fluids that are in continuous motion by means of bodily circulation. Then the metaphor appeared: When these humors are in balance (*eucrasia*), health is the result, when that balance, for one reason or another, is upset (*dyscrasia*), illness results. (The English word *balance* itself comes, via Old French, from the Latin *bilanx*, meaning a two-plate scale for measuring equal portions.)

But why the metaphor of balance? Why could we not argue that the presence of, say, more and more positive humor is the key to better health? Because it does not fit the observable facts. Some people who are patently sick seem to be drowning in phlegm, so clearly, more is not always good for you. But this is an easy case; can we be sure that imbalance is always etiologic when we cannot directly observe the humors operating in the body? What was needed was a theory that generalized from observations. Health, Hippocratics argued, is a state of *natural proportion* (the Greek here is *pepsis,* from which we get *dyspeptic* and similar terms), and equality is the epitome of proportion. Hence, the four humors must be equal in quantity, and so in balance, if health is to result.

The humors and the balancing metaphor not only bore a great deal of theoretical weight, but they also offered a wealth of practical guidance. Asthma, for example, was thought to be caused by an imbalance of phlegm, which cools the heart and lungs, making it difficult to take in air. The imbalance may have resulted from a radical change in diet or changes in weather or some other environmental cause. But cause is not as important as treatment. The theory suggests that treatment should aim to limit the production of phlegm, by diet or warm baths and compresses, to reduce the body's store of that humor. Undoubtedly, trial and error was the true source of the proposed treatment, but the background theory justified it.

Significantly, from the outset, the theory of humor was intended to apply to both body and mind. A person who suffered from *melancholia*, it was taught, had an excess of black bile; a person with an excess of yellow bile was *bilious*. Six centuries later, the Roman Galen (131–201 CE) made an obvious extension to the humors theory by arguing that not only does humoral imbalance lead to emotional problems, but emotional imbalance can lead to bodily imbalance, or rather to physical symptoms that mimic those one would expect from humoral imbalance (Akiskal & Akiskal, 2007).

The "passions and perturbations of the soul" are also part of the stuff of which humans are made, and they too must be kept in balance, an account furthered in detail by the 12th-century rabbi and physician Moses Maimonides, who, anticipating Robert Burton's *The Anatomy of Melancholy* and centuries of folk psychological and "spirituality" advice, proposed regimes whereby the "movements of the psyche... can be kept in balance" (Maimonides, 1964, p. 82).

ARISTOTLE: MEAN AND BALANCING

For Hippocrates and Galen, a life in balance was not a determinant of health, a sign or symptom of health, or even a cause of health. Rather, balance was health and well-being. The intuition seems to have been that a life in balance is a good thing because it is a whole and healthy life, a life of maximal well-being. But why should this be? Hippocrates and Galen could only say that balance—equal proportions of humors—is natural, whereas disease (imbalance) is unnatural. But this explains nothing. A causal link between balance and health was not suggested until Aristotle saw the need to do so (Vinci & Robert, 2005; Shampo & Kyle, 1982).

Born in 384 BCE at Stagira in northern Greece, Aristotle was the natural successor to his teacher, Plato, and became the teacher of Alexander the Great. Returning to Athens in 335 BCE, Aristotle set up his own school at the Lyceum and spent the rest of his life developing the first systematic body of philosophic work in the Western tradition. Although a great deal of this work survives, sadly most of it is in the form of student notes from his lectures, and this is probably only a fraction of what he actually produced. We do know that one of the most important themes that went through all of Aristotle's work was that the culmination (and ultimate rationale) for philosophy was political practice, which Aristotle took to be the only plausible means that social animals like humans could employ to reach the good life.

How did Aristotle conceive of the good life? He argued—carrying on an ancient cultural tradition— that human well-being is ultimately a matter of harmony. The harmonious life brings all of the disparate parts of human existence into balance, a fact that Aristotle found in biology and the natural world. To be sure, in the *Republic,* Plato also relied on a psychological image of human harmony—the rational charioteer striving to keep the twin horses of passion and animal strength from going in different directions. But when he seeks metaphors to express the virtuous human or the virtuous state, Plato looked always to mathematical proportionality and equality. Aristotle is more down to earth. He wants to ground his concept of the good life in actions and virtues (dispositions to act in certain ways). For Aristotle, ethical matters are practical not theoretical.

In his primary ethical work, the *Nicomachean Ethics* (Aristotle, 1928), Aristotle writes that a person must study ethics to be able to live the good life, to know what is best, and to do it. Like Plato, Aristotle grounded ethical behavior in ethical virtues—justice, courage, loyalty, honesty, temperance, and the like—which, again like Plato, he thought of as complex rational, emotional, and social skills. But, unlike Plato, Aristotle thought that virtues were dispositions to act that could only be learned through practice, not theoretical investigation. The moral individual is wise in practice not in theory, or rather, the wise individual's theory arises from practice rather than being antecedent to it.

What does it mean to be *practically wise?* Aristotle rejects the notion that mortal behavior is a matter of learning general rules or commandments and following them despite sacrifices or consequences—a notion that was to become a central pillar of the Judeo-Christian approach to morality. Aristotle insists that the right thing to do is highly dependent on the circumstances of the situation and the consequences of acting one way rather than another. Because morality is a matter of doing what is right rather than merely knowing what is right, morality is a matter of developing skills that allow one to discern the right course of action *and* do it. Along the way one slowly becomes virtuous and the wisdom such virtue brings is precisely the wisdom to know what a virtuous person would do in those circumstances. The virtuous life—the life of acting in accordance with practical wisdom—is the good life.

Aristotle's teaching seems circular (i.e., being virtuous is doing what a virtuous person would do because being virtuous gives one the knowledge of what is virtuous). It is rescued from this fate by what in effect is the methodology of practical wisdom, namely the *doctrine of the mean.* The doctrine is another example of Aristotle's view that virtue is a way of acting, not of knowing how to act. For Aristotle, the doctrine of the mean is merely a restatement of the operating methodology of any practical craft or skill (Aristotle, 1998, 1106a26–b28): A good craftsman is like a virtuous person; he or she knows how to avoid excess and deficiency to produce a product that is, by the standards of the art form, just right. So too, the person with the virtue of courage will judge some dangers to be worth facing and not others. His or her behavior lies between that of a coward—who judges every danger to be excessive and flees—and the foolhardy or rash person—who judges every danger worth facing and has no fear.

For Aristotle, the heroic figure of the fearless warrior, outnumbered and facing insurmountable odds—while making for classic American theatre—is not his ideal when the dangers faced are simply not worth the risk. Rambo would have seemed the fool to Aristotle. He believed that virtue was essentially about balancing risks against potential gain. If the risks outweigh the gains, the virtuous person cuts and runs, waiting for a more favorable balance. This kind of careful calculus, weighing costs and benefits, is what distinguishes Aristotle as the master of the less idealistic and more situational notion of virtue. He does not rely on the black-and-white terms used by his predecessors. Virtue always depends on a practical calculation in particular contexts. Hence, Aristotle is the philosophical patron saint of the role of life balance in the discourse on virtue. This leads to the following curious paradox that flows naturally from Aristotle's thinking: The courageous person sometimes walks (or even runs) away.

Aristotle's doctrine of the mean can be easily misunderstood as recommending a kind of bland, unexciting middle-of-the-roadism, a case of supreme emotional control and temperance. To this, Aristotle would point out that the middle path of virtue is entirely determined by the circumstances of the situation requiring one's response or attitude. In some circumstances, strong feelings and direct action may be called for. Sometimes the right amount of anger is a great deal of anger indeed (short of irrationality, of course). Moreover, the virtuous person is not one who avoids earthly pleasures entirely but rather one who indulges in the full range of pleasures—not too much, but not too little either. Aristotle was no puritan.

The doctrine of the mean can be criticized for lacking the capacity for decision making in all but the simplest cases. Aristotle invites this criticism by succumbing to the ancient Greek fascination with numerical examples, suggesting that the mean may be calculated arithmetically. But it would be nonsensical to suggest that complex moral dilemmas could be subject to quantitative solutions. On the other hand, in what sense is the doctrine a methodology for decision making at all? Aristotle avoids this question by saying that the virtuous person, like the skilled craftsman, would just know, in particular circumstances, where the mean lies. There is no moral rule book, just trial, error, and practice, and the virtuous person "sees the truth in each case" (Aristotle, 1928, 1998, 1113a32–3). Aristotle remarks that this is how we understand all crafts, even the very difficult ones such as medicine, playing an instrument, or navigation (Aristotle, 1928, 1104a7–10).

Is this a clue that Aristotle is following the tradition of Hippocrates and arguing that harmony and balance constitute health? Perhaps, but what is decidedly not part of Aristotle's picture is the more modern conflation of health and well-being. As far as we can tell, for Aristotle, health is neither a necessary nor a sufficient condition of human well-being; at most it is one, among many other, components of a life that is going well. A healthy individual may utterly fail to lead a virtuous life, and a virtuous person may well be unhealthy. Aristotle insists, however, that if the life of an unhealthy person is otherwise going well, it would be *even better* if she or he were healthy. But then, he argues in the *Nicomachean Ethics,* the virtuous life would be better if the individual was beautiful, wealthy, and had lots of friends as well (Aristotle, 1928, 1098a31–b6). Well-being, happiness, a life that goes well—these are highly complex, multidimensional, and robust notions for Aristotle.

That being so, and because the doctrine of the mean is obviously a version of the ancient Greek notion of harmony and balance and is so central to Aristotle's ethical writing, it remains to ask how he identified the ethical roots of balance and answered the question: Why is a life in balance a good life? Aristotle's answer takes us to a very different and surprising domain. It is at this point, undoubtedly, that the ancient Greek mind radically departs from our own, modernist understanding of balance.

In a central passage of his *Ethics,* Aristotle explains that the good person's motivation to act according to virtue is for the sake of *kalon,* which is to say, the beautiful, fine, or noble. The contrast with the Judeo-Christian tradition could not be starker. The Greek is not obliged—by the gods, by rules or commandments—to do the right thing; the Greek does it out of respect for the aesthetic value of righteous acts. The good life, he continues, is like a work of art. The great artist will strive to produce a work from which nothing should be taken away and to which nothing further should be added (Aristotle, 1928, 1106b 5–14). The harmony and the balance that underwrites the good life are ultimately aesthetic.

But there is more. In book I of his *Ethics*, Aristotle asks us to compare three kinds of lives that might be thought to be especially attractive: one devoted to pleasure, another to doing good works in politics, and the third to the solitary contemplative life of pure knowledge and understanding. Rather than three separate lives, Aristotle may also be comparing three parts of a single life, lived in series. The eight books that follow describe the political life—the life of good deeds, social conscience, sympathy, and a desire for peace and prosperity for the whole community. This resonates with the other dominant ancient Greek theme of the importance of the political and the virtues of solidarity, friendship, and fellow feeling. It also resonates with our ordinary sense of the virtuous person, the person whose life is in balance.

But at the very end of the *Ethics,* in Book X, Aristotle makes an unexpected move. He takes us back to the three lives and argues that though the political life is generally the best life to lead, it is the contemplative life that is the best of all (or, it is the life that the truly wise person will end up with). Given all he has said about the practical nature of ethics, many scholars have wondered how, in the end, he would wish to opt for what, for most of us, is the ultimately *impractical* life of pure theory. But there is no inconsistency here. The best life—the happiest life—is life as a work of art, and, given the contingency of day-to-day life, that can only exist at the level of pure theory, not practice. The good life is practical, achievable, and balanced—but the very best life of all is theoretical, most likely ideal, rarely achievable, and, on its face, imbalanced. For Aristotle, the ultimate standard by which the good life is assessed is not the mechanical one of balance, but the aesthetic one of purity, abstraction, and wholeness.

METAPHOR OF BALANCE

If our cultural acceptance of balance and harmony as the operating metaphors of health and happiness are derived from these ancient Greek traditions—both medical and ethical—something profound happened between then and now. For Aristotle at least, balance and harmony are aesthetic notions at bottom: The good life is a work of art, or as Aristotle puts it, a life in which nothing more needs to be added or taken away, a life of integrity, wholeness, and meaningful completion.

Needless to say, the eccentric and the bohemian outliers notwithstanding, we no longer think in these terms, or if we do it is restricted to very circumscribed areas of our life. It is more likely that our understanding of balance takes into account what philosophers call the *deontological understanding* of ethics and value, namely doing what is right, doing one's duty, and fulfilling one's obligations. The roots of this understanding of the good life are very deep indeed but are very different from the ancient Greek tradition, which, of course, we have also absorbed.

Roughly, the deontological or duty-based approach to ethics flows from our basic Judeo-Christian heritage. Certainly in the Jewish tradition, the key to the good life are the *mitzvoth*. These are divinely sanctioned and instituted rules of conduct that are written down and systematized as the *Halakha* and recorded in the so called classical rabbinic literature of the *Mishnah* and the *Talmud.* The Christian Ten Commandments and their development through the ages also follow this tradition. In the history of philosophy, Immanuel Kant (1724-1804), himself scornful of Christianity, was responsible for conceptualizing deontological ethics into its present philosophical format. In the last two centuries modern ethics has revolved around the contrast between deontological or rule-based ethics and *consequentialism* (the most prominent example of which is the English 19th-century political and ethical theory called *utilitarianism).*

The deontological approach we have inherited from our Judeo-Christian heritage (which at this point in history has to be thought of more as a sociocultural heritage than just a theological one) is an emotional and intellectual gravitational force that is nearly impossible to resist. Leading a good life is leading a moral life. At its core, this means doing what is right and avoiding what is wrong, which in turn means following, not violating, moral rules, laws, and commandments. Nearly all aspects of what ethical theorists call the *logical framework* of ethics—such as the rule that one can only be held to account for the deeds he or she does consciously, voluntarily, intentionally, or at least knowingly—derive from this model of good conduct. When we read in Aristotle's *Ethics* that a man who is handsome and carries himself nobly is morally superior to the man who is ugly and slovenly (Book X), we wonder how Aristotle could believe that physical traits over which humans have little control can count for or against their moral worth. The reason is that Aristotle's good life is aesthetic, not deontological.

With these contrasts in mind, recall the three questions we suggested need to be answered before "life balance" could be a workable, operational notion:

- Why is the life in balance better than a life not so?

- In what manner, precisely, is the life in balance better?

- What is being balanced in the balanced life?

For the Greek mind, the metaphor of balance reflects the value of harmony of disparate elements of the human, viewed either organically and biologically, or more broadly socially and ethically. For Aristotle in particular, the foundation of the metaphor is aesthetic. A life in balance is better for the same reason that a good work of art is better than a bad work of art: Nothing needs to be added, nothing needs to be taken away. But, given his conclusion about the best life of all, Aristotle does not believe there is a precise way of decomposing the human life and recomposing it in a single formula for the optimal life balance. The point is wholeness and integrity, not the disparate parts in equipoise. The life of pleasure is less balanced than the political life because some of the virtues—solidarity, justice, temperance—are not taken into account in the life of pleasure. But we need to move beyond that as well. The life of contemplation is best of all, because it constitutes the best of which humans are capable: pure rationality.

Why then, do we persist in thinking that the good life requires balancing of particular and disparate life components? Likely because for us, immersed in the Judeo-Christian rather than the ancient Greek tradition, balance is grounded, not in aesthetics, but in deontology. We must balance work and family for the simple reason that fulfilling one's family roles is part of a moral code and as such, is one of our duties as a moral being. We are obliged to have family as part of our life. By contrast Aristotle's philosopher, the person living the best of all human lives, is the ultimate workaholic: all contemplation, no family life. Such an individual is a problem for us in the Judeo-Christian world because the components of our lives are deontologically set for us. We are obliged to do all our duties. (Significantly, the notions of *duty* and *obligation* have no obvious translation into Aristotle's Greek.)

Where does that leave us? For one thing, it shows why we ought to be concerned about medicalizing life balance because doing do is essentially turning an ancient and persistent moral tradition into a model of health. Aristotle gives us a competing model, one in which "balance" is either not a human good or is radically different than the notion ingrained in us from our heritage. On the Aristotelian view, balance is a matter of wholeness and integrity (which he associated with philosophical contemplation); in the Judeo-Christian view, balance is a matter of equipoise or *détente* between incompatible, incommensurable but equally valuable components of the well-being.

Aristotle could plainly envision the imbalanced life of the solitary scholar as one of perfection and value because the balance he sought was completion, not equal representation of countervailing components of well-being. To insist he was wrong about this—and worse, to insist as a matter of the science of human health that he was wrong—presumes a more encompassing account of the valuable life in terms of which the two versions of balance should be compared and adjudicated.

At this point in our human history, we lack that grander account; indeed, there may not be such an account. But, at the end of the day, what we must resist is the very human temptation of discounting variations by turning them into problems, especially, as we have argued, medical problems. For all we know, the imbalanced outlier—the hermit, artist, or scholar—may have it right.

REFERENCES

Akiskal, H. S., & Akiskal, K. K. (2007). In search of Aristotle: Temperament, human nature, melancholia, creativity, and eminence. *Journal of Affective Disorders, 100,* 1–6.

Aristotle. (1928). *Nicomachean Ethics* (W. D. Ross, Trans.). Claredon: Oxford University Press. (Original work published 350 B.C.E).

Aziz, S., & Zickar, M. J. (2006). A cluster analysis investigation of workaholism as a syndrome. *Journal of Occupational Health Psychology, 11,* 52–62.

Bryden, P., & McColl, M. A. (2003). The concept of occupation, 1900 to 1974. In M. A McColl, M. Law, D. Stewart, L. Doubt, N. Pollock, & T. Krupa (Eds.), *Theoretical basis of occupational therapy* (pp. 27–37). Thorofare, NJ: SLACK Incorporated.

Callahan, D. (1982). The WHO definition of "health." In L. Beauchamp & L. Walters (Eds.), *Contemporary Issues in Bioethics* (2nd ed.). Belmont, CA: Wadsworth.

Eikhof, D. R., Warhurst, C., & Haunschild, A. (2007). Introduction: What work? What life? What balance?: Critical reflections on the work–life balance debate. *Employee Relations, 29,* 325–333.

Frone, M. R. (2001). Work–family balance. In J. C. Quick & L. E. Tetrick (Eds.), *Handbook of occupational health psychology* (pp. 143–162). Washington, DC: American Psychological Association.

Golden, T. D., Veiga, J. F., & Simsek, Z. (2006). Telecommuting's differential impact on work–family conflict: Is there no place like home? *Journal of Applied Psychology, 91,* 1340–1350.

Grawitch, M. J., Gottschalk, M., & Munz, D. C. (2006). The path to a healthy workplace: A critical review linking healthy workplace practices, employee well-being, and organizational improvements consulting. *Psychology Journal: Practice and Research, 58,* 129–147.

Grawitch, M. J., Trares, S., & Kohler, J. M. (2007). Healthy workplace practices and employee outcomes. *International Journal of Stress Management, 14,* 275–293.

Kenny, D. T., & Cooper, C. L. (2003). Introduction: Occupational stress and its management. *International Journal of Stress Management, 10,* 275–279.

Maimonides, M. (1964). Two treatises on the regimen of health (A. Bar-Sela, H. E. Hoff, & E. Faris, Trans.). *Transactions of the American Philosophical Society, 52,* 4.

Mills, C. W. (1959). *The sociological imagination.* New York: Oxford University Press.

O'Driscoll, M. P., Poelmans, S., Spector, P. E., Kalliath, T., Allen, T. D., Cooper, C. L., et al. (2003). Family-responsive interventions, perceived organizational and supervisor support, work–family conflict, and psychological strain. *International Journal of Stress Management, 10,* 326–344.

Quick, J. D., Henley, A. B., & Quick, J. C. (2004). The balancing act—At work and at home. *Organizational Dynamics, 33,* 426–438.

Roberts, K. (2007). Work–life balance—The sources of the contemporary problem and the probable outcomes: A review and interpretation of the evidence. *Employee Relations, 29,* 334–351.

Shampo, M. A., & Kyle, R. A. (1982). Aristotle. *Journal of the American Medical Association, 248,* 89.

U.S. Census Bureau. (2008). *Historical income data.* Retrieved February 11, 2009, from http://www.census.gov/hhes/www/income/histinc/histinctb.html

Vinci, T., & Robert, J. S. (2005). Aristotle and modern genetics. *Journal of the History of Ideas, 66,* 201–221.

Whybrow, P. C. (2005). *American mania: When more is not enough.* New York: W. W. Norton.

Worrall, L., & Cooper, C. L. (2001). *The quality of working life: Survey of managers' changing experiences.* London: Chartered Management Institute.

Wulff, H. R. (1999). The concept of disease: From Newton back to Aristotle. *Lancet, 354* (Suppl.) SIV50.

Zola, I. K. (1972). Medicine as an institution of social control. *Sociological Review, 20,* 487–504.

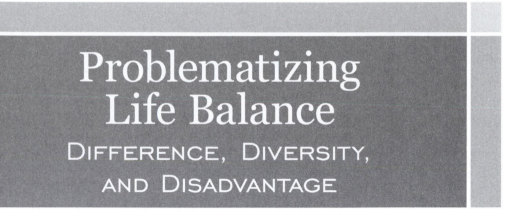

Problematizing Life Balance
DIFFERENCE, DIVERSITY, AND DISADVANTAGE

GAIL ELIZABETH WHITEFORD

INTRODUCTION

Life balance, as it is presented and discussed in the academic literature and within policy documents, is a construct underpinned by a number of tacit assumptions that have not, to date, been fully interrogated from different experiential perspectives or knowledge traditions. Indeed, life balance, as it is popularly understood, has largely been shaped by a particularly Eurocentric discursive tradition and the labor-market issues associated with late (post-20th-century) Western capitalism. In this chapter, life balance is critiqued and problematized, with a number of key issues discussed, including whether the pursuit of life balance is a universal, cross-cultural value; whether life balance is attainable or even relevant in the face of significant forces that work against it; and finally, whether balance is always desirable. A case study, drawn from South Africa, including narrative data, informs the discussion.

BACKGROUND: IDENTIFYING THE PROBLEMS

Achieving balance among the numerous demands on the time of individuals and families in resource-rich countries has become part of a broader social consciousness in which an evaluation of fundamental values has become prevalent. It is, for many in postindustrial capitalist societies, a zeitgeist in which an apparent new paradigm is emerging: a move away from consumerist culture to lifestyles in which meaning and relatedness are more central. Terms such as *down shifters*, *sea changers*, and *tree changers* have become part of everyday colloquial language in many countries. Their incorporation points to the social and geographic responses indicative of the scale of this paradigm upheaval. In particular, it seems, people are seeking a new relationship with work.

Clearly, this not an overnight phenomenon. Nor can it be viewed in isolation; rather it may be seen as part of a complex interplay among numerous forces, most of which are supra-individual. This makes the extent to which individual choice and control are being exercised in this social phenomenon somewhat questionable (Kay, 2003). Indeed, the broad discursive arena of work–life balance has developed over several decades in different countries relative to different governments and their attendant policy orientations (Duncan, 2002) as well as relative to economic and demographic trends. As Dean (2007) points out, work–life balance discussions cannot be separated from labor-market policies concerned with maximizing participation of a shrinking workforce through enhanced flexibil-

K. Matuska & C. Christiansen (Eds.)
Life balance: Multidisciplinary theories and research (pp 23–32)
© 2009 SLACK Incorporated and AOTA Press

ity. Neither can the idea of life balance be separate from the growing process of deinstitutionalization, in which the major institutions in society assume responsibility for their members). It is a process

> supported by other social institutions such as the state and market, and underpinned by economic change, specifically the change from mass production to more flexible forms of production and employment... changes in social policy also reflect this de-institutionalisation... moving towards supporting families with two adult earners, thereby relating to individuals as wage earners rather than as individuals as gendered family members. (Charles & Harris, 2007, p. 293)

Although, as suggested above, the new policy orientations associated with deinstitutionaliza-tion tend to reduce individuals to the status of *wage earner*, gender has been a fundamental aspect of the work–life balance debate and policy development over time and will most likely continue to be so (Abrahamson, 2007). Issues relating to everything from accessible and affordable child care (Human Rights and Equal Opportunity Commission [HREOC], 2007) to the impact of caregiving responsibilities on women's ability to participate in the labor market (Evandrous & Glaser, 2003) to the feminization of managerial regimes (Dean, 2007), have informed national and interna-tional discussion and debate. These issues have, in many instances, contributed to national policy reforms (Houston, 2005; HREOC, 2007). Such reforms have been implemented to address the reality in many countries that women still face greater challenges in achieving work–life balance because of their additional roles or "second shift" (Duncan, 2002).

Gender is not the only problematic and potentially divisive aspect of the work–life balance discourse. Significantly, it seems that work–life policy and rhetoric tends to reinforce divisions in society along socioeconomic lines (Dean, 2007). While a full discussion of this complex sce-nario is beyond the scope of this chapter, essentially, as Kay (2003) suggests, work–life policies are experienced by *work-rich* (those with access to secure and well-paid work) and *work-poor* (those without access to secure and well paid work) families very differently. As a corollary, there is a difference in the ability of each group to interact with the policy environment.

While highly educated workers in professional occupations may be relatively well positioned to negotiate favorable working conditions, low-skilled employees in insecure employment usually have less scope to do so. Work-rich and work-poor households, therefore, differ in their level of dependency on policy or external intervention to address this disparity (Kay, 2003, p. 232).

This difference is also evident in the extent to which employers invest in valued workers and in which workers take advantage of flexible arrangements. Managerial discretion in this respect has actually been identified as a key cause of discrimination by women from minority ethnic backgrounds in the workplace (Bradley, Healy, & Mukherjee, 2005).

Professionally, concerns with the life balance and lifestyles of individuals has been an area of focused attention and, in some instances, has become a growth industry, leading to new interven-tions such as *lifestyle redesign*. In occupational therapy, a discipline that has had a stated concern with *occupational balance* since its inception, the notion of *balance* developed over time and became enshrined within a number of practice models (Iwama, 2006; Kielhofner, 2002; Townsend & Polataijko, 2007). Fundamental to this centralization of balance are tacit beliefs concerning the relationship between balance and well-being: that achievement of a balanced lifestyle will result in optimal levels of health and well-being. Indeed, as Christiansen and Matuska (2006) have identified, there is quite a bit of evidence that points to the negative health impacts of work stress–related disorders and, among other things, a lack of balance in time use.

However, in occupational therapy, as with the general literature on work–life balance, the con-ceptual development to date has been relatively uncritical. It remains underpinned by tacit value systems, ideologies, and simplistic constructions that fail to problematize difference, diversity, and disadvantage. Life balance, as it appears in the literature, reflects a particular ontological standpoint of late, Western, capitalist, affluent countries. When we begin to consider what life balance may mean from other ontological standpoints, the issues include the following:

- Work is considered as "other" than life.
- Categorizations of time use, which classically include work, rest, and play, are overly simplistic and do not reflect different cultural or socioeconomic contexts.
- Care and caregiving occupations are sometimes considered work and sometimes considered life.
- Balance may be irrelevant or a low priority in the face of issues of survival and the processes associated with the construction or reconstruction of civic society or the enactment of citizenship by disadvantaged sub-groups.

As well as being evident in the extant literature, these issues of life balance reflect my own experiences as a clinician, researcher, and educator in various cultural and national contexts, where I have interacted with people from very disadvantaged backgrounds. In my experience, historical, sociocultural, religious, and other contextual factors, such as politics and economics, have a profound impact on how time is perceived and used. Different cultural experiences of being and time and the orchestration of the numerous occupations of life within it have been an enduring interest of mine both personally and professionally for many years. For this reason, I have chosen to explore these issues, not just theoretically, but also relative to a specific site and with a specific group of people facing what can only be described as extreme conditions: sub-Saharan Africa and those living with the HIV/AIDS epidemic.

CONTEXT: SUB-SAHARAN AFRICA AND HIV/AIDS EPIDEMIC

That sub-Saharan Africa has a major challenge in the face of HIV/AIDS is not news. It is the region most affected in the world, with an estimated 22.5 million people infected and 1.7 million people newly infected in 2007 alone (Joint United Nations Programme on HIV/AIDS [UNAIDS], 2007). This is compounded by the fact that 80% of those who are infected don't know they are HIV positive; in sub-Saharan Africa, only 12% of men and 10% of women have been tested and collected the results of their tests (World Health Organization [WHO], 2005). South Africa has the highest population of people infected, though rates vary by region—for example from 39% in Kwa Zulu Natal to 15% in the Western Cape (South African Department of Health, 2007). UNAIDS (2007), however, reports a slowing in the rate of increase, particularly in pregnant women ages 15 to 24 years—a trend apparently linked with greater use of condoms in both men and women in this age group.

One of the particularly tragic outcomes of the HIV/AIDS epidemic is the number of children orphaned each year. WHO's formal definition of an AIDS orphan is a child who has had either the mother or both parents die from AIDS before the child turns 15. Global estimates are that the number of AIDS orphans will reach 41 million by 2010, and 90% are currently in sub-Saharan Africa (WHO, 2005). As the major caregivers, women particularly carry the burden of this devastating phenomenon, which has economic and social impacts.

GRANDMOTHERS AGAINST POVERTY AND AIDS

I first heard about Grandmothers Against Poverty and AIDS (GAPA) when visiting South Africa for the first time in 2004, attending a conference at which Lionel Davies, formerly incarcerated on Robbin Island along with Nelson Mandela, was due to speak. Although Davies was an uplifting speaker, it was the presentation made by this group of grandmothers that was most inspiring. Their presentation was made even more powerful by their songs: Singing is a powerful cultural vehicle that they use to do everything from delivering educational messages, to lobbying politicians, to reinforcing their connection to and support of one another.

GAPA's story is set against a backdrop of hardship, alienation, and relative occupational deprivation (Whiteford, 2000, 2004). Founded in 2001 by Alicia Mdaka in conjunction with occupational therapist Katherine Broderick and a number of other grandmothers, GAPA was established as a response to the impoverishment and burden experienced by the grandmothers in caring for their grandchildren after their parents died from HIV/AIDS. They created a small business through which craft items made by the women are sold, thus providing a means of direct income generation. GAPA has also become a supportive space for the women, many of whom have faced prejudice and social stigma because of their connection to HIV. It is estimated that to date, more than 900 grandmothers have been involved in the project. The project is housed in the township of Khayelitsha, north of Cape Town. It is a town with relatively limited facilities and resources but a deep sense of resilience and hope in the face of daunting odds.

One of the most important elements of GAPA is that, from its inception, it was oriented to developing skills required for income generation, and as a corollary, opportunities for the women to earn money. The importance of having a source of income in the face of extreme poverty cannot be overstated and is central in the women's perceptions of the value of the organization. The organization has also created a space in which "nested occupations" (Bateson, 1996; Wiseman, 2007) can be performed. In essence, this means that the women can engage not only in craft production work, earning money per piece, but also in linked occupations such as caring for children (in this case grandchildren), food production, education, and supportive socializing. This is significant, as it is an environment in which structurally and practically, production, care, obligation, and relatedness happen in a culturally meaningful, naturalistic, and meshed way. In such a space, the work/life dichotomy that pervades international discourses becomes fairly meaningless.

For this reason, I wanted to explore the relevance of life balance, or work–life balance, through interviews with the women of GAPA and also to gain a sense of the priorities in the women's lives, given the many challenges they face every day. Rather than frame such discussions within the rubric of formal research, the women and I agreed that we would enter into a conversation. The women agreed (and, indeed, were proud) to share their stories and answer questions as they arose. Almost more important, the time and input of the women was acknowledged through my donation of materials to the craft-work business and a cash donation to the organization as a whole to cover any organizational costs associated with my visit. I had a South African colleague with me who was both the negotiator of the visit and, to some extent, cultural informant, though not herself a resident of Khayelishta. Our visit was also approved and managed by Vivienne, the relatively new and dynamic director of GAPA. She allowed me to speak to a large group of women assembled for a training and education day (many with children and grandchildren) and describe myself and my goals in conversing with the women.

One of the desired outcomes expressed by both Vivienne and the women was to promote the work of GAPA internationally through making their stories available broadly through publication. This of course, was agreed upon (and remains a subobjective of this chapter). Once there was a collective agreement by all that my intentions were acceptable, I was then directed to meet individually with three women: Alicia, Violet, and Constance. The women agreed to have our conversations recorded to avoid me having to write copious notes. It was also useful because one of the women became an interpreter for one of the others who was not so confident in English. I present Alicia's story here in full, just as she told it to me. The rationale for this is that any attempt to edit it or reduce it would be to diminish the rich contextual detail and the very power of her life story. It is a story of personal and collective transformation.

There are numerous elements in this account worthy of discussion. However, for the purpose of an exploratory critique of life balance as a construct and its importance across sociocultural, socioeconomic, and political contexts, I will focus on gender, collective need, nested or "meshed" occupations, and situatedness.

ALICIA'S STORY

Let me introduce myself, I am Alicia Mdaka, I'm doing my 68th year this year. I was married in Eastern Cape and my husband died in 1976...I was with the children—that time I had six children, three boys and three girls, and then after that I had to come back to Cape Town again to work for those children, then I got another boyfriend, I had another two boys, so that made eight—I've been the mother of eight: five boys and three girls.

And then the tragedy came to my house, it was a really heavy time for me. My first daughter died in 1999 from HIV and AIDS—leaving me with her three children...I have to raise those children. In 2000, my granddaughter died of HIV/AIDS—she was born with it, by her mother. That time, when my granddaughter died, her mother was fully blown with it. The day of the funeral I had to go to the hospital and ask to see her just to know how the coffin could get done so they can come and fetch it—it was very, very painful for me 'cause I had to bury that granddaughter of mine with my family, and the next door neighbors didn't come to the funeral, they said they are not going every day and every month to a funeral of HIV/AIDS.

And they were calling me some names—saying my home is an HIV home, they won't even let my grandchildren play with their children, they say that they will infect them. In 2001 I lost another child to HIV, before she died, my shack was burnt with all of my belongings: and when that shack was gone, I had no place for the funeral—[I thought] what am I going to do? I had to go to that place where they are making scrap to get some cardboard so at least I can make it warm, and to have a place for the funeral to take place. The neighbors also didn't come to the funeral. At that time I was asking myself some questions—why me? How am I going to cope with this? What about my grandchildren, how am I going to live a life like that—with nobody and no friends because I have an HIV home? I was thinking of killing myself.

Every day, I watched the train coming up and one day I said to myself it's better to go to the station and throw myself on the railway lines so that the train must just crush me down, but while I was standing there on the pavement waiting at the station, there came another woman, and she just shook me on my shoulders, and she said, "why are you looking like that, looking so sad? Come here, I want to buy you some Coke—and we can go together to drink it," and when I sat down I realized that the woman was sent by God—so I didn't go to the station again. But I was [still] crying day after day and not going out, and at that time and then I found out my other daughter had AIDS—and she was crying. So I'm not sleeping at night worrying about my life and my mother who also has nothing—she has nothing, no clothes, and no food—she can't go out 'cause she has no clothes—because all of her belongings were burnt. She has nothing, even though she worked hard before; now she just has to stay in bed. So that's why I'm worried, and also about the children and how they are after their mother died—I don't know what to do. Then the social worker said, "You must come to the support group and bring your mother," but I am too ashamed to tell my story. But the social worker takes me into her office and *makes* me tell her my story.

And she says, "It's not the end of the world—God is with you. You mustn't think of killing yourself—you are going to survive if you give your hope to God—and he is the only one. After night is dawn—you must bear in mind those words—and you must live for those children. If you are thinking of killing yourself, who will look after the children? You must think of this. God—she is going to help you." So I realized that yes, I am a child of God, I must not lose hope, I must pray. Then I realized there were other grandmothers there, and they said you must come every day, so I did, it was at the back of the hospital for the support group, so we decided to start GAPA. There were seven grandmothers who started it, then three more came, and we started. Kathleen Broderick was with us, she then got some scraps of material, and we did patchwork so we sewed; but first thing was to sew for ourselves 'cause I had nothing, even this dress was made from scraps, 'cause I had no money to go to Woolworth's so I had to make everything for myself.

And then we started small and then after that we said OK—we've got a workshop, so we must go to the community and recruit other trainees, so they must come and join with us, 'cause us as each has HIV in their house. But they hide it, nobody wants to talk about it, but we must. Then we started support groups in our houses. These 10 grandmothers formed GAPA, to help people talk about HIV; how to talk to your children when they are diagnosed, and supporting each other, and then we were united. What I saw is that we need friends, you can't do it yourself, you can't lock yourself indoors, you must have others, it makes you stronger and gives you courage—you must be ready for any action. These people, they are victims of HIV/AIDS so we must give them hope, I sit down and talk to women and give good counseling.

Here at GAPA I'm a counselor and support group leader and also a facilitator of bereavement here at GAPA. To me, GAPA is my *home*. When I'm here, I'm here because I was just a mess, but when I joined GAPA, I felt that I'm not hopeless. Now I've been working for GAPA, and I've been to places: I've been to Malta, and I've been twice to Canada talking about HIV. I'm standing up now; no more tears. I can stand up and tell my story 'cause GAPA has healed this wound. Which was so bad—I don't know how to explain it.

[Here] we do crocheting, sewing, we teach each other and we are teaching others how to care for your grandchildren, and we run aftercare for those whose mothers are working late; we are making sure they are not raped, we are keeping them safe; we are teaching them how to knit, to have skills, to make things. We have a shop here where we sell things, we have donations of old clothes, we sew some things and do bead working also. Doing things with my hands is healing because I know that if I'm thinking, "how are my grandchildren going to have bread?" I know that if I sew an apron, then at the end of the day that kid will have bread. It's making life easier for me. Also I got some money to buy some electricity. It's [GAPA] healing and helping me a lot, I can't be without GAPA as I know that if I have a problem I call one of my sisters here and ask that she will give me good advice—my scar has healed.

Now I can stand on my own feet—I am not depending on any man. I am a man myself. I am mother, father, and grandfather to those children and in that house. And as I have been staying in a little shack with those children, I was thinking, "how am I going to get out of that shack which will one day again be burnt down?" So I decided that I have got this pension money of mine, and I said to this daughter of mine, "how we can get out of here?" And she said, "we must get a small loan, it will be the start of a brick house." And then we went to the office and got a loan of 5,000 [Rand], and we have made a start, and I am doing my house bit by bit. So, GAPA has done a lot for me; she has given me a green light. I'm taking it more easy, and my body is free when I come here, my body shakes free, here... I am an example to other women.

DISCUSSION

Local, solidarity-based, bottom up, collective strategies…provide an alternative, sustainable and democratic form of development through which poor women as workers are recognized and enabled to participate as citizens in their own development. (Hill, 2001, p. 22)

The routine of Alicia's life reflects all the occupations that are important and meaningful for the collection of women, for the grandchildren, for the business of GAPA, and for Alicia. It is evident that the orientation of GAPA is not toward the individual women, though each is acknowledged in their own right and relative to her particular situation and needs, but to the collective. Therefore what "I" need to do each day is closely meshed with what "we" do here: The occupations are transactional rather than individually predicated (Cutchin, Dickie, & Humphrey, 2006). In this milieu then, *balance*, as a construct, seems irrelevant, if not entirely alien. My interpretation of this space in which the women gather, work, and provide care is that it is represents a place in which need, environmental demands, gender, and culture are inextricably linked. In short, there are just more pressing things to be concerned about, like getting food for the grandchildren, than striving for life balance as an individual.

Gender is particularly significant in Alicia's story and of course as a pillar of GAPA itself. Clearly, it is the work of women, by women, and for women and children—an enactment of care through collective agency. It is a response that reinforces the view that, although women are often those most burdened by poverty and disease in resource-poor settings (Hill, 2001), they are often the leaders of social change and transformation at a grassroots level (Thibeault, 2007). It is a response that also reinforces more recent constructions of women's responses to stressful conditions, which, as opposed to fight/flight, has been dubbed "tend/befriend" (Taylor et al., 2000). Taylor and colleagues claim that in the tend/befriend model, the enactment of care and the drive toward being with others has a positive impact on levels of wellness. In Alicia's particular case, she states that she has become "father and grandfather" to her children and grandchildren, an important position, not only in her eyes but within her specific sociocultural milieu. In traditional Xhosa society, males would traditionally hold more power, property, and capital wealth than women. In this regard then, her role and status as a new property owner define her as being comparatively empowered relative to other women: As she says, "I don't need a man." Relatively speaking then, in her particular context, it would seem that she is very possibly better off than she may have been in a traditional marriage.

From another perspective, gender seems to underpin the way that the women go about performing the numerous daily occupations requisite to GAPA. There is some evidence that women perform tasks differently from men, with a heightened ability to engage in multiple tasks simultaneously, what has otherwise been referred to as *nested* or *meshed occupations* (Bateson, 1996). This concurrent performance of everyday activities is evident in Alicia's account of what she does at GAPA, but was also very evident when I spent time there.

In the midst of an education and training session for new women attending GAPA, children and grandchildren were supervised while they slept or played, food was prepared, craft work was done, and supplies were ferried in and out of the building. As an observer, I found it impossible to distinguish work from nonwork. Indeed, I am not convinced it would be a useful differentiation in this context. The only differentiation made by the women seemed to be which of these occupations represented income generation. One of the women said to me that she hoped I didn't mind she was making something (a teddy bear apparently destined for a Norwegian designer décor store) while we spoke, as finishing the bear represented "another 30 Rand, which will make dinner better."

From both cultural and economic standpoints, the close nexus between these occupations is significant, especially between production and caregiving. In postindustrial countries, of course, tensions between parenting and work are central to the experience of many families (Kay, 2003). This has, to some extent, driven policy initiatives, such as tax credits for caregivers (Nolan, 2006) and systems in which family caregivers in some countries are paid for their time. In a comparative study of five countries, Austria, France, Italy, the Netherlands, and the United Kingdom, Ungerson and Yeandle (2005) found that there were both benefits and risks associated with such systems. Ultimately, their findings were that each of those systems "problematises a simple work–life dichotomy and heightens the complex ways in which paid employment impinges on other areas of life" (p. 261).

For the women of GAPA, however, this dichotomy did not exist—there was no so-called "care gap" (Lewis, 2006), and even for the women of the township who did have to work elsewhere, there was a safe and supportive care environment for their children, especially the after-school care as described by Alicia.

When I was visiting GAPA, a new care facility was being built, with funding from an international nongovernmental organization, that indicated the women's plans to extend this important aspect of the organization. In this respect, the women may be seen as investing in the social capital of their town, Khayelitsha, and also in the development of the capacity of its inhabitants—at least the women. It may also be read as a way through which the women engaged as citizens, building civic society in a space with numerous challenges at many levels.

But what does it mean to be a citizen in such a context, and what is the intersection with issues of life balance? Politically and economically, South Africa has numerous significant issues with which to contend in the near future. While I was there, an imminent change of political leadership was the topic of debate, and some uncertainty, among black and white South Africans. This was particularly true in the face of a looming energy crisis that looked to have a negative impact on the gross domestic product. Energy issues notwithstanding, the arenas of health and education also represent significant pragmatic challenges (United Nations Development Program [UNDP], 2007). The provision of adequate health care for all is made difficult by the costs of dealing with the HIV/AIDS situation, a pressing concern discussed earlier in this chapter. Education is no less a national concern, with clear indicators that a concerted effort is required to develop a skilled workforce to meet labor-market requirements in the next two decades. Poverty and disadvantage are still significantly linked to levels of skills and education nationally (UNDP, 2007).

In South Africa at this time then, there are real and seemingly overwhelming problems. For the women of GAPA, their collective, grassroots response to their situation was to act for change at many levels. At one level it was to change attitudes and behavior of the mean and women in their community with respect to HIV/AIDS. At another it was to change their social and economic status. At yet another, they enacted processes of change that were ultimately about the creation of a civic society in which capacity and hope were being developed in equal measure. Given the scope of the change required and these women's orientation to collective rather than individual concerns, it seems that life balance is not a priority: Social transformation and an everyday commitment to it is.

CONCLUSIONS

Life balance is a loaded term. As a construct, it has tacit historical, sociopolitical, and cultural baggage that has only relatively recently begun being systematically critiqued from different perspectives. In this chapter, I have explored what life balance may mean in a specific context to a particular group of people and asked, is life balance significant here? Is it even relevant?

Through attempting to understand a cultural milieu in the form of a women's organization, GAPA, developed to counteract the burden of HIV/AIDS and through the presentation of one woman's story about her life and the organization, two things were evident. First, that the work–life dichotomy is in itself confounding: In the setting considered, work, care, life, and civic development all took place in a relatively seamless way. Second, life balance may be seen as a cultural and socioeconomic construct, perhaps a luxury, with respect to a desired quality of life relevant to those with adequate resources: fiscal, material, and educational. For the women of GAPA, it seemed that they had more important, extrapersonal concerns.

REFERENCES

Abrahamson, P. (2007). Reconciling work and family life in Europe. *Journal of Comparative Policy Analysis, 9*, 193–209.

Bateson, C. (1996). Reflections on orchestrating a life. In R. Zemke & F. Clark (Eds.) *Occupational science: The evolving discipline.* Philadelphia: F. A. Davis.

Bradley, H., Healy, G., & Mukherjee, N. (2005). Multiple burdens: Problems of work-life balance for ethnic minority trade union activist women. In D. Houston (Ed.), *Work-life balance in the 21st century,* (pp. 211–229). Hampshire, UK: Palgrave Macmillan.

Charles, N., & Harris, C. (2007). Continuity and change in work–life balance choices. *The British Journal of Sociology, 58*, 277–295.

Christiansen, C., & Matuska, K. (2006). Lifestyle balance: A review of concepts and research. *Journal of Occupational Science, 13*, 49–61.

Cutchin, M., Dickie, V., & Humphrey, R. (2006). Occupation as transactional experience: A critique of individualism in occupational science. *Journal of Occupational Science, 13*, 83–93.

Dean, H. (2007). Tipping the balance: The problematic nature of work life balance in a low income neighbourhood. *Journal of Social Policy, 36*, 519–537.

Duncan, S. (2002). Policy discourses on reconciling work and life in the EU. *Social Policy in Society, 1*, 305–314.

Evandrous, M., & Glaser, K. (2003). Combining work and family life: The pension penalty of caring. *Ageing & Society, 23*, 583–601.

Hill, E. (2001). Women in the Indian informal economy: Collective strategies for work-life improvement and development. *Work, Employment and Society, 15*, 443–464.

Houston, D. (Ed.). (2005). *Work-life balance in the 21st century.* Hampshire, UK: Palgrave Macmillan.

Human Rights and Equal Opportunity Commission. (2007). *It's about time: Women, men, work and family* [Final paper]. Sydney: Author.

Iwama, M. (2006). *The kawa model. Culturally relevant occupational therapy.* London: Elsevier.

Joint United Nations Programme on HIV/AIDS. (2007). *HIV/AIDS epidemic update.* Retrieved February 22, 2008, from http://data.unaids.org/pub

Kay, T. (2003). Work life balance in social practice. *Social Policy and Society, 2*, 231–239.

Kielhofner, G. (2002). *A model of human occupation. Theory and application* (3rd ed.). Baltimore: Lippincott Williams & Wilkins.

Lewis, J. (2006). Employment and care: The policy problem, gender equality and the issue of choice. *Journal of Comparative Policy Analysis, 8*(2), 103–114.

Nolan, P. (2006). Tax relief for breadwinners or caregivers? The designs of earned and child tax credits in five Anglo American countries. *Journal of Comparative Policy Analysis, 8*, 167–183.

South African Department of Health. (2007). *National HIV and syphilis antenatal prevalence survey 2006.* Pretoria: Author.

Taylor, S. E., Klein, L. C., Lewis, B. P., Gruenewald, T. L., Gurung, R. A. R, & Updegraff, J. A. (2000). Biobehavioral responses to stress in females: Tend-and-befriend, not fight-or-flight. *Psychological Review, 107*, 441–429.

Thibeault, R. (2007). Globalisation, universities and the future of occupational therapy: Dispatches from the majority world. *Australian Occupational Therapy Journal, 53*, 159–165.

Townsend, E., & Polataijko, H. (2007). *Enabling occupation II: Advancing an occupational therapy vision for health, well-being and justice through occupation.* Ottawa: Canadian Association of Occupational Therapists.

Ungerson, C., Yeandle, S. (2005). Care workers and work-life balance: the example of domiciliary careworkers. In D. Houston (Ed.), *Work-life balance in the 21st century,* (pp. 211–229). Hampshire, UK: Palgrave Macmillan.

United Nations Development Program. (2007). *United Nations Development Program in South Africa 2007–2010.* Retrieved February 26, 2008, from http://www.undp.org.za

Whiteford G. (2000). Occupational deprivation: Global challenge in the new millennium. *British Journal of Occupational Therapy, 64*, 200–210.

Whiteford, G. (2004). When people cannot participate: Occupational deprivation. In: C. Christiansen & E. Townsend (Eds.), *Introduction to occupation: The art and science of living* (p. 221–242). Upper Saddle Creek, NJ: Prentice Hall.

Wiseman, L. (2007). *Retirement as an occupational transition for rural men.* Unpublished doctoral thesis, Charles Sturt University, Albury NSW.

World Health Organization. (2005). *HIV/AIDS Country information.* Retrieved February 23, 2008, from http://www.who.int.hiv/countries/en/index/html

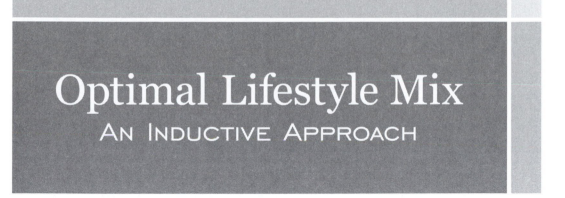

Optimal Lifestyle Mix
AN INDUCTIVE APPROACH

RUUT VEENHOVEN

INTRODUCTION

There are three approaches to assessing life balance: (1) assessing how well the reality of a person's life fits preconceptions of what a balanced life should be, (2) assessing how balanced people think their own life is, and (3) assessing which lifestyle mixes yield the most happiness. In theory, these approaches can yield quite different results, and the available evidence shows that they also do so in practice. In case of conflict, there are good arguments for favoring the last approach, but the policy process is best served with making the differences explicit.

CONCEPTS OF LIFE BALANCE

The notion of *life balance* figures in several contemporary discourses, particularly in the discourses on working hours in modern market economies and on division of household tasks between members. In these contexts, the term denotes mostly that there is an imbalance that should be corrected. The term is typically used for rhetorical purposes and for that reason is not sharply defined. In this chapter, the focus is on the analytic use of this notion, which requires that we be more specific.

Life Balance as a Property of Lifestyle Mix

The word *balance* denotes that different things weigh against each other. When used in combination with life, it refers mostly to major life domains, such as working life and private life. The term is also used for major activities, such as work versus leisure, or within domains, for example, the shares of leisure time spent alone versus time spent socializing. As such, the term life balance conveys a judgment about the composition of someone's way of life or *lifestyle*.

An imbalanced life then, is a lifestyle in which one or more components have too much weight at the expense of other components, typically too much paid work and as a result too little time at home with the family. A balanced life is a lifestyle where components are in proportion relative to each other. In proportion may mean that there is nothing wrong with the relative weights, but it may also mean that the weights are the best possible. When referring to the best possible weights,

K. Matuska & C. Christiansen (Eds.)
Life balance: Multidisciplinary theories and research (pp 33–42)
© 2009 SLACK Incorporated and AOTA Press

the term denotes an optimal lifestyle. In this chapter I will consider the entire range, from imbalanced to optimal.

In sum: A lifestyle is a composition of habitual activities, and this composition or mix can be more or less appropriate. The term *life balance* denotes the degree of aptness, which can vary from inapt (imbalanced) to optimal (balanced).

Assessment of Balance

How do we assess how apt a lifestyle mix is? Traditionally, there are two approaches: (1) the *objective* approach, based on explicit criteria of aptness that can be applied by an outside observer, and (2) the *subjective* approach, based on mostly implicit criteria of the individual concerned. In addition, I will propose a third approach with both objective and subjective elements, in which aptness is judged ex post facto on the basis of its observed consequences.

These three approaches can also be seen in other fields of inquiry, such as nutrition research. The objective way of assessing whether a diet is balanced requires checking if the required amounts of various nutrients appear on the table. However, minimum levels can be specified better in the case of nutrition than in the case of lifestyle components. The subjective way of assessing diet is asking people whether they think their diet is balanced. Research in this line has shown that people are often ignorant about serious deficiencies in their eating habits. The third way is assessing the consequences of eating patterns on long-term health and longevity. This latter approach is common practice in large-scale follow-up studies such as the 36-year follow-up study on effects of energy intake by Willcox et al. (2004).

ASSUMED LIFE BALANCE

The objective approach is based on preconceptions of what is balanced or not. Such preconceptions may be based on ethics of fairness, for instance the idea that fathers and mothers should take an equal share in child care. Preconceptions may also derive from a theory about reality, for instance the idea that working more than 10 hours a day puts our health at risk. There are several problems with this approach. One problem is that axioms about a proper mix are often disputable. Is the 50/50 share in child care really the most fair? That is the case only if parents have the same preferences for child rearing and other home tasks. Likewise, one may doubt the rule that 10 hours of work a day is too much for everybody.

A second problem is that preconceptions tend to conflict. For instance, a 50/50 split in child care may be fair, but not economical, therefore leading to more hours of work and less time for family life. The problem of conflicting preconceptions can be solved in theory; if utility functions are known and interpersonal, comparison of these is possible. Yet in practice this does not work, with preconceptions of a proper lifestyle mix being as comparable as apples and oranges.

A third problem is measuring the degree to which the appropriate lifestyle balance is met in practice. This is often more difficult than it seems at first. For instance: how to assess the share of child care of fathers and mothers? Simply clocking time does not suffice, since there is also variation in emotional investment and pedagogical effectiveness.

All these problems make the objective approach impractical when applied to the entire lifestyle mix. The objective approach can only be used in the simple one-issue comparisons that dominate rhetoric. It falls short in an empirical assessment that takes more components into account.

SELF-PERCEIVED LIFE BALANCE

The subjective approach assesses balance in the eye of the beholder. In this approach, a life is balanced if the person leading that life thinks it is balanced. This method bypasses the above-mentioned problems of the objective approach but runs into different ones.

The subjective approach is often defended with the argument that nobody is better informed than the people concerned, yet people are often unaware of the reasons for their view about their

Table 4-1

FOUR QUALITIES OF LIFE

	OUTER QUALITIES	*INNER QUALITIES*
Life chances	Livability of environment	Life ability of the person
Life results	Utility of life	Satisfaction with life

life balance. Criteria of aptness are often implicit or lacking, and as a result, people know better *how* they think of the balance in their life than *why*. Researchers have learned that perceptions draw on more sources than reality alone and that this is particularly true for intangible things such as balance in one's life. Because clear reality anchors are lacking, perceptions of this matter are likely to be largely shaped by preconception and wishful thinking.

As a result, perceptions of life balance can be flatly wrong: You can think that your life is imbalanced, while in fact you lead the best possible life. One reason for such misunderstandings may be the tendency to think that the grass is greener on the other side of the fence. Another reason may be in faulty attribution, such as the case of the neurotic man who attributes his misery to his workload rather than to his personality. On the other hand, defense mechanisms can make you think that you lead a balanced life, while most people around you say you do not.

A clear advantage of this approach is that balance can be easily measured using self-reports. For that reason the subjective method dominates in the research literature.

APPARENT LIFE BALANCE

The third approach is to look at the consequences of lifestyle mixes for overall happiness. In this approach *aptness* of lifestyle mix is seen functionally as leading a happy life. If people live happily with a certain mix of activities, then that mix is apparently apt, even if it does not fit preconceptions of good balance, or if people think that their life is imbalanced.

In this chapter, I explore the third way of inferring aptness of life balance from the consequences of different lifestyle mixes on happiness. I do so by assessing long-term effects of lifestyles on happiness. This requires an explanation of what is meant by happiness and why happiness is used as an outcome criterion.

HAPPINESS

When used in a broad sense, the word *happiness* is synonymous with quality of life or well-being. In this meaning, it denotes that life is good, but does not specify what is good about life. The word is also used in more specific ways, and these can be clarified with the help of the classification of qualities of life presented in Table 4-1.

Four Qualities of Life

The classification of meanings in Table 4-1 depends on two sets of distinctions. Vertically, there is a difference between chances for a good life and actual outcomes of life. Chances and outcomes are related but are certainly not the same. Horizontally, there is a distinction between external and internal qualities. In the first case, the quality is in the environment, in the latter, it is in the individual. Together, these distinctions mark four qualities of life, all of which have been denoted by the word *happiness*.

LIVABILITY OF THE ENVIRONMENT

Livability of the environment, the top-left quadrant, means good living conditions. Often the terms *quality of life* and *well-being* are used for this particular meaning, especially in the writings of ecologists and sociologists. Economists sometimes use the term *welfare* for this meaning. *Livability* is a better word because it refers explicitly to a characteristic of the environment and does not carry the connotation of paradise. Politicians and social reformers typically emphasize this quality of life.

LIFE ABILITY OF THE PERSON

Life ability of the person, the top-right quadrant, means inner life chances, that is, how well we are equipped to cope with the problems of life. This aspect of the good life is also known by different names. In biology, the phenomenon is referred to as *adaptive potential*. On other occasions, it is denoted by the medical term *health*, in the medium variant of the word. Sen (1992) calls this quality-of-life variant *capability*. I prefer the simple term *life ability*, which elegantly contrasts with *livability*. This quality of life is central in the thinking of therapists and educators.

UTILITY OF LIFE

Utility of life, the bottom-left quadrant, refers to the notion that a good life must be good for something more than itself. This presumes some higher value, such as ecological preservation or cultural development. In fact, there are myriad values on which the utility of life can be judged. There is no current generic for these external results of life. Gerson (1976, p. 795) referred to these quality-of-life concepts as *transcendental*. Another appellation is *meaning of life*, which then denotes true significance instead of mere subjective sense of meaning. I prefer the simpler *utility of life*, admitting that this label may also give rise to misunderstanding. Moral advisors, such as pastors, emphasize this quality of life.

SATISFACTION WITH LIFE

Finally, *satisfaction with life*, the bottom-right quadrant, refers to the inner outcomes of life. That is, the quality in the eye of the beholder. As we deal with conscious humans, this quality boils down to subjective appreciation of life. This is commonly referred to by terms such as *subjective well-being; life satisfaction;* and *happiness,* in a limited sense of the word. There is no professional interest group that stresses this meaning, which seems to be one of the reasons for the reservations surrounding the value of happiness.

Which of these four qualities of life should be used as an outcome criterion in our assessment of consequences of lifestyle mixes? Clearly not the top quadrants of life chances because life balance itself belongs in this category. The focus should be at the bottom quadrants of life's outcomes.

Should we judge the life balance by the final utility of life? This is very difficult, because utility can be hard to grasp. A life may have many different consequences on the environment over different periods of time, and one can only guess at the long-term balance of effects. Moreover, this criterion can lead to counterintuitive results, such as the life of a workaholic turning out to be the most useful in the long run. Satisfaction is a better criterion, because it concerns outcomes for the person and, as such, indicates how well a lifestyle mix works for the person who lives that life.

Four Kinds of Satisfaction

This brings us to the question of what *satisfaction* is precisely. This is also a word with multiple meanings and again we can elucidate these meaning using a simple scheme. Table 4-2 is also based on two sets of distinctions—vertically, between satisfaction with parts of life versus satisfaction with life as a whole, and horizontally, between passing satisfaction and enduring satisfaction. These two bipartitions yield again a four-fold taxonomy.

Table 4-2

FOUR KINDS OF SATISFACTION

	Passing	*Enduring*
Part of life	Pleasure	Part satisfaction
Life as a whole	Peak experience	Life satisfaction (happiness)

Pleasures

Passing satisfaction with a part of life is called *pleasure*. Pleasures can be sensory, such as a glass of good wine, or mental, such as reading this text. The idea that we should maximize such satisfactions is called *hedonism*.

Part Satisfaction

Enduring satisfaction with a part of life is referred to as *part satisfaction*. Such satisfactions can concern a domain of life, such as working life, and aspects of life, such as its variety. Sometimes the word *happiness* is used for such part satisfactions, in particular for satisfaction with one's career.

Peak Experience

Passing satisfaction can be about life as a whole, in particular when the experience is intense and oceanic. This kind of satisfaction is usually referred to as *top experience*. When poets write about happiness they usually describe an experience of this kind. Likewise, religious writings use the word happiness often in the sense of a mystical *ecstasis*. Another word for this type of satisfaction is *enlightenment*.

Life Satisfaction

Enduring satisfaction with one's life as a whole is called *life satisfaction* and also commonly referred to as happiness. I have delineated this concept in more detail elsewhere (Veenhoven, 1984).

Which of these kinds of satisfaction should we use for assessing apparent balance in life? By looking at the satisfaction taxonomy, it is clear that we should use overall life satisfaction or happiness. A life full of short-lived pleasures is not necessarily a balanced life, and neither is a life with incidental peak experiences. Likewise, satisfaction in particular domains of life does not denote balanced living, such as high job satisfaction that accompanies the cost of low satisfaction with family life. Balance is best reflected in satisfaction with life as a whole, that is, in happiness.

Significance of Happiness

There are many misgivings about the value of happiness, such as that happiness is mere contentment and that it typically results from an unrealistically rosy view of reality. In this context, I cannot go in the details of these qualms. Suffice to say, that in assessing how happy we are, we use our mood as the prime source of information, and that mood reflects the degree to which basic needs are met. As such, happiness signals how well we thrive biologically (Veenhoven, in press). Consequently, happiness is strongly linked with physical and mental health and also is predictive of longevity (Veenhoven, 2008). Happiness exerts also beneficial effects on productivity and social bonds (Lyubomirsky, Diener, & King, 2005) and tends to "broaden" our action repertoire and "build" up resources (Fredrickson 2006). As a result, happiness appears to be contagious, your personal happiness tends to enhance the happiness of your family members and friends (Fowler &

Christakis, 2008). In this context, it is not surprising that happiness is also highly valued all over the world (Diener & Oishi 2004).

ASSESSMENT OF APPARENT LIFE BALANCE

Having established that life balance must result in happiness, we can now proceed to find out what kinds of lives are more and less balanced. The first step is to chart lifestyle mixes, the second step is to assess happiness, and the third step is to assess the effect of the former on the latter.

Measurement of Lifestyle Mix

Most studies on life balance focus on specific aspects of lifestyle, such as the number of working hours (Faganini & Letablier, 2004) and having child-care responsibilities (Tausig & Fenwick, 2001). Obviously, that does not provide a comprehensive view of the lifestyle mix. Time-use studies are better suited for that purpose.

Time-use studies differ in sophistication, and some of their weaknesses are discussed in Christiansen and Matuska (2006). The simplest ones only ask respondents to record the time spent on a set of activities on a typical day. Another approach is to have respondents keep a time dairy for a week or so. A recent variant in this line is the day recall method (Kahneman, Krueger, Schkade, Schwarz, & Stone, 2004), which will be discussed below.

Time-use studies provide the following pieces of information about lifestyle mix: (1) the number of waking hours, (2) the proportion of time spent on productive activities and leisure, (3) the variation in activities, and (4) the nature of activities. Typologies can be constructed on the basis of these strands.

Measurement of Happiness

Happiness was defined as subjective enjoyment of one's life as a whole. Because that is something people have in mind, it can be measured using questioning. Different ways of questioning about happiness are being used.

GLOBAL SELF-REPORTS

The most common way to measure people's happiness is using single direct questions, such as the following standard item in the World Values Surveys (2008): All things considered, how satisfied are you with your life as a whole these days?

1   2   3   4   5   6   7   8   9   10
Dissatisfied   Satisfied

This question is well understood all over the world. Typically less than 1% of respondents choose the "don't know" option, and there is remarkable consistency in distribution and patterns of correlation in successive surveys. Although quite valid, these measures are not too reliable. A person may check 7 today, but 6 tomorrow. This is no problem when aggregates are compared, but it does hinder comparison of the same people over time. Another limitation of these measures is that they tap a cognitive evaluation of life that may be influenced by defensive distortions. Happiness can also be measured using multiple questions, such as the Satisfaction With Life Scale (Diener, Emmons, Larsen, & Griffin, 1985). Yet many such inventories involve items that do not quite fit the previous definition of happiness.

AFFECT BALANCE SCALES

Another category of measuring happiness focuses on hedonic level of affect. One variety in this kind is the Affect Balance Scales (Bradburn, 1969). These are lists of questions on positive and negative feelings in the recent past (eg, whether one has felt "blue" or "cheerful" in the past week). Ratings are summarized in scores for positive affect and negative affect, the difference of which is the affect balance score. An advantage of this approach is that the experience is less cognitively filtered, but a disadvantage is that the week on which the respondent reports may be atypical. Hence this method works best when repeated over time.

EXPERIENCE SAMPLING

A radical variant of this approach is focusing on happiness of the moment and asking people repeatedly "How happy or unhappy do you feel right now?" Such multimoment assessments use beepers that call for responses at several times during a day. Often respondents note their answers on a palmtop computer or a cell phone. An advantage of this method is that the respondent can also note what he or she is doing at that moment, which is particularly relevant in this context. This method is discussed in more detail in Schimmack and Diener (2003).

Assessment of Effect of Lifestyle on Happiness

The next step is to assess the outcome of different lifestyle mixes on happiness. This is usually done with cross-sectional analysis, such as studies that compare working mothers with full-time homemaking mothers. For example, Veroff, Douvan, and Kulka (1981) found homemaking mothers to be happier than working mothers. Obviously, this difference can be due to other things than lifestyle, such as having higher earning husbands. To some extent, such intervening variables can be controlled in a multivariate analysis, but the best way to get the effect on happiness is to follow-up with the same people over time. This requires panel studies that involve measures of lifestyle and happiness.

Effects are probably not the same for everyone; for example, a speedy lifestyle may be more satisfying for young adults than for seniors. Hence studies must either focus on specific categories or use samples that provide a sufficient number of cases in subgroups.

Combination Study: Lifestyle and Life-Satisfaction of Retirees

Several of the above-mentioned approaches are combined in a study by Lyanda Vermeulen and myself among people ages 50 years or older in the city of Rotterdam in the Netherlands. This study focuses on retirees who adopt new lifestyles and follows what they do and how they feel. Data are gathered using our Web-based Yesterday's Diary, on which respondents first note their activities for the previous day and then rate how much they enjoyed each of them (Veenhoven & Vermeulen, 2007). An example is presented in Figure 4-1.

Respondents complete this diary one day a month. The study plan is to have respondents do so the entire 4 years of the study. If this works as designed, it will result in a detailed view of participants' habitual activities, from which much information about their lifestyle mix can be inferred. It will also provide detailed information about how happy they feel, providing an accurate estimate of their average happiness and also information about enjoyment of particular activities. The sample is focused on a specific category and quite sizable.

SOME ILLUSTRATIVE FINDINGS

Attempts to assess the effects of lifestyle on happiness are few as yet. The section "Lifestyle and Happiness" in the World Database of Happiness contains only a handful of research findings (Veenhoven, 2007). Most of these findings are cross-sectional, but there are also a few findings from longitudinal studies.

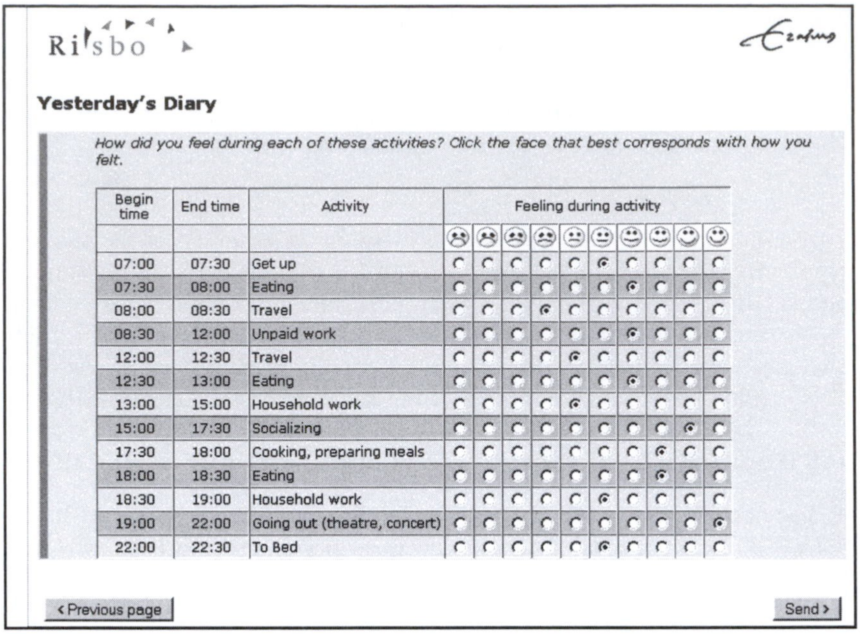

Figure 4-1. Final web-page of Yesterday's Diary.

Yesterday's Diary

How did you feel during each of these activities? Click the face that best corresponds with how you felt.

Begin time	End time	Activity	Feeling during activity										
07:00	07:30	Get up	○	○	○	○	○	●	○	○	○	○
07:30	08:00	Eating	○	○	○	○	○	○	●	○	○	○
08:00	08:30	Travel	○	○	○	●	○	○	○	○	○	○
08:30	12:00	Unpaid work	○	○	○	○	○	○	●	○	○	○
12:00	12:30	Travel	○	○	○	○	●	○	○	○	○	○
12:30	13:00	Eating	○	○	○	○	○	○	●	○	○	○
13:00	15:00	Household work	○	○	○	○	●	○	○	○	○	○
15:00	17:30	Socializing	○	○	○	○	○	○	○	○	●	○
17:30	18:00	Cooking, preparing meals	○	○	○	○	○	○	○	●	○	○
18:00	18:30	Eating	○	○	○	○	○	○	○	●	○	○
18:30	19:00	Household work	○	○	○	○	●	○	○	○	○	○
19:00	22:00	Going out (theatre, concert)	○	○	○	○	○	○	○	○	○	●
22:00	22:30	To Bed	○	○	○	○	○	●	○	○	○	○

< Previous page   Send >

Working Hours and Happiness in Nations

There is much concern about growing imbalance between work life and private life in modern society. Exemplary books are Julian Schorr's (1992) *The Overworked American* and Robert Lane's (2000) *Loss of Happiness in Market Democracies*. Cross-national studies indeed show more working hours in the most advanced economies, and comparison over time reveals a slight rise in hours worked. Yet these differences are not accompanied with a decline in happiness. Average happiness rather tends to be higher in nations where reported time pressures in work are highest ($r = +.50$!) and appears to be unrelated to incidence of complaints about time stress (Garhammer, 2002). Moreover, the slight rise in working hours in modern nations is typically paralleled with a slight rise in average happiness (Veenhoven & Hagerty, 2006).

Remarkably, this pattern coexists with rising complaints about time stress (Garhammer, 2002). This illustrates that the subjective approach to assessing life balance can yield different results than the present approach of assessing "apparent" balance. A possible explanation for the paradox is that doing more than we want may be good for us, as long as it keeps us vital. This fits the theory that we feel best when functioning optimally (Csikszentmihalyi, 1997), and from an evolutionary perspective, one can imagine that we are designed to live in a challenging environment.

Working Mothers

As mentioned previously, an early cross-sectional study in the United States found working mothers to be less happy on average than full-time homemaking mothers. This finding is replicated in a recent large-scale follow-up study in Germany. Using the German Socio Economic Panel, Stutzer and Frey (2003) followed the happiness of people from 10 years before marriage to 10 years after. They observed a rise in happiness from singlehood to marriage and a gradual decline after marriage. That decline is strongest in couples with children and sets in earlier in dual-career couples (thick dotted line of no specialization in Figure 4-2) than in couples where one works and the other (typically women) is a full-time homemaker (thick line of full specialization in Figure 4-2). This difference exists for about 5 years and roughly equates to the preschool period. The average difference is about half a point on the 0–10 Life-Satisfaction Scale.

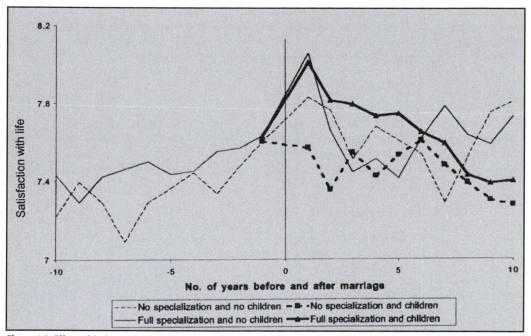

Figure 4-2. Effects of dual careers on happiness. *Note*: The graph represents the pattern of well-being after taking respondent's sex, age, parenthood, household size, relation to the head of the household, labor market status, place of residence, and citizenship into account. Data source: GSOEP. Specialization = both have a full-time job; no specialization = one person is a full-time homemaker and the other has a full-time job outside the home. From "Does Marriage Make People Happy or Do Happy People Get Married?" by A. Stutzer and B. Frey, 2006, *Journal of Socioeconomics, 35*, p. 340. Copyright © 2006, by Elsevier. Reprinted with permission.

This case illustrates the difference between the objective approach to assessing life balance and the present approach of assessing apparent balance. On the basis of ideological preconceptions of what a balanced life is, one can say that the lives of working mothers are more balanced, their role being more equal to their husbands' and their tasks being more varied. Yet this ideology has a price; a loss of half a point of happiness during 5 years is comparable to 1 year of mild depression.

CONCLUSION

The term 'life-balance' is used in three different meanings: (1) meeting preconceptions of what a balanced life is; (2) thinking that one lives a balanced life; and (3) leading a life that is apparently balanced, because one thrives well. This latter meaning is not very prominent in the discourse as yet but marks a promising approach to evidence policy making.

REFERENCES

Bradburn, N. (1969). *The structure of psychological well-being.* Chicago: Aldine.

Christiansen, C. H., & Matuska, K. M. (2006). Lifestyle balance: A review of concepts and research. *Journal of Occupational Science, 13,* 49–61.

Csikszentmihalyi, M. (1997). *Finding flow: The psychology of engagement in everyday life.* New York: Basic Books.

Diener, E., Emmons, R. A., Larsen, R. J., & Griffin, S. (1985). The Satisfaction With Life Scale. *Journal of Personality Assessment, 49,* 71–75.

Diener, E., & Oishi, S. (2004) Are Scandinavians happier than Asians? Issues in comparing nations on subjective well-being. *Asian Economic and Political Issues, 10,* 1-25.

Faganini, J., & Letablier, M. T. (2004). Work and family life balance: The impact of the 35-hour laws in France. *Work, Employment and Society, 18,* 551–572.

Fredrickson, B. L. (2006). The broader-and-build theory of positive emotions. In: M. Csikzentmihalyi & I. S. Ciskzentmihalyi (Eds.), *A life worth living. (pp.* 85 –103). New York: Oxford University Press.

Fowler, J. H., & Christakis, N. A. (2008). Dynamic spread of happiness in a large social network: Longitudinal analysis over 20 years in the Framingham Heart Study. *British Medical Journal, 337*:a2338.

Garhammer, M. (2002). Pace of life and enjoyment of life. *Journal of Happiness Studies*, 3, 217–256.

Gerson, E. M. (1976). On quality of life. *American Sociological Review, 41,* 793–806.

Kahneman, D., Krueger, A. B., Schkade, D. A., Schwarz, N., & Stone, A. A. (2004). A survey method for characterizing daily life experience: The day reconstruction method. *Science, 306,* 1776–1780.

Lane, R. (2000). *The loss of happiness in market democracies.* New Haven, CT: Yale University Press.

Lyubomirsky, S., Diener, E., & King, L. A. (2005). The benefits of frequent positive affect: does happiness lead to success? *Psychological Bulletin, 131,* 803–855.

Schimmack, U., & Diener, E. (Eds.). (2003). The experience sampling method. *Special Issue of the Journal of Happiness Studies, 4,* 1.

Schorr, J. B. (1992). *The overworked American.* New York: Basic Books.

Sen, A. (1992). Capability and wellbeing. In M. Nussbaum & A. Sen (Eds.), *The quality of life.* Oxford: Clarendon Press.

Stutzer, A., & Frey, B. S. (2003). *Does marriage make people happy, or do happy people get married?* [Working Paper No. 143] Zurich, Switzerland Institute for Empirical Research in Economics .

Stutzer, A., & Frey, B. (2006). Does marriage make people happy, or do happy people get married? *Journal of Socioeconomics, 35,* 326–347.

Tausig, M., & Fenwick, R. (2001). Unbinding time: Alternate work schedules and work-life balance. *Journal of Family and Economic Issues, 22,* 101–119.

Veenhoven, R. (1984). *Conditions of happiness.* Dordrecht: Springer.

Veenhoven, R. (2007). *World Database of Happiness, Collection of Correlational Findings.* Retrieved January 2, 2009, from http://worlddatabaseofhappiness.eur.nl.

Veenhoven, R. (2008). Healthy happiness: Effects of happiness on physical health and the consequences for preventive health care. *Journal of Happiness Studies. 9,* 449–464.

Veenhoven, R. (in press). How do we assess how happy we are? Tenets, implications, and evidence for three theories. In: A. Dutt & B. Radcliff (Eds.), *Happiness, economics and politics.* Northampton, MA: Edward Elger Publishers.

Veenhoven, R., & Hagerty, M. (2006). Rising happiness in nations, 1946–2004: A reply to Easterlin. *Social Indicators Research, 79,* 421–436.

Veenhoven, R., & Vermeulen, L. (2007). *Onderzoek naar succesvol ouder worden* [Investigation on successful aging]. Retrieved December 8, 2007, from http://www.risbo.org/levensstijl/info/

Veroff, J., Douvan, E., & Kulka, R. A. (1981). *The inner America: A self-portrait from 1957 to 1976.* New York: Basic Books.

Willcox, B. J., Yano, K., Chen, R., Willcox, D. C., Rodriguez, B. L., Masaki, K. H., et al. (2004). How much should we eat? The association between energy intake and mortality in a 36-year follow-up study of Japanese-American men. *Journals of Gerontology Series A: Biological Sciences and Medical Sciences, 59,* B789–B795.

World Values Survey. (2008). Retrieved December 1, 2007, from http://www.worldvaluessurvey.org/

CHAPTER 5

Multiple Roles and Life Balance
AN INTELLECTUAL JOURNEY

STEPHEN MARKS

INTRODUCTION

For over 30 years I have been thinking about balance, and I want to share my process in the form of a personal narrative. The issues I have struggled with arose within my own biography, but they were also embedded in a historical, social, and intellectual context. In some ways, I feel that I plugged myself into a kind of current, and I think you will understand the ideas in a deeper way by knowing something about that current. The chapter begins with my graduate school experience in the 1960s, when the magic of the classic sociological tradition converged with the social upheavals exploding around me, and my intellectual passions began to take a shape and direction. I show how a simple emerging conviction—that human energy and even time might be far more expansive than we think—became the animus for my career-long exploration of balance. Along the way, several research projects trained my focus on some core issues, and I summarize the thrust of each of these projects and the conclusions to which they led me.

EARLY INFLUENCES

When I began my graduate studies in 1964, I was most drawn to the classic tradition in sociology. I devoured the works of that venerated European triumvirate Karl Marx, Emile Durkheim, and Max Weber. I saw myself as a pure sociological theorist, and eventually I wrote a theoretical dissertation on Durkheim's theory of *anomie*. I embraced Durkheim's conviction that society was ill, as evidenced by the spiraling rates of suicide in his time and the social upheaval of my own era. I also embraced his vision of the sociologist as a sort of societal doctor who diagnoses the illness and proposes an effective remedy. The job of social science, I agreed, is to teach us that personal problems are often social problems and to show us how to solve them. From Durkheim I also learned an implicit theory of *life balance*: People thrive best when they have a balance of self-oriented and other-oriented tendencies—when they are neither too egoistic nor too altruistic. Similarly, they flourish when there are rules and limits that guide them counterbalanced by some release from rigid rules and constraints; people should be neither too anomic nor too fatalistic.

I was hungry for *achievement*—one of the buzzwords of the time. My father was a self-made Jewish doctor, totally absorbed in his profession and determined that his only son should follow in his footsteps. I rejected a career in medicine because I hated my chemistry and anatomy courses,

K. Matuska & C. Christiansen (Eds.)
Life balance: Multidisciplinary theories and research (pp 43–58)
© 2009 SLACK Incorporated and AOTA Press

but I held fast to the desire to distinguish myself through professional achievement. It was an ambivalent relationship, achievement and me. I wanted to throw myself into it and protect myself from it at the same time. That ambivalence was probably rooted in my father's story—in the anxiety of desperately wanting approval yet fearing that I could never win it on my own terms.

Reading Weber's thesis in *The Protestant Ethic and the Spirit of Capitalism* (1958) was an epiphany for me, because it demonstrated how arbitrary and historically unique this obsession with career success is. Weber showed that for Reformation leaders, nothing but hard work in one's occupation was worthy in the sight of God. The Calvinists insisted that one's "calling" was the only thing in daily activity that mattered, and in America they sought the freedom to practice this ascetic ideal. Weber's analysis gave me a deeper understanding of my urgency to carve out a professional identity and my career-obsessed mentality. The words at the end of *The Protestant Ethic* about the continuing legacy of Calvinism utterly haunted me. "Today," Weber wrote, "the idea of duty in one's calling prowls about in our lives like the ghost of dead religious beliefs" (p. 182). I did not realize it then, but Weber was squarely focused on broad-scale issues of life balance, and he was documenting the lack of such balance in the post-Reformation Judeo-Christian world.

As my graduate studies moved through the turbulent 1960s, the explosive energy of the counterculture pulled me out of my head and into the upheaval. The continuation of the civil rights movement, the growing protest over the war in Vietnam, resurgent feminism, the hippie movement, the emergence of spiritual alternatives to conventional religion, the messages and sounds of folk and rock musicians, the vision of a more freely flowing sexuality—we were scrutinizing, challenging, and often rejecting everything our parents had made for us. I became strongly identified with all these currents, but I was especially drawn to the expressive and sensual exuberance of the hippies and intrigued by the experiments in communal living that were springing up in both rural and urban settings. In retrospect, I think I was again searching for life balance. The popular bumper-sticker slogan "make love, not war" crisply summed it up. Peacefulness could balance aggression; spontaneity could balance control and discipline; sensuous feeling could balance reason; play could balance work. Careers became suspect because they epitomized the Calvinistic elevation of work above everything else in life.

I almost "dropped out"—the ultimate refusal in the 1960s to collude with the evil "establishment." Although my wife Joan would have welcomed a communal adventure, I decided to stay the course of my graduate program and get my PhD. At the time I reasoned that I could become an academic professional and keep my counterculture values without "selling out," but I now recognize that my fear of losing my middle-class privileges was surely an important piece of it. Perhaps I was also guided by my interest in balance. My intellect was a gift that had often brought me joy. Did I really want to deal with the split between reason and feeling by abandoning one side of the polarity to favor the other? I wanted both in my life, and I recommitted myself to my studies and to my career, determined to find answers that could lead to experiencing life more fully. Early in 1968, Joan and I took up Transcendental Meditation, attracted to the simplicity of Maharishi Mahesh Yogi's message: Human energy is potentially infinite, and through meditation, every person can make direct contact with the energy and intelligence that permeate the universe.

EARLY EXPLORATIONS OF BALANCE: SOCIETY "VERSUS" THE INDIVIDUAL

I started teaching in Maine and continued my studies, focusing especially on the relationship between society and the individual. Do societies thwart the most creative impulses of individuals or might they not promote and encourage them? I was troubled by the early American sociologist W. I. Thomas's sharp contrast between society's desire for security and the individual's desire for new experience. Thomas (1923) wrote,

> There is…always a rivalry between the spontaneous definitions of the situation made by the member of an organized society and the definitions which his society has provided for him. The individual tends to a hedonistic selection of activity, pleasure first; and society to a utilitarian selection, safety first. Society wishes its members to be laborious, dependable, regular, sober, orderly, self-sacrificing; while the individual wishes less of this and more of new experience. (p. 42)

I soon discovered that this alleged conflict between the individual and society was a centerpiece of Sigmund Freud's work in psychology. It appears in his contrast between the pleasure principle and the reality principle and again in his concepts of id, ego, and superego—the cornerstone of his personality theory. Perhaps its most dramatic expression came in *Civilization and Its Discontents* (1930/1961), the little book that is surely one of the most provocative treatises of the 20th century. Freud suggested that civilization "does not like sexuality as a source of pleasure in its own right" (p. 52) because of the ever-present potential of lovers to withdraw into their couple bond. Their intense pleasure together threatens to steal away the energy that any civilization needs to carry out its projects. The books, buildings, highways, and manufacturing and the careers in which these achievements are embedded all get accomplished via energy that is borrowed from sexuality. Great civilizations are direct evidence of sublimation and sexual repression, simply because the sum total of *libido,* or human energy, is too little to go around.

Freud's artful and seductive exposition of his theory was almost irresistible, but I did not want to believe it, and I groped for some ammunition against it. Maharishi's position about human energy was more appealing to me. His argument was that energy is something we open to, something we can plug into and make contact with. It is not anyone's private possession. A fully developed person has boundless energy to work, play, love, and to enjoy life the way it is meant to be lived. I wanted Freud to be wrong and Maharishi to be right, in large part because I wanted both a career filled with creative achievement and a family and private life filled with love and pleasure.

HUMAN ENERGY AND TIME: SCARCE, ABUNDANT, OR BOTH?

I continued to bring these internal rumblings into my reading. I began to pay close attention to how social scientists were writing about human energy and time, and I soon noticed that virtually everyone was appealing to a scarcity theory. We have very limited time and energy resources, they were saying, as if scarcity is something that is built into the human condition. They never offered any direct evidence of this scarcity. They simply inferred it whenever they needed a convenient explanation of why people run into difficulties managing their multiple roles: There is not enough time and energy for all of one's responsibilities, they claimed, and that is why people regularly experience role conflict and overload. Sociologist William Goode's (1960) theory of role strain is still the best-articulated statement of this scarcity position. He wrote that the individual has "a finite sum of role resources" with regard to "role energies, time, emotions, [and] goods" (pp. 488, 495), and that this scarcity condition runs up against

> a wide, distracting, and sometimes conflicting array of role obligations. If [the individual] conforms fully or adequately in one direction, fulfillment will be difficult in another. Even if he feels lonely and would like to engage in additional role relationships, it is likely that he cannot fully discharge all the obligations he already faces. He cannot meet all these demands to the satisfaction of all the persons who are part of his total role network. Role strain—difficulty in meeting given role demands—is therefore normal. In general, the *individual's total role obligations are overdemanding.* (p. 485, italics original)

Does this scarcity theory adequately express the way people experience their everyday lives? When I thought about my own life, I came to some provocative conclusions. My energy does not seem to function as a sort of payout, with each successive activity costing me some of my scarce daily supply. Rather, my energy seems to wax and wane throughout the day, and at any given point it might just as easily wax as wane, no matter how big my "expenditures" were earlier in the day and no matter how many role obligations I am trying to meet. When I am interested in what I am doing, I perk up, become charged with attentiveness, and my energy flows. When I lose interest in doing something or listening to someone, my energy slackens. When I read a book that does not engage me, I may quickly feel so drained of energy that I am ready to fall asleep, no matter how energetic I felt moments before. If I drop that reading to do something of greater interest to me (even a different book), I can suddenly find energy in abundance.

As part of this self-survey, I thought of the many long car trips I had taken to my parents' home in Miami Beach, Florida, over the years. I recalled the long nights driving; the youthful, dogged determination to press onward regardless of how tired I was; and the monumental struggle to stay awake after some 15 or more hours on the road. And I recognized an invariant phenomenon that was part of this experience: No matter how tired I was, as soon as my destination began to feel within reach, I became a person transformed. My energy surged, my excitement grew, and my interest became reengaged with everything around me. Where did all this energy come from?

I now had the rudiments of a new approach to human energy, role strain, and multiple roles, although it took me several more years to work it into a published paper (Marks, 1977). My starting point was simple enough. When sleep and food intake are sufficient, human energy is perpetually produced and renewed by human beings; it is not simply consumed by activity. Moreover, in some conditions, energy resources seem to expand, while in other conditions they seem to contract. The trick is to identify the conditions that give rise to feelings of expansion and abundance in contrast to those that give rise to feelings of scarcity, depletion, and drain.

The early and simple version of the theory was that commitment to an activity generates an expansion of both the energy and the time for it. The more highly committed we are, the more we want to do it. Lack of commitment to an activity generates a feeling of drain and depletion, and the less committed we are to it, the less we want to do it. If we are strongly committed to everything we do, we find ample time and energy for all our activities and the role partners we encounter within them. Role strain is neither normal nor inevitable. Time and energy shortages are not due to some human condition of scarcity but are the product of our own interests, our likes and dislikes, and our patterns of commitment that grow out of them. It never takes us very long to find the time and energy for whatever we really want to do.

Although I had no doubt that I was on the right track, I needed to resolve one very thorny contradiction to the argument I was making. If it is true that we produce ever-expandable amounts of time and energy for any endeavor to which we are highly committed, why is it that so many people who are fired up about some activity feel that they are in a constant state of overload? They may love their job activity, but they report having too little time and energy to get it all done, and their intimate partners complain, in turn, that they wind up with little more than crumbs. According to my theory that energy expands endlessly for anything we like, this scarcity situation is not supposed to happen!

It took me several more years to find a resolution that satisfied me, and it came from a synthesis of sources. Once again, I drew some of my inspiration from Weber. Plainly, the legacy of Calvinism is not simply a very high commitment to work. There is often a driven, compulsive quality about it, something unhealthy about the person–work connection, something unbalanced. In careers, many people are chronically anxious about their work performance. All too often, they deal with that anxiety by working still more feverishly, a process that leaves them feeling overloaded, drained, and exhausted. One insight about the contradiction, then, was that perhaps there are certain conditions of high-level commitment that drain time and energy rather than expand it.

Another source of inspiration came from the humanistic psychologist Maslow's work on self-actualization. Abraham Maslow insisted that psychology should refocus its attention away from the average "deficiency-motivated" person to learn from "self-actualizers" about a more optimal level of human functioning. Growth-motivated people, Maslow (1971) suggested, are filled with aliveness, richness, effortlessness, and meaningfulness, and he came to understand the absence of these qualities as "meta-pathology," marked by deadness, grimness, fatigue, strain, "loss of zest in life," and "loss of interest in [the] world" (1971, pp. 318–319). Here, then, was another piece of the puzzle. Perhaps the Calvinist mentality robs people of an effortless engagement in their work. It creates excessive strain and grimness, and it throws people out of balance with their other activities. Away from work, they mark time and feel dead by comparison, having sacrificed their interest in "comprehensiveness" to the altar of career achievement, or to simply earning as much income as they possibly can.

A final source of inspiration came from a search for cultural alternatives to the Calvinist approach to life. I discovered a study of the Bruderhof, a Christian Anabaptist intentional community in Woodcrest, New York, where sociologist Benjamin Zablocki (1971) spent several months collecting observational data. Zablocki portrays the Bruderhof as a "joyful community" whose religious culture enjoins them to "become an empty vessel" and "bear witness" to the presence of the Holy Spirit in everything they do. He notes "the dignity accorded to simple pleasures: lighting a candle, wearing a garland, dancing, singing, hiking, visiting, greeting visitors" (p. 41). Zablocki writes that he "was especially impressed by the loving care with which the most routine jobs were done" (p. 34), and he sees a parallel with the Zen Buddhist perspective on life: "What they have in common is the desire to destroy the notion of a secular sphere of life. The message is that there are no activities, however trivial, that cannot be permeated by the divine spirit" (p. 31).

I now had alternative models for how people might approach their total round of daily activities, or in sociological language, their multiple roles. In one model—the Zen Buddhist and the Bruderhof—everything one does is deemed worthy of a person's full and careful engagement ("nothing special," as the Zen paradoxical understatement goes). In the other model—the Calvinist—just one activity does become the special one; all other activities become relegated to a subordinate position. In my first publication about these issues (Marks, 1977), I gave these two models technical names—a type 1 system of equally positive commitments and a type 3 system of uneven commitments, which I called a system of overcommitments and undercommitments. I also suggested the possibility of a type 2 system of equally negative commitments—a pattern in which nothing in one's everyday life feels worth doing, resulting in lethargy, apathy, depression, a sense of meaninglessness, and diffuse alienation.

This was a thrilling period of my research, and the synthesis I emerged with (Marks, 1977) has stayed with me in its essential features for over 30 years. My typology of commitment patterns made it possible to acknowledge opposite experiences of time and energy. First, the type 1 people: Fully and positively engaged in everything they typically do, they are the joyful ones. Their lives are rich, meaningful, and relatively effortless. They are not plagued by role strain. Except for instances of having to deal with some situational crisis or emergency, they never seem to run out of time or energy. They do not have a concept of "wasted time" because in their experience everything they do is well worth doing. All their role partners enjoy being with them because they get quality time. It is an unmistakably good feeling when someone you are interacting with is fully and positively engaged in being there with you. Finally, type 1 people are usually "good choosers," a notion I borrow from Maslow's description of self-actualizers. Determined to make time for every one of their activities and role partners, they avoid involvements in greedy organizations or with individuals who are prone to a never-ending barrage of demands on them. They are careful and thoughtful about taking on any new role because they need to know that it will not encroach too much on the rest of their role system. And if they should happen to make a mistake, they will ride it out as long as they have to, and then make adjustments to bring their role system back into balance.

The type 3 situation is more complex because it is two-sided; it entails both an overcommitment and a set of undercommitments. First the overcommitment: Type 3 people single out just one of their roles and elevate it into a privileged position. In some instances, they simply become passion driven about something they do and the self-experience they get from it, perhaps involvement with a child, a job, a lover, a scientific project, a recreational interest, a volunteer activity—it could be almost anything. In other instances, the privileged role is fuelled by anxiety or fear. Here, the driving animus is the worry that if they do not throw themselves into this one activity, they will lose something they desperately want to keep, or they will fail to get something they desperately want to attain. The Calvinists' anxiety about their salvation and their belief that success in their calling could be the only possible sign of their chosen status is a formula for this fear-driven privileging of just one activity. Recently, I have developed a hunch that the overcommitments driven by fear or anxiety may be more pernicious in their impact on the person than the ones driven by passion. I have never looked for evidence of this possibility, but it could make for a fascinating research project.

Whether passion or fear driven, overcommitments beget undercommitments. The favored role receives the lion's share of a person's identity investment, and this leads to an expansion of the activities in that role, because this is where the person feels most validated. As projects keep expanding, they begin to encroach on the remaining activities in one's total role system, including activities that may previously have been given a very high priority. These other activities may remain positively valued, but they do not generate as much "buzz" in the person as the favored activity does. Workaholics may say, "My family is what matters most to me," but their actions belie their claims: They keep expanding the time and energy they put into work and contracting the resources they put into family. This is the scarcity situation, the one that generates a feeling of role strain. The passion-driven overcommitter is having an affair with the favored interest (e.g., "my career thrills me with new and exciting challenges every day"). The fear- or anxiety-driven overcommitter simply feels stuck (e.g., "If I don't study all the time and get all As, I will never get into a good graduate school." "If I don't work two jobs, my family will not have enough to get by.").

Several different responses to type 3 people are commonly found among the role partners to whom they are undercommitted. One response is *supportive acceptance:* Overcommitters are stars, and it is their partners' duty, even their pleasure, to suppress their own claims and eagerly pay homage to the stardom. A second response is *expedient indifference,* typically found among role partners who themselves are overcommitted to something outside of this particular relationship. "You do your thing, and I'll do mine" is a formula for this pattern. A third response is *resistance.* Unhappy with what they are getting, resistant role partners may begin to press for more of their fair share. In turn, the overcommitters may honestly feel that they wish they could give them more. It is almost impossible for them to do so, however, because the ever-swelling projects within their overcommitted interest keep on beckoning them. Appeals to scarce time and energy may then come to the rescue, handed out to those role partners who have begun to feel cheated. These excuses will be honored if the overcommitment is promoted by the overall culture. In Western societies with a Calvinist legacy, excuses because of overwork are most likely to be honored, and they are the ones that are most frequently offered. Indeed, people with some other overcommitted interest will sometimes appeal to overwork, knowing that this is the premier honorable excuse.

Although my types of commitment have sometimes been interpreted to mean personality types, I never intended this kind of framing. I am a sociologist and a social critic, not a personality theorist. I strongly agree with sociologist C. Wright Mills' (1959) principles about the sociological imagination. We should ask, "What varieties of men and women now prevail in this society and in this period?…In what ways are they selected and formed, liberated and repressed, made sensitive and blunted?" (p. 7). Like Mills, I see personality types more as the dependent variable, an outgrowth of culture, social structure, and history. If Goode was right about role strain being "normal" in the United States, this is only because type 3 people are the ones most promoted at home, at school, and at work, the ones most "selected and formed" by our culture.

There is nothing inevitable about role strain, however, as type 1 people also appear among us. Like Maslow's self-actualizers (and they are likely the same people), these more evenhanded folks are able to resist the lure of what the culture promotes, along with "the honors, the status, the popularity, the prestige, and the love" [that others] can bestow" (Maslow, 1970, p. 162). Although Maslow was suggesting that self-actualizers seem to have become independent of their culture's rewards, I felt he was too quick to rule out the possibility that some cultures might actually encourage rather than inhibit such people from appearing. In a piece I published in the *Journal of Humanistic Psychology* (Marks, 1979), I paid homage to Maslow's work, and I suggested that Maslow himself waffled on the relationship between culture and self-actualization. Late in his career, he wrote approvingly of anthropologist Ruth Benedict's work on *high-synergy* cultures, and when he visited the Blackfoot Indians, he was impressed with the growth-promoting tendencies that seemed to pervade their culture. The clear implication is that some cultures may not need to be resisted, and I offered my comparison between type 3 and type 1 cultures to show that our experiences of energy and time are in part culturally driven. They are not purely idiosyncratic tendencies that spring from some presocial and precultural property of individuals.

QUALITATIVE STUDY OF BALANCE IN MARRIAGE

My next project was a study of long-term marriages (Marks, 1986). I had been intrigued by a well-known qualitative study of middle-aged couples with demanding and challenging careers (Cuber & Harroff, 1965). Most participants had utilitarian marriages, with the couple's lives subordinated to work, but a minority had intrinsic marriages and vibrant relationships, even though they had the same kinds of high-profile careers as the participants with utilitarian marriages. I reasoned that if I could oversample the intrinsic types, I might wind up with a preponderance of people with type 1 systems of role organization. I could then explore in greater detail how they accomplish this more balanced arrangement of their life pattern, even though they go against the cultural grain.

In the early 1980s, I interviewed each partner of 57 couples. My sampling strategy did not turn up as many intrinsics as I had hoped, but my rich data provided good material for thinking about types of role-system management. Around this time, I had been reading family-systems literature. Psychiatrist Murray Bowen's work (1978) suggested that family members often get fused into a stuck-togetherness. This fusion generates tension and anxiety in one or both partners, which they often ineffectively deal with—emotional distancing, having frequent conflicts, acting out, or projecting the anxiety onto the most vulnerable family member. I was most taken with the concept of *triangulation*: Tensions arising in a relationship may ease through a one-to-one communication process, but failing that, one or both partners will often "triangle in" a third party. This person may be a friend, a child, a lover, an extended family member, a therapist, or any convenient listener with a shoulder available for support services. Triangulation may temporarily ease the tension, but the problems in the fused twosome remain unresolved.

I then worked out a modification of Bowen's framework. I began to see the self-system of a person in a couple as a three-cornered arrangement. The first corner—the inner corner—is one's private drama with its internal dialogue and its storehouse of yearnings, hopes, fears, and strivings. The second corner—the partnership corner—is the part of the self that is constantly coordinating one's own relational needs with the partner's expectations, needs, moods, and whereabouts. And the third corner is a complex of interests—a child, a job, a hobby, a lover, a friendship, God, a volunteer activity, and so on—that turn one's focus away from one's intimate partner.

My concept of triangulation was inspired by Bowen, but it is different in important ways. I began to see it as something perfectly normal that everyone does all the time, not something that is simply a response to rising tensions. Everyone in a couple focuses some energy and attention away from their partner. The question is how much of their focus goes elsewhere and how much

Figure 5-1. Romantic fusion (1st = inner corner, 2nd = partnership corner, 3rd = third corner). Adapted from S. R. Marks (1989). Toward a systems theory of marital quality. *Journal of Marriage and the Family, 51,* 19-26.

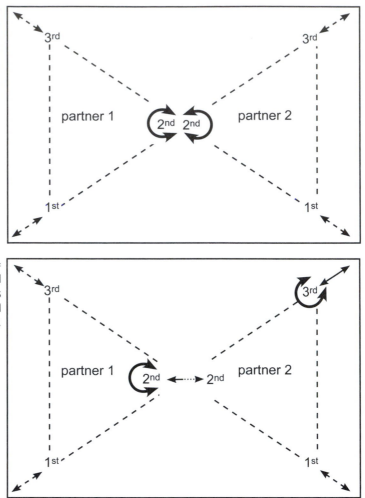

Figure 5-2. Dependency distancing (1st = inner corner, 2nd = partnership corner, 3rd = third corner). Adapted from S. R. Marks (1989). Toward a systems theory of marital quality. *Journal of Marriage and the Family, 51,* 19-26.

goes to the partner. And how does the partner apportion her or his own focus? Thinking about my data, I concluded that couple dynamics are driven by the collision of each person's triangle-management, and triangulation is the mover and shaker of these dynamics.

I arrived at several different couple configurations. Early in a relationship, some couples get into a *romantic fusion,* or *dyadic withdrawal* (Figure 5-1). Each person fuses with the partner part of themselves (their second corners) and distances from their third corners. This arrangement can be exciting and wonderful until the lure of some third-corner interest begins to beckon one or both of them, a development that is no doubt inevitable.

If one partner then remains fused with their second corner while the other one increasingly triangulates into some third corner, the relationship becomes unsettled and uncomfortable. I call this pattern *dependency distancing*—dependency on one side, distancing on the other (Figure 5-2). The dependent one feels deprived because everything is riding on the relationship, and the fact that the distancer's energy is focused elsewhere is a constant source of anxiety. In turn, the distancer may feel nagged—constantly charged with not caring enough, giving enough, or being available enough. The relational power is lopsidedly in the hands of the distancer, as less interest in the relationship always means more power, along with the opportunity to exploit the more interested partner's dependency.

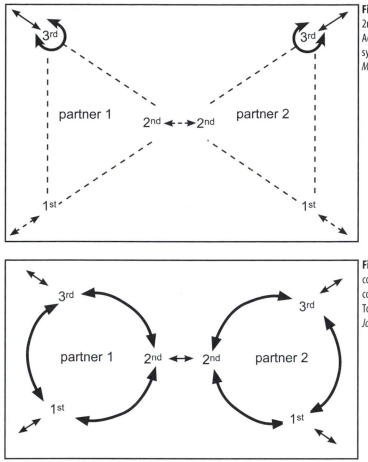

Figure 5-3. Separateness (1st = inner corner, 2nd = partnership corner, 3rd = third corner). Adapted from S. R. Marks (1989). Toward a systems theory of marital quality. *Journal of Marriage and the Family, 51,* 19-26.

Figure 5-4. Balanced connection (1st = inner corner, 2nd = partnership corner, 3rd = third corner). Adapted from S. R. Marks (1989). Toward a systems theory of marital quality. *Journal of Marriage and the Family, 51,* 19-26.

Separateness is a third pattern (Figure 5-3). In some instances this pattern is a resolution of the tensions and discomfort of dependency distancing, as if the dependent one has decided "If you can't beat 'em, join 'em," and proceeds to distance into a third corner of his or her own. In other instances, the pattern suits both partners' preferred inclinations. We see this pattern in traditional couples with children, when the husband is married to his job and the wife is married to their children, and we also see it in some dual-career couples when both partners have exciting jobs and want very little from each other.

Whatever the pathway to it, separateness is a lot more comfortable than dependency-distancing, and it remains comfortable unless or until one partner begins to triangulate more intensely than the other or decides to de-triangulate and bring more energy into the partnership corner.

A fourth pattern is *connection*. Although this pattern has several subtypes, here I will summarize only one of them—*balanced connection* (Figure 5-4). The basic pattern is that the energy flows throughout the triangle, around each corner, and over to the partner. There is no fusing with any corner and no distancing from any corner. Both partners have vigorous third-corner interests. Some of these interests are shared and jointly enjoyed, and others are pursued separately. Their separate interests enhance rather than threaten the relationship, because when both partners have a lot of energy swirling around their partnership corners, they make certain to tell each other about what has happened to them while they are apart. They are likely to be proud and supportive of one another's third-corner involvements. This is in sharp contrast to separateness, in which both partners treat their third corners as closely guarded secrets and act as if the other either is not interested or will ruin it for them if they get wind of what is going on.

In retrospect, it is amazing to me how closely my marriage study had reinvented my earlier theoretical framework about human energy. Fusion and distancing were alternate concepts for overcommitment and undercommitment in a type 3 system. In romantic fusion, the partners are overcommitted to their relationship role and undercommitted to everything else. In separateness, the overcommitments and undercommitments trade places: The third corner gets the overcommitted focus and both partners are undercommitted to their relationship. *Connection*, on the other hand, was an alternate name for partners who maintain a type 1 pattern of commitments. All the parts of themselves are energized. They are highly and positively committed to each and everything they do, and they find ample time and energy for doing it.

HOW I BECAME A QUANTOID[1]

By the 1990s, my earlier theoretical work had apparently struck a nerve. It was getting cited in many disciplines, including psychology, sociology, management, health, aging, nursing, and counseling. My work was in some ways the beneficiary of women's increasing entry into the labor force, beginning in the 1970s and accelerating through the 1980s. Back then there was a widespread concern—at times it seemed to be a veritable panic—that women's work involvement was a dangerous thing. It would diminish women's health, cheat their children, bring marriages to ruin, make women into men, and deprive the universe of the comfort and care that stay-at-home women should be delighted to serve up.

In response to this panic, a number of scholars launched research projects to see what the actual impact was of women's paid work on the roles of mother and wife and on women's overall well-being. Literature reviews in this work began to have a formulaic ring to them, still seen today in studies of multiple roles. It goes something like this: There have been two perspectives on multiple roles. There is a *scarcity approach*, which suggests that bad things will come of people trying to accumulate too many roles because they have too little time and energy. And there is an *enhancement approach*, which counters that human beings are not plagued by scarcity, roles provide the person with valuable resources, and therefore the addition of a new role to one's repertoire is a good thing. Almost invariably, the scarcity approach is linked to Goode's (1960) work, and the enhancement perspective is linked to mine, as well as to a paper by sociologist Sam Sieber (1974) on the benefits of role accumulation.

As the research findings came in, most of the evidence supported Sieber and me rather than Goode. Mothers and wives were doing just fine with their expanding presence in the work force, even thriving measurably better than women without paid work. You might think that I would have felt unequivocally pleased with this triumph, but I often felt cranky about my impact. I was disturbed by the oversimplification of a lot of the research. For example, some work explored whether the simple addition of a role to one's role system is good or bad for people, and I would never have framed the issue of role strain versus role enhancement as a mere function of adding or subtracting roles. Some of the more sophisticated work explored how the quality of a given role (such as paid work) was the important factor in whether people feel strain or enhancement when they have that role or when they add it. Much as I could appreciate the importance of these role-quality findings, again I had some misgivings. The main one was that, in my judgment, the most important questions were not getting asked. The central issue for me was the way that people approach all their roles as a system. Do they believe that some things they do are more important than other things, or do they think that everything they typically do is worthy of their very best efforts? A woman who thinks her parent role is far more important than her paid work role is more likely to feel role strain than a woman who thinks that both roles are equally special, despite the fact that both women may see the quality of their work role the same.

---

[1]*Quantoid*: As used in this chapter, a scientist who studies phenomena through quantitative analysis.

The final straw came from within my own discipline of sociology. In the 1980s and 1990s, several symbolic interactionists began to explore roles as identities. They focused on how the salience of a given role identity affected their relationships, their health and well-being, and their role performance. My issue centered on an unfortunate assumption put forward by sociologist Sheldon Stryker (1980)—the notion that all people organize their role identities into a *salience hierarchy*, which means, simply, that we necessarily see some of our role-identities to be more important than others. What then happened is that researchers designed survey instruments that reproduced and reified Stryker's working assumption. For example, sociologist Peggy Thoits (1992) prompted her participants to generate a list of their identities and then to sort them into three groups—identities most important to them, identities second most important, and identities third most important. The participants did what they were told to do, which is what research subjects most often do. But whose salience hierarchy was this—the participants' or the researcher's? These participants were never given the choice *not* to have a salience hierarchy!

For me, this rhetoric about an inevitable salience hierarchy had a familiar and uncomfortable ring to it. It sounded much the same as my type 3 pattern of overcommitments and undercommitments, now applied to self-organization, and this was the very pattern that I had linked to scarce time, scarce energy, role strain, and other outcomes that people find to be troublesome. I had argued in my 1977 paper that even if this pattern does characterize most people, there is good reason to believe that it does not hold true for everyone (Marks, 1977). The important thing is to leave open the possibility of a nonhierarchical approach to one's self-system and role system, and to allow our theory and our research to discover such an approach if it is out there.

THEORY OF ROLE BALANCE

I then decided that if other folks are not interested in finding and exploring type 1, nonhierarchical, balanced approaches to role systems and self-systems, I would do it myself. I also decided that I needed to become quantitative, because that would be the most effective way of interesting other people in launching similar explorations. My friend work–family researcher Shelley MacDermid from Purdue University was willing to join me, and we published a paper in the *Journal of Marriage and Family* in 1996. In our literature review, we began by fighting back. First, we challenged the tendency to think atomistically instead of holistically about roles. Any given role is embedded in a system of roles: One's experience of that role and one's decisions and feelings about it are always implicitly mindful of what is going on in the rest of one's role system. Goode (1960) himself saw role strain holistically. For him, role strain happens because the *total* role system is overdemanding, not because of what happens in this or that particular role.

Second, we took on the notion of an inevitable salience hierarchy in the way that people organize their role systems and self-systems. We argued that the justification of this notion often rested on a misreading of psychologist and philosopher William James (1890), and we retrieved some text in James's work (located close to the often cited passage) that suggests a very different, more evenhanded approach to life than the salience hierarchy idea. Finally, we took great care in clarifying our concepts. We replaced the language of type 1 and type 3 commitment patterns with the simpler and more descriptive concepts of balanced versus hierarchical role systems. We referred to these orientations as *master cognitive–affective structures* and *internal working models*—terms that we see as nearly synonymous. We defined the *role-balance orientation* as "the tendency to become fully engaged in the performance of every role in one's total role system, to approach every typical role and role partner with an attitude of attentiveness and care" (Marks & MacDermid, 1996, p. 421).

We then constructed a single-item measure of the role-balance orientation. Our item was, "Nowadays I seem to enjoy every part of my life equally well," scored on a 5-point response scale that ranged from *strongly disagree* to *strongly agree*. Our intent with this and our later role-balance items is to get participants to call to mind their entire set of active roles and how they feel about them. We did not name specific roles, because a person's total role system could include an unnamed role (or roles) that may have a major impact on the rest of the role system, and we would have no way of identifying either the role or the impact. It does not solve this problem to recruit research participants who are all spouses, parents, and workers. They may have other roles that they assess much differently than these three, and the other roles might be major contributors to their overall life organization and experience. Again, we believe that the only way to deal with this problem is to give the job of recalling the total role system to the participants, without us trying to name its components for them.

Our next task was to see if people who score higher on our role-balance measure will report different outcomes than people who score lower, as our theory would lead us to predict. We tried our single-item measure in a study of 65 female bank workers in Indiana. All the women were wives and mothers and therefore a very busy population who certainly might be expected to experience a lot of role strain in their everyday lives. We predicted that women who scored higher on role balance would report less role strain, greater self-esteem, less depression, and more positive role-specific experiences than women who scored lower. We also predicted that these higher *balancers* would not have to depend on narrowing their role obligations to achieve these salutary outcomes. Our measure of role strain was a shortened version of an "overload" scale (Reilly, 1982), with items such as "I need more hours in the day to do all the things which are expected of me" and "I can't ever seem to get caught up."

Surely, our most important hypothesis concerned the relationship between role balance and this role strain measure, as this was the most direct way of putting Goode's theory of role strain to the test. In a sample of very busy women, could the mere fact of enjoying all of one's roles equally make a difference in the likelihood of reporting feelings of overload? To test our hypotheses, we split our sample into three nearly equal groups—those who scored highest on the role-balance measure, those who scored lowest, and a middle-level group. We then ran planned comparisons between the higher balancers and the lower balancers to see if their mean scores on our dependent variables were significantly different.

In quantitative research, there is always that magic moment long after the hypotheses have been organized, the data have been collected and entered, and the most appropriate statistical tests have been selected. You tell the computer to run the tests, and with the fond hope that the world will work the way you think it does, you wait for the results to appear on your screen. These results were indeed thrilling! Of the 11 variables on which we ran our group comparisons, all mean differences were in the predicted direction, and 8 of the 11 were statistically significant, including our overload measure of role strain. The greater balancers were less likely to report problems of overload, and they had higher self-esteem, less depression, and higher parental nurturing scores. They also reported greater closeness with their husbands and greater productivity at work. Yet, they not only reported no greater tendency to subordinate their careers, but they even reported less of a tendency than the nonbalancers to cut down on their recreational activities (for a more complete report, see Marks & MacDermid, 1996).

Fortified by this exciting confirmation, we were now ready to expand our role-balance measure beyond a single-item measure and try it out with an entirely different population. In the fall of 1993, we surveyed 333 sociology students at the University of Maine. This was another very busy population. Nearly all were full-time students, and most had paid work, were married or in a serious romantic relationship, and had active social lives. To expand our role-balance measure, we created an eight-item scale by retaining the single item and adding seven more. Examples of these additional balance items are "I try to put a lot of myself into everything I do"; "I am pretty good at keeping the different parts of my life in balance—I generally don't let things slide"; and "Work time, classes and study time, partner time, friend time, family time, leisure time—I find satisfaction in everything I do." We also created a measure of *role ease*. Just as health is more than the absence of disease, we think that the experience of ease and effortlessness in one's life pattern is more than the absence of what Maslow called "strain and striving." Our five-item role-ease measure asked how easy it was to have quality time with friends, get personal chores done, have a pleasant meal, have satisfying leisure time, and stay in contact with one's parent(s). Responses were scored on a 4-point scale from *very easy* to *very difficult.*

Our hypotheses were quite similar to those in our study of bank workers: Students who score higher on our role-balance measure report less role strain, greater role ease, higher self-esteem, less depression, and more positive role-specific experiences than students who score lower. Our strategy for analysis was to split the sample into two groups—students scoring above the median of our eight-item role-balance measure and students scoring below the median. We then conducted planned comparisons of the two groups to test our hypotheses. Once again the results were impressive, as all of our hypotheses were confirmed. In addition, we found that the more role-balancing students had significantly higher grade point averages and reported more weekly "good times with friends" than the less role-balancing students. Yet, there was no evidence that these balancers' lesser role strain and their other salutary outcomes were accomplished because they were less busy. They did not take fewer credit hours, work less hours in paid work, or report having fewer friends (for more details, see Marks & MacDermid, 1996).

ROLE BALANCE AND MARRIED COUPLES

A new opportunity for work on role balance emerged in 1994 when psychologist Ted Huston at the University of Texas invited me to include some measures in a new wave of data collection for his well-known marriage study called PAIR (*Processes of Adaptation in Intimate Relationships*). Huston had been following a sample of Pennsylvania couples for some 12 years. His data collection includes a diary strategy in which both spouses are contacted separately by phone after each of three weekdays and three weekend days. Participants are asked exactly what they did over the previous 24 hours, how long the activity lasted, with whom they did it, and how they felt in the middle of it. The chance to hook up with this rich data set was irresistible.

Once I saw the characteristics of the sample, I became especially interested in three issues. First, is role balance a social-class privilege and perquisite? Will participants who report fewer financial difficulties score higher on role balance? In my earlier work, I had suggested that this was a strong possibility. Maslow had claimed that when people feel unsafe (including their economic security), they become fixated on eliminating the deficit, even at the expense of needs and activities to which they would otherwise be drawn. Our hunch was that PAIR participants would be similar. Insufficient economic resources create a chronic sense of emergency, pushing people to keep moving other components of their role systems to the back burner. Feelings of balance will then be lessened.

Second, even when economic worries are not present, do people have to cut back on what they do to feel balanced across their remaining activities? In the student survey, we had expected that the more balanced students would report less feelings of overload, and they would accomplish this feat without having to trim their everyday activities. We never anticipated that instead of not simply cutting down on their activities as the price for feeling more balanced, the balancers apparently did more than the less balanced students. Their higher grade point averages suggests that they put more into their studies, and their reports of more friends with whom they enjoyed good times in a given week suggests an expanded social life compared with the less-balanced students. With Ted Huston's rich data set, my research team felt we now had a more fine-grained way to explore this relationship between balance and the ways that role systems expand or contract.

Third, is role balance a gendered phenomenon? We had not found any gender differences in our student survey. In the PAIR data, although wives' role balance scores were not significantly different from the husbands', it was clear from differences in work hours and leisure time with children that husbands had very different patterns of daily activity than wives. Did this mean that the correlates of husbands' role balance were different from the correlates of wives' in some predictably gendered way?

Our sample consisted of 80 white couples married for 13 years, all in their first marriages. All participants had at least one child ages 13 or younger; 35% had at least one preschooler. Our analytical strategy was to create separate models predicting wives' and husbands' balance. The fact that there was no correlation between wives' balance and husbands' balance, along with the clear evidence of different patterns of time use, gave us confidence that separate models were the way to go.

Our dependent variable, feelings of role balance, was a four-item version of the scale we had used in the student survey (the items with the highest loadings in a factor analysis). In all our models, we controlled for gender attitudes, feelings of financial strain, both partners' paid work hours, feelings of parental attachment, having at least one preschool child, and global marital satisfaction. We then entered variables reflecting the specifics of the marital relationship and patterns of leisure and network involvement.

There is not space here to detail our final models (see Marks, Huston, Johnson, & MacDermid, 2001), but I will focus on the three issues mentioned above. First, is role balance a social-class privilege and perk? The answer seems to be yes. Wives who feel more financial strain consistently report lower role balance, regardless of what else is in the model. Financial strain is one of the most robust predictors—a negative one—of wives' balance. Husbands' feelings of balance are likewise tied to economic matters, but not through feelings of financial strain. Their job income averages more than three times that of their wives, and they probably feel a lot more responsible for it. We found a direct and significant relationship between husbands' income and their role balance, even controlling for their feelings of financial strain. Notice the clear policy implications here: If we in the United States think that role balance is a good thing, it behooves us to do a better job of spreading an economic safety net under people who most need it.

Second, is cutting back on what we do the price we must pay for feeling more balanced? The answer is mixed. For PAIR wives, feeling more balanced correlates with having less of their leisure alone with their children but doing more of everything else. Wives' paid work hours are a robust, positive predictor of their balance, and this is a linear relationship, not the curvilinear one we had expected. We found no fall-off in the role balance of women who work the most hours. In addition, wives who reported any couple visits with friends scored higher on role balance than wives who reported no such visits. Similarly, wives who reported more instances of leisure with relatives scored higher on balance. As for husbands, again we found a mixed relationship between role balance and issues of role expansion and contraction, but the mix was very different than that for wives, and this brings us to our third question.

Is role balance a gendered phenomenon? The answer is a clear yes, at least in this particular sample. PAIR husbands average a 52-hour workweek, whereas wives average a 25-hour workweek. For husbands, with upward of 9- or 10-hour workdays plus commuting time, compounded by frequent weekend work time, the pathway to role balance is not going to be accumulating more roles or becoming more active in the roles they already have! Unlike wives, husbands' work hours are negative correlates of their role balance: The longer they work, the less balanced they feel. This is the exact gendered counterpart of what we found in the wives' model: The more the wives spend leisure time alone with their children, the less balanced they feel.

The story seems to be that when you do too much of any one thing, you are less likely to feel a sense of balance across the totality of what you do, and doing more of the other things will not usually add any balance to the mix. Given husbands' long work hours, doing more leisure alone with their wives could not contribute to their role balance because then they would hardly see their children. And being alone with their children could not contribute to their balance because then they would hardly see their wives. Husbands do score higher on role balance when they report more leisure with their wives and children together, but this is the exception that proves the rule. To put it baldly, they must multitask their connection with their wives and children simply to see them. Anything that expands their role system beyond that, such as visits with friends and relatives, makes no contribution to their feelings of balance.

These findings lead me to a somewhat different conclusion than I had reached earlier about the prospects for balance. When I had worried as a budding professional that Calvinistic achievement pressures might rob me of my balance in life, I did not fully appreciate what a social-class luxury that worry was. And my strategy for preserving my balance was again in some ways a social-class luxury. It was not unlike what the Beatles (Lennon & McCartney, 1967) proposed when they sang "all you need is love." When feelings of balance are not present, all you need to do is shift your internal working model so that you might fully engage in everything you do whenever you get around to doing it. "There is nothing you can do that can't be done," the Beatles sang.

Now, I am enough of a child of the 1960s to believe that we do, after all, create our own reality—and not just upper-middle-class people. I still hold to my earlier position, for the most part. In our 1996 paper, Shelley MacDermid and I were mindful of situational urgencies that can derail a person's balance in life. We wrote, "Even role-balanced people may need to temporarily postpone certain role engagements to deal with [an] emergency" (Marks & MacDermid, 1996, p. 421). We saw such postponements as just that—something temporary. Role balancers have learned a mode of functioning that simply feels better, and they will return to their baseline as soon as they can. We contrasted this situation with the tendencies of people who have a more hierarchical internal working model. In that case, we suggested, the favored role at the top of the hierarchy becomes a chronic emergency rather than a situational one. The roles lower down on the hierarchy become almost a hindrance to dispatching the more favored role.

The PAIR study findings have coaxed me to recognize how easily these chronic emergencies can overtake the lives of people who might otherwise be balancers. The need felt by PAIR husbands to work long hours so they could earn an adequate income creates a chronic emergency. So does wives' child-care responsibility when they have inadequate help with it, and there is no nationally subsidized program, such as in France, that provides free, competent, preschool day care to all who want it. Consider, too, the chronic emergency faced by millions of people who are caring for an aging or ill parent or for a child with special needs. Or consider the way we professor types create a kind of enforced, hierarchical internal working model for our undergraduate students, expecting them to prioritize every one of their too-many-courses-taken-at-once and forgetting that many of them have to work long hours simply to stay in school. The examples can easily multiply, and they add up to an inescapable conclusion: Balance in life is not always easy; sometimes it is downright fugitive, especially in the face of a public culture that does very little to promote it. And yet, despite the obstacles, and no matter how busy the sample we look at, we do find some people who score higher on balance when we attempt to measure it and other people who score lower. It continues to be a worthy challenge, then, to figure out the difference.

LOOKING FORWARD

I conclude with a few comments about work that remains to be done. First and foremost, we need to create adequate measures of hierarchically arranged role systems. Thus far we have only a workable measure for balance, not hierarchy, and we need to have both kinds of measures in the same study. It may seem logical that the same people who claim to have an evenhanded spirit of engagement will not be the ones who say that they like to do some things more than other things, but people are not logicians. Perhaps feelings of role balance and feelings of role hierarchy are separate continua, not opposite poles on a single continuum. Shelley MacDermid and I did attempt to measure hierarchical tendencies, but the scale did not work very well, and as yet we have not gone back to the drawing board.

Second, neither role balance nor role hierarchy may be singular phenomena in themselves. Perhaps our failed attempts to measure hierarchy were due to unwittingly combining different kinds of hierarchical tendencies within the same scale. Earlier in this chapter, I suggested that passion-driven overcommitments may work differently in one's total role system than fear-driven overcommitments, with different consequences for one's overall functioning. I think this is an exciting lead for future studies of hierarchical role arrangements. In general, good, smart, typological thinking is what we need here, along with measures that faithfully operationalize the types we create.

Third, like any self-respecting sociologist, perhaps I have been too quick to steer clear of personality variables as potentially important factors in role balance and how it varies. Years ago, the folks who came up with a link between type A personalities and heart disease were already offering a model of this kind of exploration, but that was about just one kind of personality configuration. Obviously, there are many other possibilities. For example, can someone have an oppositional personality and be a role balancer at the same time? Can a procrastinator be a balancer? And what about people I call "intensity junkies"—people who get so excited about anything they are doing that it becomes difficult to put it aside to engage anything else in their role system? Perhaps this is the same species as the "passion-driven overcommitter," but I see the latter's passion as focused consistently on just one thing, whereas intensity junkies get so caught up in anything they are doing that they could keep doing it forever.

Who will do any of this work remains to be seen. It may not be me, as I will soon retire, and I am currently immersed in a different project. Regardless, studies of balance are not going away, and this pleases me. Balance has become another buzzword, appearing variously as role balance, life balance, work–family balance, and work–life balance. I am proud to have been a contributor to this work, and it amazes me that across many disciplines, people still routinely cite the piece I published more than 30 years ago. It is a rare privilege to be appreciated for something you love to do!

REFERENCES

Bowen, M. (1978). *Family therapy in clinical practice.* Northvale, NJ: Jason Aronson.

Cuber, J., & Harroff, P. (1965). *Sex and the significant Americans.* Baltimore: Penguin.

Freud, S. (1961). *Civilization and its discontents* (James Strachey, Trans.). New York: W.W. Norton & Co. (original work published 1930).

Goode, W. J. (1960). A theory of role strain. *American Sociological Review, 25,* 483–496.

James, W. (1890). *The principles of psychology.* New York: H. Holt.

Lennon, J., & McCartney, P. (1967). All you need is love. On *Magical mystery tour* [record]. London: Abbey Road Studios.

Marks, S. R. (1977). Multiple roles and role strain: Some notes on human energy, time, and commitment. *American Sociological Review, 42,* 921–936.

Marks, S. R. (1979). Culture, human energy, and self-actualization: A sociological offering to humanistic psychology. *Journal of Humanistic Psychology, 19,* 27–42.

Marks, S. R. (1989). Toward a systems theory of marital quality. *Journal of Marriage and the Family, 51,* 19–26.

Marks, S. R., Huston, T. L., Johnson, E. M., & MacDermid, S. M. (2001). Role balance among white married couples. *Journal of Marriage and the Family, 63,* 1083–1098.

Marks, S. R. (1986). *Three corners: Exploring marriage and the self.* Lexington, MA: Lexington Books.

Marks, S. R., & MacDermid, S. M. (1996). Multiple roles and the self: A theory of role balance. *Journal of Marriage and the Family, 58,* 417–432.

Maslow, A. (1970). *Motivation and personality* (2nd ed.). New York: Harper & Row.

Maslow, A. (1971). *The farther reaches of human nature.* New York: Viking Press.

Mills, C. W. (1959). *The sociological imagination.* New York: Oxford.

Reilly, M. D. (1982). Working wives and consumption. *Journal of Consumer Research, 8,* 407–418.

Sieber, S. D. (1974). Toward a theory of role accumulation. *American Sociological Review, 39,* 567–578.

Stryker, S. (1980). *Symbolic interactionism: A social structural version.* Menlo Park, CA: Benjamin Cummings.

Thoits, P. A. (1992). Identity structures and psychological well-being: Gender and marital status comparisons. *Social Psychology Quarterly, 55,* 236–256.

Thomas, W. I. (1923). *The unadjusted girl.* Boston: Little, Brown.

Weber, M. (1958). *The Protestant ethic and the spirit of capitalism.* New York: Scribner's.

Zablocki, B. (1971). *The joyful community.* Baltimore: Penguin.

SECTION II

Measuring Life Balance

CHAPTER 6

Defining and Validating Measures of Life Balance

SUGGESTIONS, A NEW MEASURE, AND SOME PRELIMINARY RESULTS

KENNON M. SHELDON

INTRODUCTION

Life balance, work–life balance, and work–family balance have become increasingly trendy terms since they first appeared in the social sciences literature in the late 1980s and early 1990s, and their popularity shows no signs of abating. Indeed, an informal search of the abstract database PsycINFO using the term *life balance*, from 1996 to 2006, revealed although there was only one publication on that topic in 1996, there were 39 by 2006.

The life balance concept appears to be popular in part because it crystallizes a growing awareness in Western culture, particularly in the United States, that modern adults work too much, too hard, and too long. Notably, the concept has links to concepts of harmony and optimal living proposed in the mid-20th century (Jahoda, 1958; Maslow, 1954; Rogers, 1961), and ultimately can be traced back to Aristotelian concepts of optimal function and the benefits of moderation, virtue, and the golden mean. Thus, the life balance concept seems to be an important research topic, worthy of careful consideration and study.

In this chapter, I will first review the recent theoretical formulations regarding life balance—what, exactly, does *life balance* mean? This is a surprisingly difficult question to answer, as few researchers have supplied explicit definitions of their usage of the term. Implicitly, *imbalance* usually refers simply to a stressful lifestyle or, sometimes more specifically, to a lifestyle in which there is too much work or, sometimes even more specifically, to a lifestyle in which there is too much work and not enough family or relationships. Often, the existence of imbalance within individuals' lives is simply taken as a given—a societal, organizational, or cultural-level problem for which various programs, interventions, and policy strategies need to be created. However, balance has also been measured as an individual difference, and I will review some of the existing measures of this construct. Measuring imbalance (vs. balance) allows the construct be tested as an independent variable that predicts health and well-being outcomes and also allows it to be examined as a dependent variable that changes over time or that differs between different demographic groups (e.g., full-time vs. part-time workers; mothers vs. fathers; office workers vs. telecommuters).

After surveying extant definitions and measures, I will suggest that they are inadequate to encompass the true potential richness of the life balance concept. In addition, they are inadequate for distinguishing life balance from related constructs, like meaning, satisfaction, success, and low neuroticism. I will then propose a new assessment approach and two complementary

K. Matuska & C. Christiansen (Eds.)
Life balance: Multidisciplinary theories and research (pp 61–72)
© 2009 SLACK Incorporated and AOTA Press

measures of life balance that can be derived from this approach. One of the measures is based on numerically equivalent time use across multiple life domains, and the other is based on the correspondence (vs. discrepancy) between actual-life time use and ideal-life time use. Preliminary supporting data for this two-pronged approach will be summarized. I will conclude that life balance is a potentially important construct in its own right, and that it can be measured, but only as a system-level property of peoples' lives—an emergent state that represents more than the sum of the particular components that make up that state.

HOW TO DEFINE LIFE BALANCE?

Background

The idea that leading a balanced life is important is a familiar one in contemporary society and in both classical and contemporary psychological research. However, the idea goes back to the ancient Greeks and can also be found in many Asian and Chinese philosophies, as well as in Native American, African, and Australian aboriginal religious and cultural traditions. These differing cultural and religious traditions all emphasize maintaining a state of balance or harmony between many varying types of life elements, including life energies (*chi*), spirit forces, motivations, identities, values, roles, tasks, activities, occupations, and relationships.

As this list suggests, a bewildering variety of different life elements can be involved in some sort of balance equation. Furthermore, there are many ways to think about what "achieving balance" means. Consider *balance* as a verb: when we balance a mathematical equation, we do the same thing to both sides of the equation; when we balance the books, we reconcile monetary inputs with outputs; and when we balance on one foot, we compensate for our fluctuations away from our own center of gravity. In such terms, what are we doing when we balance our lives?

Considered as a noun, to be balanced is to be in a state of equilibrium, equipoise, or stability. However, the term balance can also refer to the mere remainder (the balance of the debt) or the predominant amount (the balance of opinion favors proposition X). In such terms, how can the presence of a state of balance within a person's life be conceptualized and quantified? Furthermore, are balance and imbalance opposite extremes of a single dimension, or are they actually somewhat different dimensions, such that a person could be both balanced and imbalanced at the same time? Also, is imbalance necessarily a state to be avoided, or can it have benefits? These are very difficult questions to answer.

Problems in Defining Life Balances

In their comprehensive review of the empirical research literature, Christiansen and Matuska (2006) noted that "although the concept of a balanced lifestyle seems implicitly understood, no consensus definition, model, or measure has emerged to guide theory development" (p. 49). Similarly, Backman (2004) stated that life balance remains "an abstract and evolving construct" that is "seldom clearly and succinctly defined" (pp. 202–203). Backman (2004) also provided a table of 12 published conceptual definitions of life balance, which were noteworthy primarily for their diversity. As examples, balance has been defined in terms of the perceived impact of daily occupations on each other (Christiansen, 1996, p. 436), the extent one's environment supports multiple occupations (Llorens, 1984, p. 30), the extent of agreement between the individual's goals and abilities and the demands of the environment (Jonsson, Moller, & Grimby, 1999, p. 355), perceived success in balancing work and personal life concerns (Tausig & Fenwick, 2001, p. 105), and being underoccupied or overoccupied in one's time (Townsend & Wilcock, 2004, p. 253).

To begin their review, Christiansen and Matuska (2006) proposed their own working definition of life balance from the perspective of occupational therapy: "a consistent pattern of occupations that results in reduced stress and improved health and well-being" (p. 50). Thus, balance is defined in terms of its purported outcomes or effects: greater health, mood, and life satisfaction, and reduced stress (and presumably reduced strain, conflict, and overload also). Although one can sympathize with the comprehensiveness and holistic appeal of this definition, unfortunately, it does not provide clues for conceptualizing balance as something distinct from the positive outcomes it presumably causes. Is life balance just a synonym for *psychological well-being* or *mental health*? If so, researchers might question whether the term is really needed (we might call this the *no-new-information problem*). Similarly, defining balance in terms of its effects is conceptually problematic: how do you know a person is balanced? Because he or she is healthy. How do you know a person is healthy? Because he or she is balanced (we might call this the *circularity problem*). Indeed, the circularity problem is even more directly evident in several of the definitions reviewed by Backman (2004): *balance* refers to "the relative balance across… areas of self-care, productivity, and leisure" (Law, Polatajko, Baptiste, & Townsend, 1997, p. 38) or "balance among self-care, work/productive activities, play or leisure, and rest" (Nurit & Michal, 2003, p. 228). Here, *balance* is defined as balance.

To further illustrate the problems, and also to point the way toward a possible solution, consider that Christiansen and Matuska (2006) organized their empirical review around four overarching perspectives on balance they found in the literature: (1) that it involves optimal time use, (2) that it involves successfully performing multiple social roles, (3) that it involves having a lifestyle that meets one's psychological needs, and (4) that it involves being synchronized with one's own biological rhythms and physiological clocks. A wide variety of research and conceptual issues were discussed under this four-fold framework. However, I suggest that the second, third, and fourth definitions are all compromised by the no-new-information problem. We already have a large literature on role conflict, role strain, and role performance, a literature which (arguably) does not need the balance concept. Similarly, we already have a large literature on psychological need satisfaction, which may have nothing to gain from a balance concept (but see Sheldon & Niemiec, 2006, discussed below). Finally, we already have a large literature on the effects of being synchronized (or not) with one's biological rhythms, a literature that may also have no need for balance concepts.

Reasons for Focusing on Time Use

I suggest that basing the concept of life balance on the first perspective, optimal time use, provides the most solid foundation for the concept. There are several reasons for this. First, a focus on time use has already been a major thrust within the work–life and work–family balance literature, as researchers consider the competing demands of work, family, and leisure. Indeed, the idea that time is a resource of increasing scarcity likely is the chief motivator of contemporary interest in the concept of balance, not only within public discourse but also within a variety of research literatures, including economics, occupational therapy, sociology, vocational psychology, stress psychology, and industrial–organizational psychology. Again, from this perspective the problem is that we have too much to do and too little time in which to do it. As a result, we experience much conflict and pressure within our lives, and important restorative experiences are crowded out (Frey, 2001) or permanently foregone.

A second advantage of a time-use definition of balance is that it allows us to examine a person's life as a total system, including all of his or her moments of experience. In one sense, time is the most important "stuff" of peoples' lives, the moving window of awareness that we fill via our daily choices (Csikszentmihalyi, 1988). Arguably, an inability to properly apportion this essential stuff across the different days and domains of our existences is precisely indicative of an imbalanced life. A third advantage of basing the concept of life balance on time use is that time is (at least potentially) objectively and precisely quantifiable. Such measurement characteristics are desirable, in part, because they help eliminate shared method variance from candidate balance measures and the subjective outcome measures (e. g., mood, satisfaction, happiness) that we might predict from a balance measure.

Considerable research has already used time-based methodologies to measure balance, focusing on the total hours spent in work and nonwork activities (Camporese, Freguja, & Sabbadini, 1998; Holman & Jacquart, 1988), the relative allotment of time and energy across work and nonwork life domains (Judge, Boudreau, & Bretz, 1994; Tenbrunsel, Brett, Maoz, Stroh, & Reilly, 1995), and the proportion or ratio of time spent in a particular category (such as work) relative to the total time available (Greenhaus, Collins, & Shaw, 2002; Gutek, Searle, & Klepa, 1991). Such studies have used both *retrospective recall methodologies*, in which participants indicate their recent or typical allotment of time across categories, and *time-diary* or *activity-log methodologies*, in which these quantities are measured throughout a period of time rather than retrospectively (Juster & Stafford, 1991).

Problems With Time-Use Definitions of Balance

Still, there are some apparent problems with time-use methodologies and approaches. First, time-use studies sometimes yield weak or inconsistent results (Christiansen & Matuska, 2006), limiting the appeal of this methodology (although I will suggest some potentially more powerful ways to use such methodologies below). Second, retrospective methodologies may be biased by memory or motivational processes, which distort such estimates (although ongoing time-diary studies overcome most of these problems; Zuzanek, 1998). Moreover, comparisons of cumulative diary data and retrospective data have shown that retrospective measures are not necessarily biased or inaccurate (Sandvik, Diener, & Seidlitz, 1993). Third, much of the prior time-use research has focused on only one or two categories (e.g., work and nonwork), ignoring the many other categories in which people can and do spend their time (although there is no reason not to expand the list of categories to be examined; Warren, 2004). Fourth, it is not always clear what categories to use when asking people to allocate their time; should they divide their time up by role categories (e.g., worker, parent, child), goal categories (e.g., relationship, financial, community), functional categories (e.g., work, chores, recreation), physical location categories (e.g., home, work, car, health club), or categories of their own unique devising?

As a fifth problem, time-use methodologies do not capture how people feel about the way they use their time and the meaning of the time they spend in various places. For example, Backman (2004) points out that cooking may have very different meanings as a work occupation than as a household chore, and shopping may have very different meanings as a burden versus as a source of recreation. Similarly, Christiansen and Matuska (2006) have suggested that estimating the hours allocated to various life domains does not provide information about the contextual or qualitative features of time use, such as perceived enjoyment or meaning of the time spent. In short, counting hours may be an overly simplistic (Spencer, 1989) approach to the complex issues of harmony and overall systemic functioning that are implied by the life-balance construct.

I suggest that the "meaning" problem is the most difficult one for time-use approaches to surmount. Indeed, merely counting hours does seem to miss the potential richness of the life balance concept. Unfortunately, incorporating participants' ratings of meaning of their time allocations into a life balance measure begins to raise the no-new-information problem, because we already have measures of meaningfulness, fulfillment, satisfaction, and the like that are applied across multiple life domains. Also, if feelings of meaning and satisfaction are incorporated centrally into the definition and measurement of life balance, then we are back to the circularity problem; the person is balanced because life is meaningful and satisfying, and life is meaningful and satisfying because the person is balanced.

Thus one key, it seems, is to define life balance in a way that allows the construct to stand on its own, as something that has not already been studied by another name. Insisting on such discriminative validity should help the overall cause of psychological science, in which terminological redundancy and overlap remain a huge problem (Staats, 1999). However, a second key, it seems, is to somehow incorporate meaning into the definition so that the participants' subjective construals of their time can be addressed—but not in such a way that the balance construct is reducible to existing meaning constructs and measures. My proposed approach to these two goals will be considered shortly. First, however, I will briefly review some existing measurement approaches, to better illuminate the advantages of the definition and measure I will propose.

EXISTING MEASURES OF LIFE BALANCE

Work Dominance

As suggested by the many extant conceptual definitions of life balance (Backman, 2004), researchers have employed a variety of individual-difference measures of the construct. Some measures, such as those based on time use, have already been considered above. Scrutiny of other measures reveals a number of possible problems. One problem is that some measures refer merely to overwork. For example, although Loretto et al. (2005) showed that work–life imbalance uniquely predicted employee well-being in a UK National Health Service survey, the imbalance measure was only a measure of work dominance: items included "How often do you work at home, think about work at home?" "How often are you too tired because of work to interact with family and friends?" and "How often does work schedule conflict with family/social life schedule?" Similarly, Dex and Bond's (2005) seven-item measure addressed overwork alone—"I usually work long hours," "I have to take my work home," and "There isn't much time to socialize/relax." Although it may be reasonable to operationally define *life imbalance* as occurring in part when one works too much, ideally the construct could be measured with reference to the person's life as a whole, not just work (Backman, 2004). Thus, just as in the time-use studies mentioned above, these studies may focus overmuch on just one domain. Also, the meaning of a dominant work life is not addressed by these measures; we can all think of people who work long hours but who nevertheless are engaged and satisfied by their vocation, despite not being balanced according to researchers' intuitions. Indeed, many of our greatest and most fulfilled innovators and performers can be characterized as workaholics (Simonton, 1984).

Other life balance measures also focus on work and nonwork, but they take a somewhat broader conceptual focus. For example, Podratz (2004) defined balance as a second-order factor that reflected five first-order factors found within a lengthy Likert questionnaire: work-to-personal-life conflict, work-to-personal-life facilitation, personal-life-to-work conflict, personal-life-to-work facilitation, and values attainment. Fisher (2002) directly assessed perceptions of work–life balance via a 21-item Likert measure, finding three underlying dimensions: work interference with personal life, personal life interference with work, and work and personal life enhancement. Notably, these approaches still focus on only two life domains and not on life more broadly construed. Also, they begin to deconstruct the overall balance concept into a suite of component parts. This can be desirable if this suite is indeed "carving nature at its joints," but not so desirable if it is missing important components.

Subjective Life-Domain Evaluations

Another general approach to assessing life balance is to rely on peoples' subjective evaluations of the positivity or negativity of various features and issues within their lives. For example, Backman (2001) measured balance by asking participants to rate how satisfied they were with the time spent on work, self-care, leisure, and rest. As another example of the satisfaction approach, Warren (2004) defined balance in terms of satisfaction ratings regarding eight different life domains, including, among others, leisure time, social life, job, health, and spouse or partner. Although these approaches expand the measure beyond mere work and nonwork, the focus on "satisfaction" within various life domains may be problematic because life-satisfaction measures already exist with a similar multiple domain focus (Cummins, 2005). Also life-satisfaction measures typically do not invoke balance concepts in their formulation and definition; instead, life satisfaction is more often treated as a dependent variable, that which might be predicted by a balance measure. Thus, the satisfaction approach may lead to the circularity problem, in which the predictor and the outcome are measured or conceptualized in the same way.

As a further illustration of the tendency of researchers to measure balance via subjective evaluation, recall from above that balance has been defined (and thus measured) in terms of the rated impact of occupations on each other (Christiansen, 1996), the rated extent one's environment supports multiple occupations (Llorens, 1984), the rated agreement the individual sees between their goals and abilities and the demands of their environment (Jonsson et al., 1999), and the rated success in balancing work and personal-life concerns (Tausig & Fenwick, 2001). All these measures of imbalance rely on participants agreeing with negative portrayals of their life and situation or disagreeing with positive portrayals.

Finally, a more general problem with using participants' positive versus negative assessments of their lives is that such ratings may be reducible to simpler personality constructs such as neuroticism, extraversion, or temperament (Fortunato & Goldblatt, 2002). A dispositionally unhappy person might score high on imbalance, not because their time is out of whack but rather because everything looks bad. If this is the case, then again, the measure may tread into already-known territories (the no-new-information problem), and the complex concept of life balance may be unnecessary to explain the data. In short, subjective evaluation-type measures may confound balance measures with other theoretical predictors or with important outcome measures, threatening the discriminant validity of the construct.

PROPOSED DEFINITION AND MEASURE OF LIFE BALANCE

I propose a two-pronged definition and measure of life balance: first, that balance represents an equitable distribution of time across one's actual time-use profile, and second, that this distribution is also non-discrepant from one's ideal time-use profile. In this definition, a *balanced person* is one who is able to spread time fairly evenly across the different domains, with the feeling that this particular time-use profile is the ideal profile for him or her. I will talk about each of these prongs below but will first talk about an overall assessment approach that permits measurement of the two aspects of balance, the Discrepant Time-Use Profile (DTUP).

Discrepant Time-Use Profile

The first step of the DTUP assessment is to ask participants to consider a 24-hour period. This period could be participants' most recent day (i.e., the last 24 hours) or the participants' typical day. Typical days might refer to weekdays or weekend days, workdays or vacation days, or whatever suits the researcher's purposes. Participants should be presented with a range of major time categories and asked to apportion the 24 hours of the day across those categories—the only constraint being that the numbers must add up to 24. In our preliminary research (Sheldon & Cummins, 2007), we have used the time categories sleeping, working, commuting, studying, doing chores, and recreating and also the categories of health/self-maintenance, community, personal relationships, and spirituality/religion. In some studies, we have also included an "other" category, so that participants can write in any major category that seems missing from the list and indicate the time they spend in that category.

After apportioning their actual 24 hours, participants are then asked to apportion 24 hours again, this time considering their ideal time apportionment—that is, how much time they would like to spend sleeping, working, on personal relationships, and so on, (the total amount is still constrained to add up to 24). This allows participants to tweak the amounts to their liking, envisioning what a more balanced time-use profile would be, from their own perspective.

There are several possible uses and advantages of such data. The first is that they enable the simple amount of time spent in each life domain to be considered as single variables. Does the person spend 0, 4, 8, or 12 hours a day working? How much sleep does he or she get? How much time does he or she spend on relationships or community compared to work and school? What about potentially aggravating life domains—chores and commuting—how much time is spent there? In a large-sample study, simply being able to look at the simultaneous association of each of these single variables with outcomes could be quite valuable. It could also be valuable to look at the relative strength of effects—for example, the effects of the amount of time spent working, while controlling for the amount of time spent in other domains of life (e.g., commuting). Perhaps apparent negative work effects are really due to the inordinate time that is spent getting to and from work. Given the weak time-use effects that have sometimes been reported in past time-use studies (Christiansen & Matuska, 2006), we might expect these single-domain effects to be mostly small or nonsignificant.

Computing a Balanced Time-Use Variable

However, it is the further uses of such data that are most promising. Ideally, we would like an imbalance measure to represent more than "not enough sleep" or "too much work"—that is, it will somehow address and summarize the entire life configuration or time profile of the individual in a way that represents and relies on the specific domains that comprise the measure but goes beyond these specifics. And indeed, this is possible with the DTUP. In our preliminary data, we have computed a balanced time-use variable, operationally defined as having a low standard deviation across the 10 actual hour estimates made across the 10 life categories. Thus, the more evenly distributed the 24 hours are across the 10 or so categories, the more balanced the person is considered to be, with an impossible ideal of a 0 standard deviation representing exactly 2.4 hours in each category. Although this computation may be crude in some ways, it may also be effective. For example, it addresses a central intuition of much work–life balance research: that work can become all-consuming and crowd out other areas of life. Victims of such processes (e.g., workaholics), with 10 or 12 hours in the work category and 0 hours in several other categories, should be represented by high standard deviations as measured by the DTUP.

Computing a Nondiscrepant Time-Use Variable

But what about a person who is evenly distributed across categories but wants to have a more uneven distribution? One example is somebody who only sleeps 5 hours a night and would like to sleep 8 hours. Another is a person who would like to work full-time but has only succeeded in finding a part-time job. How can such desires be accommodated? More generally, how can we get at the subjective meaning of the time spent? Although most people dislike commuting, for some people it may represent a chance to relax on the bus with the paper or to reconnect with friends on the train. Maybe some would prefer to spend *more* time commuting. The same is true of cooking (Backman, 2004)—maybe some would rather spend more time on this household activity.

This is where an actual-ideal discrepancy measure can be useful. By summing the absolute values of the 10 discrepancy scores (i.e., ideal sleep hours – actual sleep hours + ideal work hours – actual work hours, and so forth), one arrives at a single global discrepancy measure that represents the extent to which the person would rearrange his or her life schedule as a whole, given the opportunity. Presumably, this measure allows consideration of the meaning or quality of time use. The important aspect of this measure is to be spending time as one wants—not too little or too much—across all of the different areas of life. Notably, some previous balance researchers have employed a discrepancy approach. For example, Jacobs and Gerson (2001) used an actual/ideal work-hours discrepancy approach, finding that on average, participants work more than their ideal (although a considerable number worked less than their ideal). However, they did not consider other domains besides work and did not treat the measure as a variable to be correlated with other variables.

The general characteristics and advantages of discrepancy measures are worth further consideration. Discrepancy theories and measurement approaches have a long history and pedigree within psychology, going back to early humanistic and self theorists (Lecky, 1951; Rogers & Dymond, 1954), continuing on to early cognitive personality theorists (Higgins, Bond, Klein, & Straumann, 1986; Straumann & Higgins, 1987), and thriving through the present (Dittmar, 2005; Petrocelli & Smith, 2005). An advantage of well-constructed discrepancy measures is that the participant does not directly rate the discrepancy, that is, there is no self-rating ranging from "no discrepancy" to "much discrepancy." This helps the measure avoid the pitfall of possible overlapping method or conceptual variance shared with satisfaction, meaning, neuroticism, or negative affectivity. Instead discrepancy is a computed variable, a quantity that is derived from independently produced sets of data. For example, in the Selves questionnaire (Higgins et al., 1986), discrepancies (e.g., between actual and ideal self or ideal and ought self) are derived by counting the number of common descriptors that appear across separately generated lists. In the DTUP approach suggested in this chapter, discrepancies are computed by summing the 10 differences between actual and ideal time-use allotments in each category, derived from two separately generated time profiles. Yet another advantage of discrepancy approaches is that discrepancy assessment is more of a method than a theory (especially when a traditional actual vs. ideal approach is taken). Thus, life balance as assessed by a discrepancy approach does not encroach on other theoretical literatures, avoiding the no-new-information problem.

To illustrate an existing application of a discrepancy methodology to the life–balance issue, I, along with Christopher P. Niemiec (2006), examined balance within the domain of psychological need satisfaction. Although our focus on need satisfaction threatened to raise the no-new-information problem discussed earlier, we solved this problem by creating a new type of measure, specifically, the overall disparity between the levels of satisfaction of three presumed psychological needs (autonomy, competence, and relatedness). We did this by summing the three pair-wise differences between the three needs, yielding a measure almost identical to a measure derived via a standard deviation approach (as above). We also showed (2006) that this measure of balance predicted well-being above and beyond the large main effects of each of the three satisfaction variables themselves.

For example, according to the data, a person with a balanced 5–5–5 profile of autonomy, competence, and relatedness, need satisfaction is slightly (but significantly) happier than a person with a 6–6–3 need satisfaction profile, even though both sums totaled 15. Our research provides part of the rationale for the current suggested assessment approach based on time use. This finding that unbalanced (discrepant) need-satisfaction was detrimental to well-being, independent of the 3 constituents of the measure, suggests that unbalanced (discrepant) time use might also be detrimental to well-being, independently of the 10 constituents of the measure.

Validating Measures of Life Balance

Controlling for Constituent Time Usage

As the last observation suggests, I believe it is important to show that candidate life balance measures have effects that are demonstrably more than their constituent parts. The concept of life balance pertains to an emergent and holistic organization of life and activity, which should substantively transcend the particular elements (such as time spent working or sleeping or in recreation) that make it up. Practically, this entails controlling for the 10 actual hour amounts within the regression equation when testing the effects of the balanced-time and nondiscrepant-time measures. This procedure has two advantages: (1) It shows that the effects of these two compound computed variables are not reducible to one or more of the variables that compose it (e.g., the effects of the life–balance measure are not just due to variations in sleep time), and (2) it directly shows what effects (if any) the component parts themselves have in relation to each other. For example, perhaps the problem is not so much that people work too long but rather that they socialize too little. Many such issues can be addressed at the same time that effects of aggregate balance are examined.

EXAMINING MULTIPLE OUTCOMES

To validate new measures of life balance, it is also important to show that they are associated with a wide variety of positive outcomes construed to be indicative of flourishing or thriving (Keyes, 2007). Such outcomes might include mood, need satisfaction, and meaning and might also include objective variables such as stress reactivity, vocational performance, and even longevity.

CONTROLLING FOR RELEVANT KNOWN PERSONALITY DISPOSITIONS

Also, one would ideally control for relevant dispositional or trait variables (such as neuroticism or conscientiousness) to show that balance effects are also more than the effects of these known personality constructs (Fortunato & Goldblatt, 2002). In the next section I will review evidence that both the balanced time-use measure and the nondiscrepant time-use measure, computable from the DTUP, predict positive outcomes—while controlling for the constituent time-use variables that go into the measures; controlling for other relevant constructs such as neuroticism and extraversion; and examining various indicators of thriving, such as mood, satisfaction, and happiness.

PRELIMINARY DATA USING THE DTUP

In this section I will briefly summarize the results from two studies applying the DTUP to predict various measures of subjective well-being (Sheldon & Cummins, 2007). One study is a sample of 196 University of Missouri undergraduates, most around age 20, and the other is a sample of 1,109 Australian adults of widely varying ages. The Australian data were collected as part of the Australian Unity Wellbeing Index Longitudinal Survey ARC 14 conducted by Cummins in 2007. Although both groups were administered the DTUP, the Missouri group was not provided with an "other" category for the actual and ideal hour apportionments, and the Australian group was. Also, the Australian group was not provided with a "school (time studying and in class)" category. Thus, the Missouri sample evaluated time sleeping, in school, working, doing chores, participating in groups/community, recreation, commuting, relationships, health, and religion/spirituality; the Australian sample evaluated time sleeping, working, doing chores, participating in groups/ community, recreation, commuting, relationships, health, religion/spirituality, and "other."

Also, the subjective well-being (SWB) measures varied in the two samples: The Missouri sample received positive affect and negative affect from the positive affect/negative affect schedule (Watson, Tellegen, & Clark, 1988) and the Diener, Emmons, Larsen, and Griffin (1985) life-satisfaction measure. The Australian sample received a single global life-satisfaction item (Cummins, 2005), the Rosenberg self-esteem scale (Rosenberg, 1965), and a two-item measure of general happiness. Finally, the Missouri sample completed the measures in an online survey format, which forced the hour apportionments to add up to 24 (or else the participant could not proceed). In contrast, the Australian sample completed the measures at the end of a paper-and-pencil survey, and a number of participants did not complete the apportionment task correctly (in that the hours listed did not add up to 24). I retained all members of the Australian sample for whom the actual hours listed ranged between 20 and 28, indicating basic understanding of the task with modest arithmetical errors (84% of the sample).

The general procedure for the analyses involved regressing the chosen SWB variables on 9 of the 10 actual hours variables at step one (at least one of the 10 hours variables had to be omitted to avoid multicollinearity. The "other" category was omitted in the Australian sample, and the "religion" and "work" categories were omitted in the Missouri sample, the latter two because most participants rated "0" hours in these two categories). At step two, either the balanced time-use variable or the nondiscrepant time-use variable was entered into the equation. The hypothesis was that the two balance measures would each predict SWB, controlling for the constituent domain variables.

This hypothesis was confirmed in both samples. In the Missouri sample, non-discrepant time use was positively associated with life satisfaction and positive affect and negatively associated with negative affect (βs = .18, .23, and −.21, respectively, all ps < .05). Similarly, balanced time-use was also associated as expected (βs = .18, .21, and −.21, respectively, ps < .05). In the Australian sample, nondiscrepant time-use was positively associated with global life satisfaction, self-esteem, and happiness, although the effects were considerably smaller (βs = .07, .07, and .08, respectively, all ps < .05). Similarly, balanced time use was also associated as expected, also with small effect sizes (βs = .10, .11, and .11, respectively, all ps < .01). The smaller effects may be because the DTUP was administered at the very end of the Australian questionnaire and also had no check on the hour amounts entered. Still, the effects were apparently quite reliable.

What about the simultaneous effects of the individual hour measures? To derive the most stable estimates of these effects, I averaged the three SWB measures in each sample to create a single aggregate SWB variable (after recoding negative affect in the Missouri sample) and included both of the balance variables in the equation. In the Australian sample, greater SWB (life satisfaction, self-esteem, and happiness) was associated with more sleep (β = .13, p < .01), more group/community time (β = .09, p < .05), more work-time (β = .21, p < .01), more relationship time (β = .19, p < .01), and more time on health/self-maintenance (β = .13, p < .01). In the Missouri sample, however, none of the specific hour measures were associated with greater SWB. At present I do not have a convincing explanation for why this was the case. Nevertheless, the take-home message is that both candidate measures of global life balance were significant predictors in their own right, in both samples.

Thus, the above data help validate the new DTUP measures by controlling for specific time-use variables and by looking at multiple measures of SWB. Recall my suggestion that relevant personality traits should also be examined as control variables. In the Missouri sample, I had a 2-item measure of neuroticism, based on the 10-item personality inventory (Gosling, Rentfrow, & Swann, 2003). Although this measure was very strongly associated with SWB in the Missouri sample analyses (β = .65), in no case did the candidate life balance measures become nonsignificant when neuroticism was included in the equation. Thus, imbalance, by both measures, appears to be something different from mere neuroticism.

CONCLUSION

Thus, it appears that life balance is a real psychological construct, with real effects on mood that are not reducible to already known concepts and constructs, such as meaning, neuroticism, or to the undue influence of particular life domains such as sleep time or work time. I hope that others will try to use, and also improve upon, the concepts and measures described in this chapter.

REFERENCES

Backman, C. L. (2001). Occupational balance: Measuring time use and satisfaction across occupational performance areas. In M. Law, C. Baum, & W. Dunn (Eds.), *Measuring occupational performance: Supporting best practice in occupational therapy* (pp. 203–213). Thorofare, NJ: SLACK Incorporated.

Backman, C. L. (2004). Occupational balance: Exploring the relationships among daily occupations and their influence on well-being. *Canadian Review of Occupational Therapy, 71*, 202–209.

Camporese, R., Freguja, C., & Sabbadini, L. L. (1998). Time use by gender and quality of life. *Social Indicator Research, 44,* 119–144.

Christiansen, C. H. (1996). Three perspectives on balance in occupation. In R. Zemke & F. Clark (Eds.), *Occupational science: The evolving discipline* (pp. 431–451). Philadelphia: F. A. Davis.

Christiansen, C. H., & Matuska, K. M. (2006). Lifestyle balance: A review of concepts and research. *Journal of Occupational Science, 13,* 49–61.

Csikszentmihalyi, M. (1988). The flow experience and its significance for human psychology. In M. Csikszentmihalyi & I. Csikszentmihalyi (Eds.), *Optimal experience: Psychological studies of flow in consciousness* (pp. 15–35). New York: Cambridge University Press.

Cummins, R. A. (2005). Instruments assessing quality of life. In J. Hogg & A. Langa (Eds.), *Assessing adults with intellectual disabilities: A service provider's guide* (pp. 119–137). Malden, MA: Blackwell.

Dex, S., & Bond, S. (2005). Measuring work–life balance and its covariates. *Work, Employment, and Society, 19,* 627–637.

Diener, E., Emmons, R., Larsen, R., & Griffin, S. (1985). The Satisfaction With Life Scale. *Journal of Personality Assessment, 47,* 1105–1117.

Dittmar, H. (2005). A new look at "compulsive buying": Self-discrepancies and materialistic values as predictors of compulsive buying tendency. *Journal of Social and Clinical Psychology, 24,* 832–859.

Fisher, G. G. (2002). Work/personal life balance: A construct development study. *Dissertation Abstracts International, 63*(1-B). (UMI No. 95014382)

Fortunato, V. J., & Goldblatt, A. M. (2002). Construct validation of revised Strain-Free Negative Affectivity Scale. *Educational and Psychological Measurement, 62,* 45–63.

Frey, B. S. (2001). *Inspiring economics: Human motivation in political economy.* Northhampton, MA: Edward Elgar.

Gosling, S. D., Rentfrow, P. J., & Swann, W. B., Jr. (2003). A very brief measure of the Big-Five personality domains. *Journal of Research in Personality, 37,* 504–528.

Greenhaus, J., Collins, K., & Shaw, J. (2002). The relation between work–family balance and family roles. *Academy of Management Review, 10,* 76–88.

Gutek, B., Searle, S., & Klepa, L. (1991). Rational versus gender role explanations for work/family conflict. *Journal of Applied Psychology, 76,* 560–568.

Higgins, E. T., Bond, R. N., Klein, R., & Straumann, T. (1986). Self-discrepancies and emotional vulnerability: How magnitude, accessibility, and type of discrepancy influence affect. *Journal of Personality and Social Psychology, 51,* 5–15.

Holman, T., & Jacquart, M. (1988). Leisure activity patterns and marital satisfaction. *Journal of Marriage, 50,* 69–77.

Jacobs, J. A., & Gerson, K. (2001). Overworked individuals or overworked families? Explaining trends in work, leisure, and family time. *Work and Occupations, 28,* 40–63.

Jahoda, M. (1958). *Current concepts of positive mental health.* New York: Basic Books.

Jonsson, A. L., Moller, A., & Grimby, G. (1999). Managing occupations in everyday life to achieve adaptation. *American Journal of Occupational Therapy, 53,* 353–362.

Judge, T. A., Boudreau, J. W., & Bretz, R. D. (1994). Job and life attitudes of male executives. *Journal of Applied Psychology, 79,* 767–782.

Juster, F., & Stafford, F. P. (1991). The allocation of time: Empirical findings, behavioral models, and problems of measurement. *Journal of Economic Literature, 29,* 471–522.

Keyes, C. L. M. (2007). Promoting and protecting mental health as flourishing: A complementary strategy for improving national mental health. *American Psychologist, 62,* 95–108.

Law, M., Polatajko, H., Baptiste, S., & Townsend, E. (1997). Core concepts of occupational therapy. In *Enabling occupation: An occupational theory perspective* (pp. 29–56). Ottawa: CAOT Publication ACE.

Lecky, P. (1951). *Self-consistency: A theory of personality.* Washington, DC: Island Press.

Llorens, L. A. (1984). Changing balance: Environment and individual. *American Journal of Occupational Therapy, 38,* 29–34.

Loretto, W., Popham, F., Platt, S., Pavis, S., Hardy, G., MacLeod, L., et al. (2005). Assessing psychological well-being: A holistic investigation of NHS employees. *International Review of Psychiatry, 17,* 329–336.

Maslow, A. (1954). *Motivation and personality.* New York: Harper & Row.

Nurit, W., & Michal, A. B. (2003). Rest: A qualitative exploration of the phenomenon. *Occupational Therapy International, 10,* 227–238.

Petrocelli, J. V., & Smith, E. R. (2005). Who I am, who we are, and why: Links between emotions and causal attributions for self- and group discrepancies. *Personality and Social Psychology Bulletin, 31,* 1628–1642.

Podratz, L. T. (2004). The nature of work-personal life balance. *Dissertation Abstracts International: 65*(11-B). (UMI No. 9901077)

Rogers, C. (1961). *On becoming a person: A therapist's view of psychotherapy.* Boston: Houghton Mifflin.

Rogers, C. R., & Dymond, R. F. (Eds.). (1954). *Psychotherapy and personality change.* Chicago: University of Chicago Press.

Rosenberg, M. (1965). *Society and the adolescent self-image.* Princeton, NJ: Princeton University Press.

Sandvik, E., Diener, E., & Seidlitz, L. (1993). Subjective well-being: The convergence and stability of self-report and non-self-report measures. *Journal of Personality, 61,* 317–342.

Sheldon, K. M., & Cummins, R. A. (2007). *Defining and testing new measures of life-balance.* Manuscript in preparation.

Sheldon, K. M., & Niemiec, C. (2006). It's not just the amount that counts: Balanced need-satisfaction also affects well-being. *Journal of Personality and Social Psychology, 91,* 331–341.

Simonton, D. K. (1984). *Genius, creativity, and leadership.* Cambridge, MA: Harvard University Press.

Spencer, E. A. (1989). Toward a balance of work and play: Promotion of health and wellness. *Occupational Therapy in Health Care, 5,* 87–99.

Staats, A. W. (1999). Unifying psychology requires new infrastructure, theory, method, and a research agenda. *Review of General Psychology, 3,* 3–13.

Straumann, T. J., & Higgins, E. T. (1987). Automatic activation of self-discrepancies and emotional syndromes: When cognitive structures influence affect. *Journal of Personality and Social Psychology, 53,* 1004–1014.

Tausig, M., & Fenwick, R. (2001). Unbinding time: Alternative work schedules and work-life balance. *Journal of Family and Economic Issues, 22,* 101–119.

Tenbrunsel, A. E., Brett, J. M., Maoz, E., Stroh, L. K., & Reilly, A. H. (1995). Dynamic and static work–family relationships. *Organizational Behavior and Human Decision Processes, 63,* 233–246.

Townsend, E., & Wilcock, A. (2004). Occupational justice. In C. H. Christiansen & E. A. Townsend (Eds.), *Introduction to occupation: The art and science of living* (pp. 243–273). Upper Saddle River, NJ: Prentice Hall.

Warren, T. (2004). Working part-time: Achieving a successful "work–life" balance? *British Journal of Sociology, 55,* 99–122.

Watson, D., Tellegen, A., & Clark, L. (1988). Development and validation of brief measures of positive and negative affect: The PANAS scales. *Journal of Personality and Social Psychology, 54,* 1063–1070.

Zuzanek, J. (1998). Time-use, time pressure, personal stress, mental health and life-satisfaction from a life cycle perspective. *Journal of Occupational Science, 5,* 25–37.

Measuring Life Balance Through Discrepancy Theories and Subjective Well-Being

ROBERT A. CUMMINS

INTRODUCTION

The concept of *life balance* implies that there is some optimal time allocation between the various forms of human activity we engage in each day. So life balance can be measured by the size of the discrepancy between how we should and how we do allocate our time.

If someone chooses to spend all of their discretionary time writing poetry, is this a balanced life? Many people would say no. They would judge such a life to be imbalanced because life is full of competing demands, and writing poetry all day means that other aspects of life are neglected. But is this just an imposed value judgment, or does the concept of a balanced life have deeper meaning? The answer must lie with whatever we use to measure the outcome. Any conclusion that balance is better than imbalance must be based on empirical evidence. So, what should be measured?

Long, long ago the measure was simple. In a feral environment, evolution uses life balance as a major determinant of fitness. The basic requirements for all feral animals are acquiring energy, avoiding predation, and procreating successfully. So animals have evolved diverse patterns of life balance that are adapted to particular ecological niches. Thus, although the actual time spent on any particular activity varies hugely between different species, the measure of optimal life balance is simple. An animal that optimally balances its time between the activities adaptive to its ecological niche will exhibit evolutionary fitness.

Humans in developed countries, however, have lost these selective pressures. Food is available on demand from the nearest fast-food restaurant, predation is no longer feared (except from certain financial institution), and successful procreation is achieved by people with serious disadvantages. So, because survival and fitness are no longer useful as measures of optimal life balance, what other measure should we choose?

The choice of measures is very broad. Indeed, because there is no longer any absolute measure of a successful life, the choice is almost infinite. It is instructive to note, however, that almost all such measures represent imposed value judgments on the basis of what is regarded as a successful human life. Such judgments may be based on notions of being responsible to others, maximizing one's potential, serving God, and so on. Therefore, with some dominant criterion of a successful life in mind, a hierarchy of activity importance could be devised that optimally fulfills this version of human success. This hierarchy would represent one version of optimal life balance.

K. Matuska & C. Christiansen (Eds.)
Life balance: Multidisciplinary theories and research (pp 73–94)
© 2009 SLACK Incorporated and AOTA Press

While such an approach allows life balance to be empirically defined, it is also problematic for all sorts of reasons. Perhaps most importantly, it does not allow for individual differences in the definition of a successful life. To determine some generic measure of life balance, a different approach is required, one that escapes the imposition of value judgments.

One alternative is to use outcome rather than process as a measure of life balance. That is, a balanced life can be identified through normative values on a global indicator of life success that transcends individual differences in process. A measure that could be used for this purpose is subjective well-being (SWB). In this scheme, normal-range SWB indicates a balanced life, below normal-range indicates life imbalance.

This idea carries positive and negative implications. On the positive side, it makes no value judgment about how people should behave to achieve life balance. It recognizes that each person has idiosyncratic needs and values, and they are free to construct their own version of a successful life in these terms. As long as their SWB is normal, their version of balance is working for them. On the negative side, this approach is clearly self-centered. It concerns the well-being of the person concerned and does not make any statement about how that person fits into, or contributes to, the rest of society. While this issue deserves debate in its own right, this chapter has a more limited scope. It concerns only understanding the essence of SWB, the use of discrepancies to measure SWB, and the theoretical usefulness of SWB as an indicator of life balance.

SUBJECTIVE WELL-BEING

The single most important property of SWB is that it is typically positive. People generally feel good about themselves, and a huge body of research has demonstrated that people are normally satisfied with their own life (Cummins, 1995; Diener & Diener, 1996; Veenhoven, 1993).

In Western nations, the average value for population samples is about 75 percentage points of satisfaction (see also Cummins, 1995, 1998). That is, on a standardized scale from 0 *(completely dissatisfied)* to 100 *(completely satisfied)* the average person rates his or her SWB at 75. Moreover, on a population basis, the mean scores are quite remarkably stable. Since 2001, a total of 17 surveys have been conducted in Australia using the Personal Wellbeing Index (PWI) to measure SWB (International Wellbeing Group, 2006). Each survey involves a new, geographically representative sample of 2,000 randomly selected adults across the nation. These survey mean scores range from 73.4 to 76.4, a fluctuation of only 3 points (Cummins, Woerner, Tomyn, Gibson, & Knapp, 2007). Why are these results so predictable?

I hypothesize that personal well-being is not free to vary over the theoretical 0–100 range. Rather, it is held fairly constant for each individual in a manner analogous to blood pressure or body temperature. This implies an active management system for personal well-being that maintains well-being at an average of about 75 percentage points. We call this process *subjective well-being homeostasis* (Cummins, Gullone, & Lau, 2002; Cummins, Lau, & Davern, in press).

These properties make SWB an interesting variable to use as a measure of outcome, because it does not show a linear relationship with degrees of psychological challenge. Due to homeostasis, people can experience a wide range of lifestyles and life difficulties yet maintain normative well-being. So any such lifestyle could be considered adaptive, or reasonably in balance, due to the normative nature of SWB. Of note, however, SWB below the normal range is indicative of psychopathology. The analogy with body temperature is apposite. Our core temperature lies in the normal range of 36–38 °C (Wikipedia, 2007), and this can normally be maintained despite considerable variations in ambient temperature. However, variation does occur within this range as various conditions cause the temperature to inhabit the edges of its normal range. Of course, extreme conditions of hot or cold will overwhelm the capacity of this homeostatic system, and body temperature will exit the normal range as a consequence.

In an analogous fashion, SWB is also held within a set-point range (Headey & Wearing, 1986; Stones & Kozma, 1991). While the width of this range is uncertain, a ballpark figure is about 12 percentage points (Cummins et al., in press). Therefore, SWB shows normal variation within this range that reflects the conditions impinging on the homeostatic system. If conditions are good, people will be more likely to be at the top rather than at the bottom of their set-point range. This means that the SWB of individuals is sensitive to change over a limited range.

Note, however, that when the level of psychological challenge becomes too great, it overwhelms the capacity of the homeostatic system to resist change, and SWB decreases. Thus, SWB may be used as a general indicator of psychological functional status. While each person has their set-point range, when a common stressor is applied to a group, the effects may be quite subtle changes in the group mean and variance. The reason for this is that people differ considerably in their resilience to challenge. These individual differences may be because some people are constitutionally weaker than others, or it may be because they are living under multiple pressures, so their system is only barely coping. For either or both of these reasons, some people have a small capacity to deal with additional levels of challenge. Thus, when a negative pressure is applied to groups, these vulnerable people quite easily succumb, and their well-being falls below the normal range. This causes the group mean to fall and the group variance to increase.

The extent of these changes will depend on the strength of the challenge and the general resilience of the group. If only a few people are defeated by the challenge, the increased variance may well be a more sensitive indicator of selective pathology than the decreased mean score of the group. However, if the challenge is strong enough to compromise a majority of the group, the group mean will fall significantly. I have detailed these progressive changes elsewhere (Cummins, 2003).

In the scheme described above, life balance could be conceptualized as a have–want discrepancy. As life balance, yielding normative SWB, gives way to life imbalance, people are increasingly likely to experience homeostatic failure. Thus, people in life balance "have" what they need, whereas people in imbalance "want" what they do not have so they can become balanced. In this view, life balance or imbalance is a function of the discrepancy between what people have and what they want. The smaller the have–want discrepancy, the more in balance the person will be, and the more likely they will have normal levels of SWB.

This seems an interesting proposition, because it provides a simple view of what influences SWB at a fundamental level. Unfortunately, the conceptualization and measurement of discrepancies is difficult territory.

Discrepancy vs. Its Two Components

The most obvious property of a discrepancy is that it contains two components. In the example already mentioned, the discrepancy occurs because what the person actually has is not enough to meet his or her wants. Thus, each component must be matched against one another in some way to yield the discrepancy. There are four approaches to doing this, which are as follows:

1. Computed Method (Simple)

The computed method is the most obvious form of measurement and was universally used by researchers prior to Michalos (1980). The discrepancy is assessed by the separate measurement of each of the two elements. For example, measuring the discrepancy between satisfaction with "your life as a whole now" and "the life you expected 3 years ago" will involve two separate measures. The discrepancy is computed by the researcher subtracting one response from the other.

This method has the advantage that the two components of the discrepancy can be investigated separately. Hence, if a researcher wishes to investigate the relationship between the computed discrepancy and self-esteem, there are three forms of dependent variable that may be used. The most parsimonious is the single variable, computed as satisfaction now minus satisfaction expected.

However, there are problems with the interpretation of this single value that will be detailed later. It is therefore very useful that the two variables have been measured separately, because they can also be used separately to yield more information. So, if the researcher feels that the power of the discrepancy to predict self-esteem is due more to variation in one variable than the other, the use of multiple regression will allow the researcher to make this determination. This is a very important strength of the computed method, as will be seen.

2. COMPUTED METHOD (COMPLEX)

The computed method (complex) discrepancy technique has been described by Sheldon (2009; chapter 6 in this volume); Sheldon & Niemiec, 2006). It involves obtaining the average discrepancy between the strength of a number of needs. This allows testing the idea that small average discrepancy scores represent a balanced life, which yields higher SWB.

3. INTRAPSYCHIC METHOD (SIMPLE)

In the intrapsychic (simple) method, using the same example as in the computed method description above, a single question is framed as "How satisfied are you now compared with 3 years ago?" So here, the two thoughts that are being compared are not separately measured; only the processed outcome from the comparison is rated by the participant.

This is a simple discrepancy judgment in that the comparison is being made over the single dimension of time. That is, the person (presumably) looks back at their life as it was 3 years ago and compares this view with their life in the present. The apparent advantage of this method is that it represents the "true" discrepancy, in that the participant provides a response that represents how the discrepancy appears to them. However, as will be seen later, the assumption that the response represents the true discrepancy is highly contestable.

4. INTRAPSYCHIC METHOD (COMPLEX)

The intrapsychic method (complex) is the method introduced by Michalos (1980) to verify his multiple discrepancies theory. Using the same example again, a single question is framed as "Considering your life as a whole, how does it measure up to what you expected about 3 years ago?" (from *far less than expected* to *far more than expected*).

I have termed this "complex" because, unlike number 3 above, the nature of the discrepancy is unclear. It involves both of the following:

1. A reference against life as a whole (in the present).

2. A variable of "expectancy," which is itself a discrepancy, involving the present and some other time, usually in the future. Here, however, the expectancy refers to the past. So respondents are being asked to recall what they expected from their life as a whole 3 years in the past and to relate that expectation to their life as a whole now.

The complexity is evident. They are not being asked to relate how their life was 3 years ago to their present life. They are being asked to recall the level of their expectation for change 3 years ago, project over the next 3 years of life, and estimate the extent to which that expectation has been met.

This seems an impossible task, and, therefore, there must be great uncertainty as to the meaning of the response to this question. This issue will be taken up again in a later section.

In conclusion, discrepancies are clearly difficult constructs to deal with and understand. They are also very appealing to theorists. The reason for their attractiveness is the intuition that much of what we think is based on comparisons of one kind or another, and these comparisons can be conceptualized as discrepancies. Because of this, discrepancies have found their way into numerous theories concerning the processes that influence SWB. These will be considered first in broad, generic terms and then in terms of specific theories.

BROAD THEORETICAL VIEWS OF DISCREPANCIES

Needs Theories of SWB

Perhaps the first point requiring clarification is that, for the purposes of this discussion, I am making no distinction between wants and needs. While an important distinction can be made between these terms, many authors use one while meaning the other. To avoid this confusion, I will deal with both terms as though they imply the perception that something is missing from life that the person wants or needs. This creates a discrepancy between the current level of some experience and its desired or perceived normative level. Analogous to the need for water, needs theories in relation to SWB make the assumption that there are universal psychological as well as physical needs and that people will experience a balanced state to the extent that these needs are met.

One of the first researchers to align happiness with needs was Wilson (1960, 1965), who proposed that the prompt satisfaction of needs causes happiness, while the persistence of unfulfilled needs causes unhappiness. While the former seems obvious, the latter leads to the possible link between chronic conditions leading to unhappiness and depression. He suggested three types of needs: (1) physiological; (2) sensory or pleasure seeking; and (3) acquired or secondary needs, such as for "affection, acceptance, popularity, status, achievement, and self-actualization" (p. 302).

In support of the last set, he reported that happiness correlated .40 with the discrepancy between need for achievement and actual achievement and .47 with the discrepancy between current self and ideal self. This presages the kinds of discrepancies used by Michalos some 20 years later for his multiple discrepancies theory.

A more recent version of needs theory has been provided by Veenhoven's (1995) livability theory. This proposes that universal human needs can be discovered by examining the characteristics of societies in which people flourish. Then a happy society will result when most of the universal needs are met.

On the surface, these ideas receive ready verification. Clearly, the basic necessities for life are essential to normal SWB, and a substantial proportion of the variance in SWB between countries can be explained by the relative provision of such commodities. However, it is notable that the relationship is strongest when the comparisons involve developing countries (see Veenhoven, 1993, 1995), where some of the basic physiological needs are obviously not being met. In the psychological sphere, the need for social affiliation, when in deficit, is one of the most powerful correlates of SWB (see Baumeister & Leary, 1995, for a review) while related needs like self-acceptance are not far behind (see Kasser & Ryan, 1993).

Arguments against this approach to the identification of universal needs have been provided by Diener and Lucas (2000). The problems they identify are as follows:

1. If basic needs can be identified only from levels of SWB, then the theory cannot be falsified. If intimate relationships are identified as a basic need because their deficit is universally linked to low SWB, then the description of the need becomes tautological.

Further doubt regarding the validity of this approach is provided by the previously discussed idea that a significant imbalance between haves and wants can be detected through abnormally low levels of SWB. However, this could not be used to identify basic needs. Homeostasis may be defeated through any source of challenge that overwhelms the capacity for adaptation. Thus, this situation might be created by moderate discrepancies of basic needs or major discrepancies of less basic needs.

2. There is empirical evidence that SWB cannot be defined simply through basic needs. For example, Diener, Suh, Smith, and Shao (1995) found that mean income in nations predicted the SWB of countries, even after basic need fulfillment was controlled.

There are other reasons to suspect that the universal needs approach will not prove very useful:

3. There are very strong correlates, even determinants, of SWB that cannot easily be classified as a basic need. An example is *core affect* (Davern, Cummins, & Stokes, 2007), which is defined as a combination of contented, happy, and alert.

4. There clearly are idiosyncratic needs that, for the people concerned, are very relevant to their SWB. The need to see their *Carassius auratus* swimming happily may be crucial to the SWB of a goldfish fancier.

In summary, there are many reasons to be skeptical that SWB theories based on needs analysis will yield much understanding beyond the obvious. That is, if someone has a major deficit in some part of their life they consider important, this will impair their ability to maintain normal levels of SWB.

Relativity Theories

There is a strong sense within the discipline of economics that the reason money is correlated with SWB is because of discrepancies of relative wealth. The more money one has, the stronger is the downward comparison with others, and so the higher becomes one's SWB.

One attraction of this belief is that it offers an explanation for a conundrum called the *Easterlin paradox*. In 1974, this esteemed economist observed that, despite the substantial rise in national wealth since the 1950s evident in most developed countries, the increased wealth had not been accompanied by a rise in population happiness (see also Easterlin, 2005). This insight has received much attention because it disputes one of the central arguments for ever-increasing national development. That is, if increasing national wealth fails to increase population happiness, the purpose of such development becomes less clear (see e.g., Chambers, 1997).

It is argued by Easterlin that SWB does not normally rise with national wealth because the rank order of wealth remains constant within the population. Moreover, because it is relative wealth that drives SWB, he argues, if all the population is becoming wealthier equally, there is no change in relative wealth, and so SWB does not change. This social-comparison hypothesis, when used to explain steady levels of happiness, is an alternative to SWB homeostasis. As such, empirical studies offering support for this power of relative wealth deserve close attention. One such recent study is that by Knight, Song, and Gunatilaka (2007). However, the authors' conclusions are flawed.

Their first error is to regard objective and subjective measurement as interchangeable. That is, respondents were asked to compute a discrepancy by comparing their current living standard with how it was 5 years ago. About 61% felt that their current standard of living was higher, and only 5% reported they were currently worse off. The authors take these discrepancy results literally and report that "60% of them now had a higher living standard and that only 5% had become worse off" (p. 3). In fact, nothing of the kind can be inferred. The natural "positive cognitive bias" (Cummins & Nistico, 2002) causes most aspects of the present life to be felt as positive, and that includes the feeling that life is better now than it was in the past. Thus, in the absence of any objective change, people will generally feel that their lives are better than they were in the past. A major exception to this is caused by depression. People who are depressed have lost this positive bias and will see the past as equivalent to, or even better than, the present. This is the "reminiscence effect," and supportive data can be readily found (e.g., Bortner & Hultsch, 1970; Cantril, 1965; Field, 1981; Shmotkin, 1991).

The underlying cause of the positive cognitive bias is *core affect* (Davern et al., 2007). This ubiquitous positive affect most strongly influences processing that concerns personal and complex feelings, such as those embodied by discrepancy questions. Thus, the results reported by Knight et al. (2007) are consistent with this type of discrepancy mainly reflecting positive bias.

Knight et al. (2007) separated their sample into three discrepancy groups: (1) feeling better-off, (2) the same, and (3) worse off than the past. The respective happiness levels were 72.0, 59.8, and 52.3 percentage points. That is, the 61% of the sample who were experiencing their normal set point (72.0 points) revealed a strong positive comparison with the past. While this percentage of 61% is much lower than would be expected from the Australian population (Cummins et al., 2007), the rural Chinese sample used by these authors had very low well-being. Their mean happiness was 2.67 on a 1–5 scale, which converts (see PWI Manual) into 55.7 points on the standard 0–100 scale (Knight et al, 2007). This mean score is extremely low and indicates that a higher than normal proportion are depressed. However, as revealed, the 61% of the sample who responded in the normal manner to the past–present discrepancy had normal range happiness (72 points).

The researchers then engage a curious logic that uses happiness as a discrepancy function of comparative wealth. Within psychology, researchers would expect to find that poverty and the importance of money would be strongly positively correlated. That is, money is very important to people who are poor, because it is a commodity that they need and do not have. These researchers, however, apparently expect to find the opposite—that people who are poor value money less. This may be based on the assumption of the "rational person," which is a common assumption in economics (see, for example, Gittins, 2005; Liu, 1976). According to this logic, people who are poor should value money less because, if they valued money highly, they would act in ways to get rich.

It seems that such an assumption allows the interpretation of results to the advantage of their relative discrepancy hypothesis. As is usual, they found that income per capita was related to happiness, with the highest quintile rating 72.3 points and the lowest quintile 60.3 points. Then they state, "In contrast to this result, we also find that income is important to those who rate their subjective well-being low" and conclude, "a possible solution to this apparent contradiction is that relative income is important for subjective well-being. People might compare themselves, or their income, either with themselves in the past or with 'relevant others,' i.e., their social reference groups" (p. 3).

This conclusion seems contrived to support the rational person assumption and to avoid the more obvious deduction, that people who are poor do, in fact, highly value money. My conclusion is that this study does not provide evidence for the discrepancy function of relative wealth. Moreover, in considering the wider literature, evidence for social comparison as a major driver of SWB seems very thin. Certainly the development of industrial economies tends to increase wealth inequality (e.g., Smith, 1991), thereby increasing discrepancies of relative wealth within such populations. Moreover, rich countries are generally happier than poor countries. However, the idea that the happiness differential is driven by discrepancies in relative wealth finds little support (see Diener & Oishi, 2000; Ott, 2005).

Importance Theories

The rated satisfaction of any life aspect can be conceptualized as the product of satisfaction with that aspect and its relative importance. Thus, satisfaction is modulated by importance. This allows a concept of life balance as the degree of congruence between these two measures. In an adaptive situation, satisfaction and importance are congruent with one another, where life aspects considered to be important attract high satisfaction. In a maladaptive situation, a life aspect that is considered very important attracts low satisfaction. Thus, both SWB and life balance are a function of the discrepancy between the rank order of satisfaction with various life aspects and their importance.

This discrepancy view has been commonly applied to the SWB literature, such that many authors have devised measurement instruments that weight rated satisfaction with importance. This procedure, which goes back at least as far as Katzell (1964), has been adopted for the Quality of Life Scale (Flanagan, 1979), Quality of Life Index (Ferrans & Powers, 1985), Schedule for the Evaluation of Individual Quality of Life (McGee, O'Boyle, Hickey, O'Malley, & Joyce, 1991),

Quality of Life Inventory (Frisch, 1992), Quality of Life Profile–Adolescent Version (Raphael, Rukholm, Brown, Hill-Bailey, & Donato, 1996), and Comprehensive Quality of Life Scale (Cummins, 1997).

All these scales combine satisfaction scores derived from multiple items. So the rationale for this weighting procedure is to overcome the problem of assuming that satisfaction derived from different items is equivalent. For example, if a scale includes satisfaction with family, then a high satisfaction score is relevant for people who consider their family important. It is much less meaningful for people who regard their family as irrelevant to their overall SWB. Therefore, so the idea goes, to equate the value of item satisfactions, both within and between respondents, each rating of satisfaction should be multiplied by its equivalent rating on importance, and the multiplicative composite used as the dependent variable. This procedure, it is assumed, will negate the problem of rank-order discrepancies between satisfaction and importance. All items will become of equivalent strength, relative to one another, through the modulating influence of importance.

Despite its intuitive appeal, this idea is regarded as theoretically untenable by Locke's (1969, 1976) range-of-affect hypothesis. This proposes that judgments of importance and satisfaction are not two independent processes but are functionally linked. Because of this, item importance has already been considered in any evaluation of satisfaction.

Locke's (1969) interest was in *job satisfaction*, which he defined as being "a function of the perceived relationship between what one wants from one's job and what one perceives it as offering or entailing" (p. 316). Thus he saw satisfaction in terms of a have–want discrepancy, in other words, a judgment of the discrepancy between one's perception of the job as it is and one's value standard for the job as it should be. While he considered this judgment to be influenced by importance, his major insight was to regard the construction of satisfaction as a dual process that involved importance. Thus, the level of satisfaction is influenced by the interaction of the have–want discrepancy with importance.

Within this formulation, the level of importance is determining the possible range over which the discrepancy can operate (hence range-of-affect). Thus, an item with high importance could produce a wide affective reaction ranging from great satisfaction to great dissatisfaction. So, for example, the person with cancer may have a have–want discrepancy of equal magnitude to the person who loves their child. Both the cancer and the child are equally important, but the former produces high dissatisfaction while the latter produces high satisfaction.

On the other hand, an item with low personal importance cannot produce either high satisfaction or dissatisfaction. Such items are only able to produce a restricted affective reaction, which approximates neutrality on the satisfaction–dissatisfaction dimension.

So for any magnitude of the discrepancy between satisfaction and importance, the range of the satisfaction is determined by the item's importance. Because of this, any rating of item satisfaction has already incorporated information regarding the item's importance, which renders weighting item satisfaction with item importance redundant.

This prediction has been confirmed by numerous authors in diverse areas of study. In relation to job satisfaction, direct cognitive comparisons between *has* and *wants* confirms that the strength of item satisfaction is determined by item importance (McFarlin, Coster, Rice, & Coopper-Alison, 1995; McFarlin & Rice, 1992; Mobley & Locke, 1970; Rice, Gentile, & McFarlin, 1991; Rice, Markus, Moyer, & McFarlin, 1991). Other results confirming Locke's hypothesis have come from studies of employee turnover (Mikes & Hulin, 1968; Waters & Roach, 1971) and global life satisfaction (Hsieh, 2003). More recently, and very convincingly, the hypothesis has been confirmed by Wu and Yao (2007) using an experimental, repeated-measures design. Thus, as predicted by Locke, satisfaction evaluations have already incorporated the judgment of importance, making the procedure of further weighting satisfaction by importance redundant.

In conclusion, the importance–satisfaction discrepancy is another false lead to understanding SWB and life balance. Perhaps another commonly used discrepancy, the process that underpins adaptation, will yield more insights.

Adaptation Theories

As noted by Lazarus (1991), *adaptation* is such a ubiquitous and fundamental part of human functioning that it is relevant to almost all human experience. In its broadest sense, the term *adaptation* is used for any facet of psychological function related to adjustment to the individual's living conditions (Schilling & Wahl, 2006). The basic concepts of psychological adaptation, reviewed as long ago as 1965 by Bevan, comprise such devices as habituation, avoidance behavior, and so-called "normative adaptation," conceptualized most prominently by Helson's (1948) adaptation level theory.

All theoretical approaches to adaptation have a common understanding based on discrepancies. That is, the adaptation mechanism is triggered by change in the individual's experience, which leads to discrepancies between some resting state and the new state, which then need to be reduced to return the organism to its previous state. Thus, through this process, the forces that cause life imbalance are counteracted by adaptation to restore life balance once again.

This theme has been taken up by many authors, who have created different kinds of discrepancy theories to account for the adaptation required to maintain SWB. Most prominent are Lawton's ecology of aging theory (e.g., Lawton & Nahemow, 1973); Michalos' (1985) multiple discrepancies theory; Higgins, Roney, Crowe and Hymes' (1994) ideas on control regulation; and the set-point model of happiness (e.g., Lucas, Clark, Georgellis, & Diener, 2003). All these concern the maintenance of life balance and will now be discussed in more detail.

INDIVIDUAL THEORIES BASED ON DISCREPANCIES

Perceptual Control Theory

An excellent review of the perceptual control theory (Powers, 1973) is provided by Abbott (2007). Powers proposed that the behavior of the organism at any moment is directed by a hierarchy of goals. These are organized in a motivational hierarchy dedicated to the self-regulation of multiple internal states. To achieve such self-regulation, or *homeostasis* (Cannon, 1932), the organism is constantly seeking to close selected discrepancies between its current state and internally determined reference levels.

The mechanisms of this regulation are twofold. At the simplest level, regulation can be achieved through physiological devices, such as cooling the body by sweating. However, such mechanisms have limited capacity to maintain homeostasis in the face of determined threat. So the second approach to regulation is through behavior. If we get too hot, we move out of the sun. By using a combination of these two approaches, the value of each internal state is held within a range that is adaptive for the organism.

The organizational hierarchy is based on the relative importance of individual discrepancies. Some goals are more important than others. Thus, simple physiological discrepancies, such as thirst, must be resolved before higher order goals, such as social engagement, can be easily undertaken. However, meeting even such basic needs requires complex behaviors to close the discrepancy. That is, the acts of locating water and drinking require much behavioral coordination. This is organized in a top-down manner through the 11 levels of Powers' organizational hierarchy.

While the mechanism of discrepancy detection at higher levels is uncertain, he follows Ashby (1952) in stating the obvious; that for any organism to assess a persistent discrepancy it must have simultaneous access to two kinds of information. These are the current value and the internal reference value. That is, the organism must have fixed reference values against which to measure the discrepancies. It is the perception of these discrepancies and therefore the control of these perceptions that give this theory its name.

One implication of this theory is that in organisms where the lower level needs are met, the higher level needs should dominate. Such individuals ought to attend most strongly to the discrepancies concerning their highest level of purpose, their life goals. Moreover, for such people, the higher level discrepancies should be important, because they are more self-defining than the lower levels (Carver & Scheier, 1990). So working toward the closure of life-goal discrepancies should bring strong feelings of self-fulfillment.

There is also evidence that progress on daily goals that serve life goals is important for emotional well-being. However, Kings, Richards, and Stemmerich (1998) found this was stronger in the negative than in the positive. While seeking life goals through low-level goals was weakly related to SWB, using low-level goals to avoid one's worst fears was more strongly, and negatively, related to SWB. Thus, having avoidance goals at the top of the needs hierarchy is detrimental to well-being.

In summary, perceptual control theory is an interesting approach with much to recommend it. It presents a rationale for an organizational hierarchy for behavior that allows the attainment of the highest level goals, which relate to an idealized view of the self. Thus, a balanced life might be seen as one that provides the means for meeting the lower level goals. Then, released from this pressure, the person experiences the maintenance of SWB within the normal range and is free to concentrate on behaviors conducive to self-enhancement.

Multiple Discrepancies Theory

Without doubt, the most influential of the discrepancy theories as they relate to SWB has been the multiple discrepancies theory devised by Alex Michalos. His classic 1985 paper (see below) has been cited hundreds of times. He first published the germ of his idea that SWB comprised discrepancies in the following terms, "I like to think of the question 'How is the quality of your life now?' as roughly equivalent to 'What is your life worth to you now, in terms of the good and bad things that might be expected?'" (Michalos, 1976, p. 36) This encapsulates the idea that subjective life quality is generated from a comparison, or discrepancy, between one's present state and some alternate recalled or imagined state. SWB is thus mainly envisaged as a product of cognitive processing.

By 1980 he had firmed his views. He reviewed the literature, already substantial on this theme, and deduced that satisfaction is a function of the perceived discrepancy between achievement and expectations. He noted the work of several researchers (e.g., Easterlin, 1973, 1974) who presented the view (discussed earlier) that people gain satisfaction from money because they have more than someone else, not simply due to some intrinsic property of money itself. These views had been reinforced by Campbell, Converse, and Rodgers (1976) who found a positive association between satisfaction with various life domains and the perceived discrepancy between current status and that to which people aspire. However, he also noted that such research tends to produce mixed results and that the problem may be methodological:

> All previous tests of the hypothesis concerning the influence of an aspiration–achievement gap on reported satisfaction have involved the calculation of the gap from separate measures of aspiration and achievement. These procedures presume that the calculations researchers make are roughly identical to the calculations respondents make. The fact that relatively strong connections have been found between gap measures thus calculated and reported satisfaction measures suggests that the presumption is not entirely unfounded. Nevertheless, from the point of view of the basic assumption behind the study of perceptual or subjective indicators, the perceived gap between one's aspirations and achievements should be more closely related to reported satisfaction than the calculated gap. (Michalos, 1980, pp. 391–392).

So Michalos proposed a new kind of measure, on the basis of his 1976 idea, such that the respondents would calculate the discrepancy themselves. Using this new technology, in his 1980 paper he proceeded to test the model proposed by Campbell et al. (1976). This group had suggested that domain satisfaction is determined by a comparison of the domain against various standards. For example, what someone aspires to, relative to what others have, produces an aspiration–achievement gap, which then determines domain satisfaction.

Campbell's group considered the implications of their model to be profound. They wrote,

> It may be necessary to distinguish between a satisfaction which is associated with an experience of rising expectations and one which is associated with declining expectations. An individual who has achieved an aspiration toward which he has been moving may be said to experience the satisfaction of success. Another person may have lowered his aspiration level to the point which he can achieve, and he might be said to experience the satisfaction of resignation. The two individuals might be equally satisfied in the sense of fulfilled needs, but the affective content associated with success and resignation may well differ. (Campbell et al., 1976, p. 10)

Indeed, this model is fundamentally challenging to the idea that levels of satisfaction are simple measures of goodness, in that more is better. While it might be expected that the "satisfaction of resignation" is adaptive, in the sense that it avoids dissatisfaction, it is not desirable because it would lead people to be less motivated to achieve much beyond their current state.

So, Michalos tested this finding using a different form of measurement. As had researchers before them, Campbell et al. (1976) used two separate questions to measure the level of aspiration and achievement for the life domains. So, for example, in relation to housing, people were asked to rate "the best house you could ever hope to live in" (p. 175) on a scale anchored by the *worst imaginable* (0) to *perfect—ideal for you* (100). They then rated the level of their achievement by indicating their level of satisfaction with their current house. Michalos (1980) combined these into a single question. In his study, the aspirational (goal)-achievement gap was measured using the following question:

> Some people have certain goals or aspirations for various aspects of their lives. They aim for a particular sort of home, income, family life style, and so on. Compared to your own aims or goals, for each of the features below, would you say that your life measures up perfectly now, fairly well, about half as well, fairly poorly, or just not at all. Please check the percentage that best describes how closely your life now seems to approach your own goals. (p. 394)

The respondents rated 12 features (domains) by using this format. They were then asked to rate the global question, "Now, considering your life as a whole, how does it measure up to your general aspirations or goals?"

Following this, respondents were asked the 13 discrepancy items again, but this time in relation to other people "of your age" and then again in relation to "your own best previous experience." Michalos then ran a series of structural equation models testing two alternatives (Figure 7-1).

He found through extensive testing that the Campbell et al. (1976) model is superior in both the prediction of global life satisfaction, as shown above, and the prediction of global happiness. Like Campbell et al., Michalos views the implications as profound:

> Human satisfaction is not just a brute fact to be accommodated like the wind and rain. It is to some extent manageable in the best sense and manipulable in the worst sense. By providing relevant experiences and information, people's goal-achievement gaps may be altered, with their satisfaction levels not far behind. Campbell et al. (1976, pp. 149–150) note that a tyrant might try to inflate the satisfaction levels of their subjects by restricting their experiences or giving them false reports about the status of their peers.

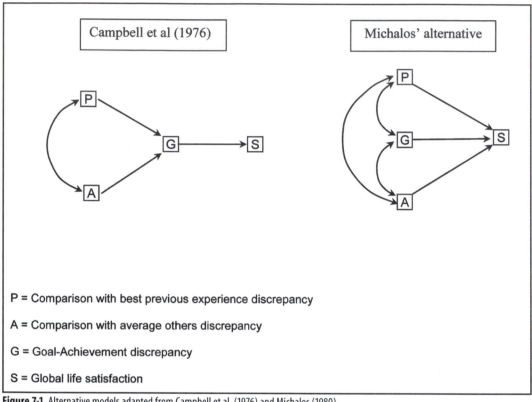

P = Comparison with best previous experience discrepancy

A = Comparison with average others discrepancy

G = Goal-Achievement discrepancy

S = Global life satisfaction

Figure 7-1. Alternative models adapted from Campbell et al. (1976) and Michalos (1980).

> Insofar as satisfaction is generated as the [Campbell] model indicates, education and individual initiative have a fundamental role to play in the development of the good life for individuals and societies. Accurate perceptions of the real world have a vital role to play in the determination of satisfaction with that world. The proverbial Fool's Paradise may be regarded as the result of experiencing uninformed or misinformed satisfaction. Thus, if knowledge is a reasonable thing (i.e., something to which principles of sound reasoning are applicable), then so is satisfaction, taste, etc. Here the dreams of all naturalistic value theorists loom large. Values may be psychologically connected to facts roughly as theoreticians have held they ought to be logically connected. (Michalos, 1980, pp. 406, 410–411)

This is all well and good, with one caveat. And that is the extent to which the goal-achievement discrepancy is, actually, responsible for levels of life satisfaction. In fact, the actual strength of this influence is slight, as will be shown in the critique of discrepancy theories in a later section.

In 1985, Michalos gave full statement to multiple-discrepancy theory:

> Reported net satisfaction is a function of perceived discrepancies between what one has and wants, relevant others have, the best one has had in the past, expected to have 3 years ago, expects to have after 5 years, deserves, and needs. (p. 347)

It may be observed that all of the mentioned needs and wants are a variation on the have–want discrepancy. All these perceived discrepancies are between the current state and some other state which can be described as "wants." Thus,

1. Relevant others have: have–wants (what relevant others have)

2. The best one had in the past: have–wants now (the best in the past)

3. Expected to have 5 years ago: have–wants now (expected to have)

4. Expects to have after 5 years: have–wants (expects to have)

5. Deserves: have–wants (deserves to have)

6. Needs: have–wants (needs).

Michalos recognized this commonality, stating, "the perceived discrepancy between what one has and wants is a mediating variable between all other perceived discrepancies and reported net satisfaction" (p. 348). Therefore, perceived discrepancies have both a direct and an indirect (mediated) effect (Baron & Kenny, 1986) on life satisfaction.

To test this, Michalos performed many multiple regression analyses, testing two forms of prediction derived from the discrepancies. One he calls the "direct effects of perceived discrepancies," meaning the prediction of satisfaction from any of the seven perceived discrepancies. The other he calls "indirect effects," by which he means prediction of the have–wants discrepancy from any of the other six discrepancies. He found both to be successful, with an overall proportion of 58% of the regressions being significant.

A crucial question at this point concerns the extent to which these discrepancies are different from one another. Or are they like the items of the Satisfaction With Life Scale, which contains five items that are all variations on the same theme?

When Michalos (1985) regressed each of the discrepancies against some dozen domains of satisfaction, he found them all to explain 50% to 58% of the variance. However, the pattern of shared variance across the domains does show differences (p. 362). Thus, the six discrepancies appear to have large amounts of shared variance but also some degree of unique variance, as might be expected.

These results will be further considered in the conclusions section of this chapter.

Dynamic Modular Model

The dynamic modular model, as proposed by Shmotkin (2005), represents one of the most recent theories to be based in discrepancies. It derives from two propositions.

The first is that SWB is not simply an outcome but a dynamic system with the role of maintaining a predominantly favorable psychological environment in the face of a hostile world. The second is that SWB operates through genetic programs that function to protect the organism from despair and add positivity to the experience of life. These programs involve affect, cognition, and controlled access to hostile-world beliefs. Through the operation of this system, SWB levels serve as a heuristic, or cognitive shortcut, for judging the world as variously benign or hostile. Thus, SWB refers to a generalized evaluation of life overall.

The model has four modules, one of which is relevant to this discussion. The experiential module involves the processing of the discrepancy between one's current state relative to relevant standards. When the standards are met, this produces positive emotions. If a discrepancy is perceived, this arouses negative emotions. It is these emotional and cognitive processes that modulate the experiential SWB. Thus, the model is based once again on have–want discrepancies.

A CRITIQUE OF DISCREPANCY THEORIES

Testing Discrepancies Against Levels of SWB

There are two major concerns in the interpretation of measured discrepancies. One serious problem in the interpretation of the intrapsychic approach is that the response does not provide information about the operating level of each component. Consider a response to "Considering your life as a whole, how satisfied are you now compared with 3 years ago?" on a 0–10 scale from *very much less satisfied* to *very much more satisfied*. Suppose the person responded much the same. Since the response is comparative, it could have been made against either of the following values that are recalled as representing satisfaction 3 years ago:

1. *A score of 3*: In this case the person probably was and remains depressed.

2. *A score of 8*: The person remains within his or her set-point range.

The interpretation of these two alternatives is very different as:

1. This person has failed to gather additional resources over this period to escape from his or her condition.

2. This person has maintained a good life balance, and his or her SWB remains with its normal range.

Thus, the response to the discrepancy question alone provides no interpretable information when considered in isolation. Any interpretation depends on a comparison with the current level of SWB, and this means that two questions must be asked. So the advantage of parsimony disappears, and ambiguity takes its place for the following reason.

In the above example 1, using the computed method and assuming equivalence between the two methods, the respondent would have rated his or her past SWB as 3. Thus, the result is simple to understand. The respondent not only views his or her current and past levels as equivalent, but the level of both equates to depression. This is not so using the intrapsychic approach. Here, the past value of 3 can be inferred only through the *much the same* response. It is not clear what advantage this procedure confers.

There is, however, a deeper problem with the intrapsychic approach, and this is that the assumption of precise cognitive processing is probably wrong. There are two main reasons. First, people do not easily recall how satisfied they were 3 years ago, so it represents a very complex task. Second, when asked such complex questions, people are very likely to respond using a heuristic, which provides them with a much simpler way of answering the question.

Heuristics and Core Affect

Information processing does not occur in a vacuum. It occurs in a sea of affect, and there is broad contemporary agreement that any evaluative response is the result of these dual cognitive–affective influences (see, e.g., Forgas, 1995, multiprocess model). Indeed, affect itself can be used as information for an evaluative response (see Schwarz & Clore, 1983, 1996). When this occurs, the response represents a heuristic—a simplified, short-cut way of making a response. Rather than engaging in a detailed analysis of all the available information, the response is made with reference to current mood.

Responses to the classic question in SWB surveys, "How satisfied are you with your life as a whole," are good examples of the heuristic process. People respond to the question almost instantly, in a highly reliable fashion, yet no one really knows what the question means. It is far too complex for cognitive processing. So, instead of attempting this, people refer to their current mood state as a reference for their reply. This mood state is held, on average, at about 75 points on a scale from 0 *(extremely sad)* to 100 *(extremely happy)*, as has been determined by asking people how happy or contented they generally feel (Davern et al., 2007). Thus, both the "life as a whole" question and the PWI yield data that approximate 75 points. The responses to both sets of questions predominantly use the affect heuristic.

Thus, heuristic and cognitive processing each represent two distinct pathways through which a judgment can be made. Whether an individual engages in one type of processing or the other depends on several factors, but the one most relevant to this discussion is complexity. Any request for complex processing that involves a feeling state is likely to be answered via a heuristic shortcut (e.g., Branscombe & Cohen, 1991; Forgas, 1995). What, then, do we know about this prevailing, positive mood state?

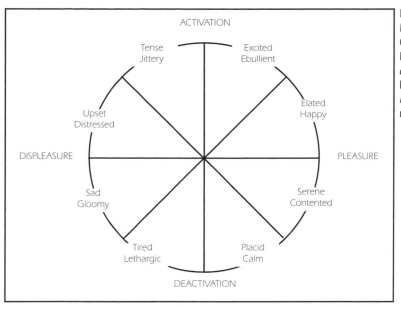

Figure 7-2. Russell's Circumplex Model of Affect. *Note.* From "A Cicumplex Model of Affect" by J. A. Russell, 1980, *Journal of Personality and Social Psychology*, 39. © 1980, by the American Psychological Association. Reprinted with permission.

In answering this, I follow Russell (2003). He described the hypothetical construct of *core affect* as a neurophysiological state that is experienced as a *feeling*. While this feeling can be consciously accessed, it is not tied to any specific object in the manner of an emotional response. Instead it is a *mood state*, which refers to how individuals sense themselves in an abstract but personal way. It can be conceptualized as a deep form of *trait affect*, analogous to felt body temperature, in that it is always there, can be assessed when attention is drawn to it, extremes are most obvious, and it exists without words to describe it. The further description of core affect calls on the *circumplex model of affect* (for a review of affect, see Cropanzano, Weiss, Hale, & Reb, 2003). This model, which has dominated affect theory for several decades, positions all affects along the circumference of a circle (Figure 7-2) (Russell, 1980).

This circle is divided into quadrants by two orthogonal axes as the *hedonic* (sad–happy) and the activated (alert–sleepy). Core affect comprises a blend of hedonic (pleasant–unpleasant) and arousal values (activation-deactivation).

As an extension of Russell's concept, Davern et al. (2007) propose that core affect is not only the affective constituent of SWB but also the basic steady-state set point that homeostasis seeks to defend. Within this concept, core affect comprises the most basic experienced feeling, being hardwired for each individual. It comprises the tonic state of affect that provides the activation energy, or motivation, for behavior. According to the results of Davern et al. (2007), core affect is most parsimoniously represented as the combined affects of happiness, contentment, and excitement. In further work we have found *alert* to replace *excited*. In any event, these affects in combination represent the activated and deactivated pleasant quadrants of the affective circumplex (Russell, 1980).

We further propose that core affect perfuses all higher process, including personality (for a review of the neurobiology of personality, see Depue & Collins, 1999), memory, and momentary experience. Consistent with this fundamental role, we suggest that the process of evolution has naturally selected individuals who experience a level of core affect corresponding to 70–80 points pleasant or positive. This level, then, constitutes the optimum set-point range for SWB, corresponding to the most adaptive range of core affect described in my theory of SWB homeostasis (Cummins, 2000, 2003).

Figure 7-3. Affective-cognitive model of SWB. The personality factors are designated as: SWB=subjective well-being; MDT=multiple discrepancies theory; N=Neuroticism; E=Extraversion; O=Openness; A=Agreeableness; and C=Conscientiousness. Note. Based on results from Davern et al. (2007).

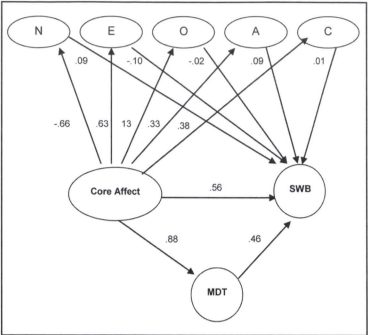

Although core affect suffuses all cognitive processes to some degree, the ones that are most strongly influenced are those rather abstract notions of the self (e.g., I am a good person). These self-perceptions are held at strength of positivity that approximates core affect. Thus, because discrepancy judgments represent complex evaluations of feelings, responses to such items are highly likely to engage heuristic processing. Thus, the intrapsychic discrepancy questions are probably answered using heuristic processing that refers to core affect as the source of information.

Davern et al. (2007) tested the relative strength of core affect discrepancies using seven items derived from multiple discrepancies theory (Michalos, 1985) and all five factors of personality, as predictors of SWB. Consistent with previous research, all three components correlated significantly with SWB and with one another. However, when the variances were controlled by structural equation modeling, it was demonstrated that affect and the multiple discrepancies theory (MDT) items are the dominant components of SWB. Indeed, after accounting for both of these, personality made only a very small contribution to the explanation of SWB variance (see Figure 7-3).

These results indicate that SWB is essentially driven by core affect and cognitive discrepancies, with the strongest influence coming from core affect. While each of the seven MDT discrepancies correlates strongly with SWB, this is vastly reduced in the presence of core affect. While the simple correlations indicate about 25% of shared variance, this reduces to about 4% when the effect of core affect is partialled out (Davern et al., 2007, table 6). In conclusion, SWB is predominantly determined by core affect, with the have–want discrepancies playing a subsidiary role.

Other Evidence of Difficulties Using the Discrepancies Approach

The example using the question "Considering your life as a whole, how satisfied are you now compared with 3 years ago?" concerns the category of discrepancies characterized as intrapsychic (complex). However, both of the other two forms of discrepancy may well create their own problems when used in analyses, as will now be demonstrated.

The computed discrepancy is the most straightforward to understand, being simply the difference between two measured variables. However, it has the potential to engender misinterpretation if results derived from the discrepancy are considered in isolation from its two components, as seen in the following example.

The Actual–Ideal Questionnaire of Nishikawa, Norlander, Fransson, and Sundbom (2007) is built on discrepancies. It is designed to measure the congruency between actual self and ideal self, for example, intelligent versus less intelligent and satisfied versus dissatisfied. The participants, Japanese and Swedish adolescents, first rated their actual self and then their ideal self. The differences between the total score of actual and ideal scales were then combined to yield an overall measure of the discrepancy between the actual and ideal self.

The authors reported that the actual–ideal self discrepancy correlates negatively with self-concept. They concluded from this that the magnitude of the self-discrepancy is therefore indicative of low self-concept, and they linked this (p. 282) with depression. However, because they did not study the two components separately, this may be a false conclusion. For example, the correlation may have been caused by the students with low self-concept having a low "actual" rating and thereby creating a large actual–ideal discrepancy. If this was so, then the major determinant of the link is the low actual correlating with low self-concept, which makes perfect sense.

In support of this simpler interpretation, they also found that compared with Swedish students, the Japanese students had overall lower ratings of self-concept, actual and ideal. However, they had a higher actual–ideal discrepancy. It seems very likely that their lower rating of actual self and self-concept explains the negative correlation between self-concept and the discrepancy.

Earlier in this chapter, I described the computed (complex) approach reported by Sheldon (2009, chapter 6 of this volume). Here, the average of three discrepancies in need satisfaction predicted SWB beyond the absolute strength of the individual levels of need satisfaction. This is a clever approach to the study of life balance and an interesting use of discrepancy data. The explanation of what the discrepancy represents in terms of functional psychological status will almost certainly extend our understanding of SWB management. It is possible, for example, that high discrepancy variance represents a weak homeostatic system.

The other form of the discrepancy has been characterized as the intrapsychic (simple). Here, respondents create their discrepancy over a single period of time. This form of discrepancy was used by Cheng and Chan (2006) in a study of *filial piety*—the respect accorded to elders and attendant care responsibilities. They asked their sample of Chinese older persons the degree to which specific filial behaviors had met their expectation for such behaviors. Using hierarchical regression, they found that the level of filial piety and the discrepancy both predicted variance in SWB. They conclude that filial piety "was most important in determining a sense of filial discrepancy and psychological well-being on the part of the elders" (p. 267). However, this conclusion cannot be validly deduced from their data.

The discrepancy in question was created from two variables, only one of which was independently measured. They measured the extent of filial behaviors but not the strength of the expectations held by the elders. Thus, it cannot be determined from their results whether the variance contributed by the discrepancy was due to the magnitude of the discrepancy or the strength of the expectations. The only way this could be resolved would be to measure the strength of the expectations as a separate variable.

CONCLUSIONS

It is clear that, despite its intuitive appeal, the use of discrepancies is fraught with practical and interpretive difficulties. If the computed (simple) method is used to generate the discrepancy, then the discrepancy itself cannot be validly interpreted without reference to the two components measured as separate variables. This makes the use of the computed discrepancies pointless.

A similar conclusion applies to the intrapsychic (simple) discrepancy. Once again, unless the variables that constitute the discrepancy are separately measured, the cause of any relationship that involves the discrepancy cannot be reliably attributed.

The intrapsychic (complex) discrepancy is more difficult to understand. When it is used to predict SWB, its power of prediction is much reduced when core affect is included. The residual explanatory variance is presumably characterized as cognitive rather than affective, and this separate component requires investigation in its own right.

The most promising approach to the use of discrepancies is the computed (complex) method of Sheldon. It is possible this can be used as a device to identify individuals who are having difficulty in their homeostatic management of SWB and so are at risk of depression.

On a comforting note, all this implies that the dark connotations of discrepancy-dominated SWB, as envisaged by Campbell et al. (1976) and Michalos (1980), are not as dire as envisaged. The level of SWB reflects the balance between a genetically determined set-point for core affect and the ability of the homeostatic system to protect the experience of that set point from negative challenges. This system dominates the construct we call SWB and cognitive discrepancies seem to play a minor role.

Finally, while the study of discrepancies seems such an obvious approach to studying life balance, the evidence from this chapter indicates otherwise. With the exception of the intrapsychic (complex) method, the discrepancies that have been discussed seem to have no advantage over the separate measurement of the two component parts. This conclusion points to a methodological simplification for researchers wishing to empirically characterize life balance.

ACKNOWLEDGEMENT

I thank Ann-Marie James for her assistance in the preparation of this manuscript and Beth Pontiff for expert editorial assistance. I am also most grateful to Kennon Sheldon and Kathleen Matuska for their comments on an earlier draft.

REFERENCES

Abbott, B. B. (2007). *A synopsis of William T. Powers' perceptual control theory.* Retrieved October 10, 2007, from http://users.ipfw.edu/abbott/pct/pct.html

Ashby, W. R. (1952). *Design for a brain.* New York: Wiley.

Baron, R. M., & Kenny, D. A. (1986). The moderator–mediator variable distinction in social psychological research: Conceptual, strategic, and statistical considerations. *Journal of Personality and Social Psychology, 5,* 1173–1182.

Baumeister, R. F., & Leary, M. R. (1995). The need to belong: Desire for interpersonal attachments as a fundamental human motivation. *Psychological Bulletin, 117,* 497–529.

Bevan, W. (1965). The concept of adaptation in modern psychology. *Journal of Psychology, 59,* 73–93.

Bortner, R. W., & Hultsch, D. F. (1970). A multivariate analysis of correlates of life satisfaction in adulthood. *Journal of Gerontology Series B, 25,* 41–47.

Branscombe, N. R., & Cohen, B. M. (1991). Motivation and complexity levels as determinants of heuristic use in social judgment. In J. P. Forgas (Ed.), *Emotion and social judgments* (pp. 145–160). Oxford: Pergamon Press.

Campbell, A., Converse, P. E., & Rodgers, W. L. (1976). *The quality of American life: Perceptions, evaluations, and satisfactions.* New York: Russell Sage Foundation.

Cannon, W. B. (1932). *The wisdom of the body.* New York: Norton.

Cantril, H. (1965). *The pattern of human concerns.* New Brunswick, NJ: Rutgers University Press.

Carver, C. S., & Scheier, M. F. (1990). Origins and functions of positive and negative affect: A control-process view. *Psychological Review, 97,* 19–35.

Chambers, R. (1997). Responsible well-being—A personal agenda for development [Editorial]. *World Development, 25,* 1743–1754.

Cheng, S. T., & Chan, A. C. M. (2006). Filial piety and psychological well-being in well older Chinese. *Journal of Gerontology Series B, 61,* 262–269.

Cropanzano, R., Weiss, H. M., Hale, J. M. S., & Reb, J. (2003). The structure of affect: Reconsidering the relationship between negative and positive affectivity. *Journal of Management, 29,* 831–858.

Cummins, R. A. (1995). On the trail of the gold standard for life satisfaction. *Social Indicators Research, 35,* 179–200.

Cummins, R. A. (1997). *Comprehensive Quality of Life Scale—Adult: Manual.* Melbourne: Deakin University, Retrieved October 10, 2007, from http://www.deakin.edu.au/research/acqol/instruments/com_scale.htm

Cummins, R. A. (1998). The second approximation to an international standard of life satisfaction. *Social Indicators Research, 43,* 307–334.

Cummins, R. A. (2000). Objective and subjective quality of life: An interactive model. *Social Indicators Research, 52,* 55–72.

Cummins, R. A. (2003). Normative life satisfaction: Measurement issues and a homeostatic model. *Social Indicators Research, 64,* 225–256.

Cummins, R. A., Gullone, E., & Lau, A. L. D. (2002). A model of subjective wellbeing homeostasis: The role of personality. In E. Gullone & R. A. Cummins (Eds.), *The universality of subjective wellbeing indicators: Social Indicators Research Series* (pp. 7–46). Dordrecht: Kluwer.

Cummins, R. A., Lau, A. D. L., & Davern, M. (in press). Homeostatic mechanisms and the quality of life. In K. C. Land (Ed.), *Handbook of social indicators and quality-of-life studies.* New York: Springer (Volume I: Theoretical and Methodological Foundations).

Cummins, R. A., & Nistico, H. (2002). Maintaining life satisfaction: The role of positive cognitive bias. *Journal of Happiness Studies, 3,* 37–69.

Cummins, R. A., Woerner, J., Tomyn, A., Gibson, A., & Knapp, T. (2007). *Australian Unity Wellbeing Index: Report 17.0—The wellbeing of Australians—work, wealth and happiness.* Australian Centre on Quality of Life, School of Psychology, Deakin University. Retrieved October 10, 2007, from http://www.deakin.edu.au/research/acqol/index_wellbeing/index.htm

Davern, M., Cummins, R. A., & Stokes, M. (2007). Subjective well-being as an affective/cognitive construct. *Journal of Happiness Studies, 8,* 429–449.

Depue, R. A., & Collins, P. F. (1999). Neurobiology of the structure of personality: Dopamine facilitation of incentive motivation and extraversion. *Behavioral and Brain Sciences, 22,* 491–569.

Diener, E., & Diener, C. (1996). Most people are happy. *Psychological Science, 7,* 181–185.

Diener, E., & Lucas, R. E. (2000). Explaining differences in societal levels of happiness: Relative standards, need fulfillment, culture, and evaluation theory. *Journal of Happiness Studies, 1,* 41–78.

Diener, E., & Oishi, S. (2000). Money and happiness: Income and subjective well-being across nations. In E. Diener & E. M. Suh (Eds.), *Subjective well-being across cultures* (pp. 185–218). Cambridge, MA: MIT Press.

Diener, E., Suh, E. M., Smith, H., & Shao, L. (1995). National differences in reported subjective well-being: Why do they occur? *Social Indicators Research, 34,* 7–32.

Easterlin, R. A. (1973). "Does money buy happiness." *Public Interest, 30,* 3–10.

Easterlin, R. A. (1974). Does economic growth improve the human lot? Some empirical evidence. In P. A. David & M. Abramovitz (Eds.), *Nations and households in economic growth* (pp. 89–125). New York: Academic Press.

Easterlin, R. A. (2005). Feeding the illusion of growth and happiness: A reply to Hagerty and Veenhoven. *Social Indicators Research, 74,* 429–443.

Ferrans, C., & Powers, M. (1985). Quality of life index: Development and psychometric properties. *Advances in Nursing Science, 8,* 15–24.

Field, D. (1981). Retrospective reports by healthy intelligent elderly people of personal events of their adult lives. *International Journal of Behavioral Development, 4,* 77–97.

Flanagan, J. D. (1979). *Identifying opportunities for improving the quality of life of older age groups.* Palo Alto, CA: American Institute for Research.

Forgas, J. P. (1995). Mood and judgment: The Affect Infusion Model (AIM). *Psychological Bulletin, 117,* 39–66.

Frisch, M. B. (1992). Use of the quality of life inventory in problem assessment and treatment planning for cognitive therapy of depression. In A. Freeman & F. M. Dattlio (Eds.), *Comprehensive casebook of cognitive therapy* (pp. 27–52). New York: Plenum Press.

Gittins, R. (2005). An economics fit for humans. *Australian Economic Review, 38*(2), 121–127.

Headey, B., & Wearing, A. (1986). *The sense of relative superiority—Central to well-being.* Melbourne: University of Melbourne.

Helson, H. (1948). Adaptation-level as a basis for a quantitative theory of frame of reference. *Psychological Review, 55,* 297–313.

Higgins, E. T., Roney, C., Crowe, E., & Hymes, C. (1994). Ideal versus ought predilections for approach and avoidance: Distinct self-regulatory systems. *Journal of Personality and Social Psychology, 66,* 276–286.

Hsieh, C. M. (2003). Counting importance: The case of life satisfaction and relative domain importance. *Social Indicators Research, 61,* 227–240.

International Wellbeing Group. (2006). *Personal Wellbeing Index* (4th ed.). Melbourne: Australian Centre on Quality of Life, Deakin University. Retrieved June 25, 2007, from http://www.deakin.edu.au/research/acqol/instruments/wellbeing_index.htm

Kasser, T., & Ryan, R. M. (1993). A dark side of the American dream: Correlates of financial success as a central life aspiration. *Journal of Personality and Social Psychology, 65*, 410–422.

Katzell, R. A. (1964). Personal values, job satisfaction, and job behavior. In H. Borow (Ed.), *Man in a world of work* (pp. 341–363). Boston: Houghton-Mifflin.

Kings, L. A., Richards, J. H., & Stemmerich, E. (1998). Daily goals, life goals, and worst fears: Means, ends, and subjective well-being. *Journal of Personality and Social Psychology, 66*, 713–744.

Knight, J., Song, L., & Gunatilaka, R. (2007). *Subjective well-being and its determinants in rural China.* Department of Economics, University of Oxford. (Discussion Paper Series No. 334). Retrieved from http://www.economics.ox.ac.uk/Research/wp/pdf/paper334.pdf

Lawton, M. P., & Nahemow, L. (1973). Ecology and the aging process. In C. Eisdorfer & M. P. Lawton (Eds.), *The psychology of adult development and aging* (pp. 619–674). Washington, DC: American Psychological Association.

Lazarus, R. S. (1991). *Emotion and adaptation.* New York: Oxford University Press.

Liu, B. C. (1976). *Quality of life indicators in U.S. metropolitan areas: A statistical analysis.* New York: Praeger.

Locke, E. A. (1969). What is job satisfaction? *Organizational Behavior and Human Performance, 4*, 309–336.

Locke, E. A. (1976). The nature and causes of job satisfaction. In M. D. Dunnette (Ed.), *Handbook of industrial and organizational psychology* (pp. 1297–1343). Chicago: Rand McNally.

Lucas, R. E., Clark, A. E., Georgellis, Y., & Diener, E. (2003). Reexamining adaptation and the set point model of happiness: Reactions to changes in marital status. *Journal of Personality and Social Psychology, 84*, 527–539.

McFarlin, D. B., Coster, E. A., Rice, R. W., & Coopper-Alison, T. (1995). Facet importance and job satisfaction: Another look at the range of affect hypothesis. *Basic and Applied Social Psychology, 16*, 489–502.

McFarlin, D. B., & Rice, R. W. (1992). The role of facet importance as a moderator in job satisfaction processes. *Journal of Organizational Behavior, 13*, 41–54.

McGee, H. M., O'Boyle, C. A., Hickey, A., O'Malley, K., & Joyce, C. R. B. (1991). Assessing the quality of life of the individual: The SEIQoL with a healthy and a gastroenterology unit population. *Psychological Medicine, 21*, 749–759.

Michalos, A. C. (1976). Measuring the quality of life. In W. R. Shea, & J. King-Farlow (Eds.), *Values and the Quality of life* (pp. 24–37). New York: Science History Publications.

Michalos, A. C. (1980). Satisfaction and happiness. *Social Indicators Research, 8*, 385–422.

Michalos, A. C. (1985). Multiple discrepancies theory (MDT). *Social Indicators Research, 16*, 347–413.

Mikes, P. S., & Hulin, C. L. (1968). Use of importance as weighting component of job satisfaction. *Journal of Applied Psychology, 52*, 394–398.

Mobley, W. H., & Locke, E. A. (1970). The relationship of value importance to satisfaction. *Organisational Behavior and Human Performance, 5*, 463–483.

Nishikawa, S., Norlander, T., Fransson, P., & Sundbom, E. (2007). A cross-cultural validation of adolescent self-concept in two cultures: Japan and Sweden. *Social Behavior and Personality, 35*, 269–286.

Ott, J. (2005). Level and inequality of happiness in nations: Does greater happiness of a greater number imply greater inequality in happiness? *Journal of Happiness Studies, 6*, 397–420.

Powers, W. T. (1973). *Behavior: The control of perception.* Chicago: Aldine.

Raphael, D., Rukholm, E., Brown, I., Hill-Bailey, P., & Donato, E. (1996). The Quality of Life Profile–Adolescent Version: Background, description, and initial validation. *Journal of Adolescent Health, 19*, 366–375.

Rice, R. W., Gentile, D. A., & McFarlin, D. B. (1991). Facet importance and job satisfaction. *Journal of Applied Psychology, 76*, 31–39.

Rice, R. W., Markus, K., Moyer, R. P., & McFarlin, D. B. (1991). Facet importance and job satisfaction: Two experimental tests of Locke's range of affect hypothesis. *Journal of Applied Social Psychology, 21*, 1977–1987.

Russell, J. A. (1980). A circumplex model of affect. *Journal of Personality and Social Psychology, 39*, 1161–1178.

Russell, J. A. (2003). Core affect and the psychological construction of emotion. *Psychological Review, 110*, 145–172.

Schilling, O. K., & Wahl, H. W. (2006). Modeling late-life adaptation in affective well-being under a severe chronic health condition: The case of age-related macular degeneration. *Psychology and Aging, 21*, 703–714.

Schwarz, N., & Clore, G. L. (1983). Mood, misattribution, and judgements of well-being: Informative and directive functions of affective states. *Journal of Personality and Social Psychology, 45*, 513–523.

Schwarz, N., & Clore, G. L. (1996). Feelings and phenomenal experience. In E. T. Higgins & A. W. Kruglandski (Eds.), *Social psychology: Handbook of basic principles* (pp. 433–465). New York: Guildford Press.

Sheldon, K. M. (2009). Defining and validating measures of life balance: Suggestions, a new measure, and some preliminary results. In K. Matuska, C. Christiansen, & H. Polatajko (Eds), *Life balance: Multidisciplinary theory and research.* Bethesda, MD: AOTA Press/SLACK Incorporated.

Sheldon, K. M., & Niemiec, C. P. (2006). It's not just the amount that counts: Balanced need satisfaction also affects well-being. *Journal of Personality and Social Psychology, 91,* 331–341.

Shmotkin, D. (1991). The structure of the Life Satisfaction Index A in elderly Israeli adults. *International Journal of Aging and Human Development, 33,* 131–150.

Shmotkin, D. (2005). Happiness in face of adversity: Reformulating the dynamic and modular bases of subjective well-being. *Review of General Psychology, 9,* 291–325.

Smith, C. L. (1991). Measures and meaning in comparisons of wealth equality. *Social Indicators Research, 24,* 367–392.

Stones, M. J., & Kozma, A. (1991). A magical model of happiness. *Social Indicators Research, 25,* 31–50.

Veenhoven, R. (1993). *Happiness in nations.* Rotterdam: University of Rotterdam.

Veenhoven, R. (1995). World database of happiness. *Social Indicators Research, 34,* 299–314.

Waters, L. K., & Roach, D. (1971). Comparison of unweighted and importance-weighted job satisfaction measures for three samples of female office workers. *Psychological Reports, 28,* 779–782.

Wikipedia. (2007). Body temperature. Retrieved October 10, 2007, from http://en.wikipedia.org/wiki/Body_temperature#Normal_human_temperature

Wilson, W. R. (1960). *An attempt to determine some correlates and dimensions of hedonic tone.* Unpublished doctoral dissertation, Northwestern University, Evanston, IL.

Wilson, W. R. (1965). Relation of sexual behaviors, values, and conflicts to avowed happiness. *Psychological Reports, 17,* 371–378.

Wu, C. H., & Yao, G. (2007). Importance has been considered in satisfaction evaluation: An experimental examination of Locke's range-of-affect hypothesis. *Social Indicators Research, 81,* 521–542.

Time Use and Balance

Andrew S. Harvey and Jerome Singleton

INTRODUCTION

Family, work, and community comprise the social environment in which people spend their time and live their lives. The ability of an individual to integrate and negotiate all three and at the same time avoid "grief, stress, or negative impact" is indicative of work–life balance (Human Resources and Social Development Canada [HRSDC], 2008, p. 1).

Economists, geographers, sociologists, and occupational scientists have all examined how people spend their time, using age, gender, and life course to study how time shifts during a person's lifetime. However, little has been done to explore time allocation in relation to both objective and subjective contextual variables. The work here will explore time allocation to activities, social space (locations), and social circle (contacts) in light of self-reported satisfaction with work–life balance, stress, and happiness.

The Canadian General Social Surveys (GSS) indicate that about one quarter of Canadians are dissatisfied with the balance between their work and family life (Statistics Canada, 1998, 2005). This finding coincides with feelings of stress and reduced levels of life satisfaction and happiness. Greater understanding of how time is allocated may provide insight into possible grounds for dissatisfaction and insight into balance and imbalance.

Christiansen and Matuska (2006) argued that knowledge of how people use time provides a useful approach for better understanding how they assign purpose and meaning to life, especially when time-use and qualitative data are combined. Zuzanek and Mannell (1998) showed, using time-use data, an objective basis for subjective feelings of time pressure. In this chapter we ask, where does time go? How is it allocated across activities, places, and people in relation to feelings about life balance? Does time allocation differ among individuals who believe their work-home life balance is satisfactory and those who believe it to be unsatisfactory, and if so, how?

We extend the literature by specifically examining objective and subjective dimensions of the relationship between perceived job and home–life balance and the allocation of time. We view allocation of time, as reflected in daily activities and the context in which they occur, in terms of its relation to perceived time balance, stress, and happiness as revealed in Canadian time-use studies.

K. Matuska & C. Christiansen (Eds.)
Life balance: Multidisciplinary theories and research (pp 95–114)
© 2009 SLACK Incorporated and AOTA Press

USING TIME-USE SURVEYS TO STUDY BALANCE

Time-use studies examine how individuals allocate their time (Szalai, 1972). They are an excellent tool to use in studying work–life balance. They show the distribution of time across activities and of activities across the study population. Activities may consist of a single event (concert) or multiple events (meals).

Time-Use Studies

Typically, the basic unit of a time-use study is an event, something that happens in time and space. The event is, in essence, a single line in a diary identifying an activity (what was done), when it started and ended, related contextual detail such as what else was done at the same time, where, with whom, for whom, and sometimes subjective impressions such as feelings and attitudes. The accepted practice in time-use research is to record sequentially all of a person's events for some fixed period (e.g., a 24-hour day).

The contextual components of an activity are commonly described in terms of time, location, and social contact. Time has several dimensions, two of which—event duration and activity duration—are routinely addressed. *Event duration* is the time allocated to a specific diary entry (e.g., how long it took to eat breakfast). Activity duration is the daily sum of diary event durations for any given activity (e.g., how many hours were spent eating meals). Location has two dimensions of interest: function (e.g., home, work) and geographic location. Geographic location is of specialized interest and seldom collected. *Social contact* refers to the presence or absence of other people during the event. Subjective dimensions, such as stress or enjoyment, are less frequently captured but highly useful when they are, as in this study.

At the level of the individual, the *classification* of activities is the interaction between objective circumstances inherent in the individual and the environment (e.g., where it takes place, with whom, for whom) and the affective circumstances (e.g., feelings, thoughts, attitudes) of the situation. Hence shopping may be a household activity undertaken as grocery shopping, a work activity such as a teacher shopping for art supplies, or window shopping. However, there is seldom sufficient detail in a study to draw such distinctions.

Virtually all time-use data can be coded into four types of time (Harvey & Pentland, 2004), and there are reasonably clear rules for assigning activities to this highly aggregated classification:

1. *Necessary time*—that required to maintain one's self in terms of eating, sleeping, and cleansing

2. *Contracted time*—that required to satisfy obligations related to paid work and education

3. *Committed time*—that devoted to one's home and family and volunteer service to others

4. *Free time*—that devoted to various discretionary, leisure, or free activities not included above

Events reported in this study are defined using the detailed hierarchical classification in the GSS (Statistics Canada, 1998, 2005).

Time Use and Context

Activities cannot be understood apart from the doer and the context. A given activity can, for an individual, be work at one time and leisure at another, or work for one individual and leisure for another (Shaw, 1985).

Contextual detail, which gives form to the social environment in which activities are undertaken, is crucial to classifying and interpreting behavior. The location where an activity is undertaken (social space), which can minimally be identified as home, workplace, or the community, and with whom (social circle), either alone or with family, friends, or others, are germane to the subjective experience of the doer and the classification process (Harvey & Taylor, 2000).

Additionally, activities and contexts can be expected to generate subjective feelings such as enjoyment, satisfaction, or stress.

Canadian General Social Surveys

This study uses information from the GSS, Time-Use Modules, Cycles 12 and 19, for 1998 and 2005. Information is also used from the American Time Use Study (ATUS), an ongoing study undertaken since 2003 by the U.S. Bureau of Labor Statistics (BLS, 2003). The GSS surveys provide an opportunity to examine the differences and similarities among individuals who claim to have balanced lives and those who feel they lack balance. Each study collected a 1-day diary per respondent. Each diary entry recorded what, when, where, and with whom something was being done.

The GSS studies also provide information on perceived work–home balance. The question used by Statistics Canada in the GSS to measure balance in 1998 and 2005 was "Are you satisfied or dissatisfied with the balance between your job and home life?" The respondents could respond *satisfied, dissatisfied,* or *no opinion.* This question was only asked of employed people; therefore, the respondents used in the analysis here are jobholders expressing an opinion. Responding jobholders indicating satisfaction are considered to be balanced; those indicating dissatisfaction are considered imbalanced.

The subjective side of daily time allocation has rarely been addressed due to lack of simultaneous time use and subjective data. The subjective dimension can be captured with information relating to enjoyment, stress, motivation, and so forth for each diary event or with global measures of well-being in relation to time allocation data. Fortunately, the GSS provides such simultaneous global data. A global measure of stress is used below to provide insight into the subjective experience of balance in the absence of event-level subjective detail. Respondents were asked to respond "yes" or "no" to a series of 10 questions to which a "yes" response was considered to be an indicator of "time crunch." A respondent could thus register from 0 to 10 "yeses." Respondents who registered 7 or higher "yeses" were considered to be experiencing high stress, and those who registered 0 to 6 were deemed to be experiencing low stress.

The Canadian study samples were 10,749 and 19,597 for 1998 and 2005, respectively (Table 8-1). The gender and marital status distributions were virtually unchanged between the two years. However, there were changes in both age distribution and reported sense of balance. The proportion of the population ages 25 to 44 years declined, while the proportion ages 45 years and over increased, reflecting the aging population of North America labeled as "boomers." Individuals indicated a greater sense of job–work balance in 2005 than in 1998.

Time Use: Stability and Change

In recent years, on average—over the whole adult population and all days of the week—one-third, or 8 hours, of every day is spent working at paid work (contracted time), unpaid work (committed time), or the two combined (productive time), as illustrated in Table 8-2. Necessary (personal) time averaged about 10.5 hours, and about 5.5 hours is allocated to free time.

The data reflect extreme stability over the several years reported in Table 8-2. Yet there is extensive literature on the issue of increasing work time versus increasing free time (see Bittman & Wajcman, 2000; Gershuny, 1999; Robinson & Godbey, 1997; Schor, 1993). However, the debate is being carried out against a backdrop of little change in the aggregate time allocation mix (see Table 8-2). On a year-to-year basis, since 2003 in the United States, and for over a decade in Canada, total productive activity (contracted + committed time) is virtually unchanged. In the United States, total productive-activity time was down 2/10ths of an hour per day in 2006 relative to 2003 and was nearly constant from 1992 to 1998 in Canada. From 1998 to 2005, Canada experienced a 1/10th of an hour increase in total productive time and a reallocation of time from committed to contracted activities. Although small in relation to the whole population, the changes can be large

Table 8-1

BASIC DEMOGRAPHICS AND SUBJECTIVE WORK–FAMILY BALANCE 1998 AND 2005 TIME-USE STUDIES

	1998		2005	
	COUNT	PERCENT	COUNT	PERCENT
Male	5289	49.2	9657	49.3
Female	5460	50.8	7534	50.7
Total	10749		19597	
Married	6592	61.4	12053	61.5
Single	4142	38.6	9469	38.5
15 to 24	1798	16.7	3264	16.7
25 to 34	2045	19.0	3285	16.8
35 to 44	2327	21.6	3795	19.4
45 to 54	1817	16.9	3663	18.7
55 to 64	1178	11.0	2625	13.4
65 to 74	927	8.6	1664	8.5
75 years and older	656	6.1	1300	6.6
Balanced	4623	74.7	9379	77.6
Not Balanced	1563	25.3	2701	22.4

Note. Data derived from Statistics Canada (1998; 2005).

for particular subpopulations, such as cohorts moving out of school, into marriage or parenthood, and those becoming empty nesters and making other life transitions (Fast & Frederick, 2004).

Time Use Over the Course of a Lifetime

How does an individual's time use change as his or her social environment changes across the life course? As people marry, start a family, become empty nesters, or lose a spouse, does their social environment (with whom, alone, family, others) affect their allocation of time use?

Studies to date have shown that time use differs among individuals at different points across their life course (Fast & Frederick, 2004; Harvey & Singleton, 1995; Zuzanek & Smale, 1999). Such studies provide insight into how time is used differently as individuals enter and leave different life stages. Over time, it can be anticipated that changes such as having children or teleworking will result in significant changes in terms of activities undertaken. Longitudinal data indicate a tendency toward behavioral stability (Crawford, Godbey, & Crouter, 1986; Elliott, Harvey, & MacDonald, 1984). Their work indicates that both the doing and nondoing of particular activities tend to be consistent over time, and change that does occur is structured and predictable in terms

Table 8-2

MAIN ACTIVITIES, SELECTED YEAR,
UNITED STATES AND CANADA

Activity Type	UNITED STATES				CANADA		
	2003	2004	2005	2006	1992	1998	2005
	HOURS PER DAY						
Personal	10.6	10.6	10.7	10.7	10.6	10.5	10.7
Committed	3.8	3.8	3.7	3.6	3.7	3.7	3.5
Contracted	4.2	4.1	4.1	4.2	4.3	4.3	4.6
Free	5.4	5.5	5.5	5.5	5.4	5.5	5.2
Total	24	24	24	24	24	24	24
Committed+Contracted	8.0	7.9	7.8	7.8	8.0	8.0	8.1
Committed/Contracted	90.5	92.7	90.2	85.7	86.0	86.0	76.1

Note. Data derived from *BLS* (2008) and Statistics Canada (1998; 2005).

of changes in roles and obligations as an individual moves through the life cycle. For example, students have virtually no committed time but much contracted time. The move out of the house to a place of their own increases committed time, as do marriage and the presence of a young child.

We (Harvey & Singleton, 1989) examined changing activity patterns across the lifespan, and it was found that age was the only significant predictor of time allocation. Other variables considered were sex, marital status, education, and whether a person resided alone across each of the four types of time, social contacts, and locations (Harvey & Singleton, 1989). We observed the existence of turning points in time use revolving around population mean ages, when deviations from mean time use switch from above to below the mean or below to above. That is, once the switch was made from above-average to below-average paid work hours, typically there was no return to the former state. For example, at age 55, contracted time fell below the all-ages mean, and the time allocated to necessary, committed, and free time increased (Harvey & Singleton, 1989). On retirement, the nature of socializing changes significantly as it moves from informal behavior around the water cooler to a more formal arranged activity.

Research has shown that from a life-cycle perspective, retired individuals spend more leisure time in fewer activities than employed individuals in all activities except paid work (Zuzanek & Box, 1988). The gender differences diminish in time spent on housework but widen in time spent in leisure activities (Zuzanek & Box, 1988). In the period of transition from paid work, women, possibly as a result of lifelong enculturation, seem to systematically revert to caring for the family and home. While men also increase their caring time, thus narrowing the gender differences, they tend to do so less systematically when viewed from a cohort perspective (Stone & Harvey, 2000). This suggests that gender differences during working life are replaced by new differences in later life. Hence, balance must be considered to exist differently for different individuals and for different individuals at different times. This indicates that as individuals age, they adapt through or with, changing the manner in which they balance time use across activity categories.

BALANCE AND TIME USE

What information in the wealth of data collected by the GSS distinguishes the characteristics of people who are satisfied with their work–life balance from those who are not? Segmentation analysis enables us to address this question.

While most analytical procedures are unable to effectively explore the complexity that exists in time use, chi-square automatic interaction detector (CHAID) analysis facilitates the concurrent examination of a wide array of situational characteristics, including environmental, demographic, socioeconomic, and affective dimensions (Andrews & Morgan, 1971).

CHAID analysis segments the data presented based on the strongest relationships, defined in terms of chi-square values, between a defined dependent variable and other variables in the data set. The dependent variable can be nominal, interval, or scale generating, as appropriate, distributions or means. First it evaluates variable values. For example, if the dependent variable is child care, all provided variables are tested against it. As a result, ages grouped in 15 5-year intervals may be regrouped into 10 groups, each of which differs significantly from the other. Each independent variable is similarly evaluated, and its values combined as necessary. Once all the variables have been evaluated internally, the dependent variable is evaluated against all of the independent variables. All independent variables that are found to significantly segment the dependent variable are then rank ordered by chi-square, beginning with the strongest relationship. The forces underlying identified relationships must then be judged on the basis of reasonableness and theory. The initial advantage of CHAID is that it is free from narrow theoretical constraints, other than any imposed through the structure and selection of the input data.

Figure 8-1 is based on the combined 1998 and 2005 samples totaling 30,346. The root box of 17,486 workers indicating their level of satisfaction with their work-life balance is 57.6 % of the total sample. The 57.6 % is comprised of 19.8% in the 1998 study and 37.9% in the 2005. Totals in each column sum to the total percentage in the previous box.

For both the 1998 and 2005 data, the CHAID analysis of perceived balance collapsed seven age groups into five (Figure 8-1). It found age groups 25–34 and 35–44 did not significantly differ from each other with respect to perceived balance. As well, age groups 65–74 and 75+ did not differ. About three-fourths of the workers (74.4% in 1998 and 77.3 % in 2005) were satisfied with the balance between work and home life. Thus about one-fourth (25.6% in 1998 and 22.7% in 2005) were not satisfied with the balance and can be considered imbalanced. The highest proportion of imbalanced were between 25 to 44 years old, an age group identified as young adulthood (Fast & Frederick, 1998). From a life–course perspective, this corresponds with their childbearing years; in contrast, individuals aged 15–24 and 55+ reported greater balance.

A slight overall improvement from 1998 to 2005 masks an apparent deterioration in balance among the older age groups. Those ages 55 years or older showed an increased proportion who registered imbalanced in 2005. This change requires further investigation.

Many demographic, temporal, objective, and subjective variables in the Canadian time-use surveys were entered into the CHAID analysis and evaluated in relation to stated balance between job and home life. The most striking observation from this procedure was the dominance of subjective dimensions as the highest ranked segmentation variables (Table 8-3). The top 14 items that emerged from the analysis were only slightly different in regard to their rank order between 1998 and 2005. However, the slight difference may have some significance.

Balance and Work Time

One cannot consider individual life balance and ignore how time is allocated in daily living. At a highly aggregated level, the overall societal allocation of time to the four major types—contracted, committed, necessary, and free time—is virtually stable (see Table 8-2). The activity mix, however, varies among subpopulations and over time for any given cohort (Apps & Rees, 2005; Zick & McCullough, 2004).

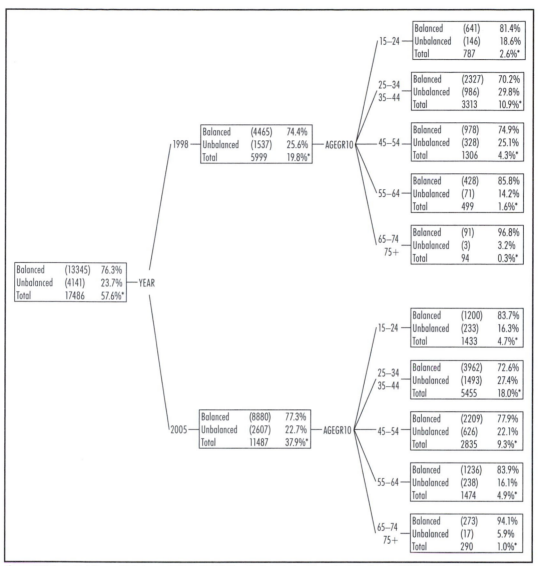

Figure 8-1. Stated job/home life balance, 1998 and 2005, Canada. Data derived from Statistics Canada (1998; 2005). Overall there was an improvement in balance between 1998 and 2005. *Note.* Percentages following total within boxes refer to the proportion of the overall time use samples in 1998 and 2005 represented by the subsamples for which work satisfaction data were gathered.

The data in Table 8-2 raise some questions. Is there a distribution of time—a time balance—that is appropriate to maintain society? If the aggregate balance is appropriate, what about those who argue that their time is not balanced and who are they?

Economists would contend that if a balance is maintained year to year, it likely is the appropriate balance; otherwise the allocation would change to achieve the appropriate balance. There are very small but consistent changes in the ratio of committed to contracted time in the United States and Canada. In the United States between 2005 and 2006, productive time remained constant at 7.8 hours a day. Contracted time became a relatively larger share of productive time, as contracted time grew and committed time declined. Thus, the United States committed/contracted time ratio dropped from 90.2% in 2005 to 85.7% in 2006. In Canada, committed time relative to contracted time dropped to 76.1% in 2005 from 86.05% in 1998, also as the result of a decline in committed time and an increase in contracted time. The net result was 1/10th of an hour's increase in productive time.

Table 8-3

SEGMENTING VARIABLES FOR "BALANCE," WORKING POPULATION, CANADA 1998 AND 2005

RANK ORDER	1998	2005
1	Time crunch	Time crunch
2	Stated stress	Stated stress
3	Time for family friends	*Feelings about main activity*
4	Spending of nonwork/family time	Constantly under stress
5	Constantly under stress	Time for family and friends
6	No time for fun	Spending of nonwork/family time
7	*Satisfaction with life as whole*	*Satisfaction with life as whole*
8	*Feelings about main activity*	*Enjoy paid work*
9	*Enjoy paid work*	Stress when not enough time
10	Trapped in daily routine	How rushed
11	How rushed	Change work hours
12	Stress when not enough time	Trapped in daily routine
13	Feelings about finances	Hours worked last 7 days
14	Unhappy	Unhappy

Note. Italics denote a direct relationship with balance.

Data derived from Statistics Canada (1998) and Statistics Canada (2005).

However, the answer to the question whether there is an appropriate time balance for society is, that we don't know, and we will not know without a great deal more research. The answer to the question about why people say their lives are unbalanced requires an understanding of how the aggregate work burden is distributed and what forces are at work distributing or redistributing it.

On a day-to-day basis, the burdens of undertaking and scheduling multiple roles and the exigencies of paid work and family create immediate stress that generates a sense of imbalance. On a lifetime basis, due to individual, family, and societal pressures, work and leisure activities and related contextual environments are segmented across the life course, which generates excessive demands at certain stages. Demands increase in volume and complexity over the early adult years with marriage and family formation, while in midlife significant changes in daily living occur with the onset of events like the empty nest and labor-force reentry (Harvey & Singleton, 1989).

To understand how time use is shaped by or impinges on context one needs to examine time use at the level of the individual through a more detailed look at activities and the contextual components.

Balance and Time Allocation to Activities

The overall change in time allocation by workers departs significantly from that of the overall population. In 2005 the amount of time that both balanced and unbalanced workers spent on work and work-related activities increased significantly. As one would expect, respondents reporting imbalanced lives spent more time at work, on travel to work, and on child care in both 1998 and 2005 than balanced workers (Table 8-4). In both 1998 and 2005, balanced respondents spent significantly more time sleeping, socializing at home, other socializing, watching television, reading books or newspapers, other passive leisure, and active sports than imbalanced respondents. In 2005, the balanced respondents also spent more time in active leisure and in education and related activities. This suggests that when time is shifted to or from one opportunity, such as work, the offset involves several activities reflecting the differing preferences of the workers who are making the shift.

Contracted time in both 1998 and 2005 and committed time in 1998 registered a significantly higher time allocation by the imbalanced (Table 8-4). However, in both years, balanced workers registered a significantly higher time allocation to necessary and free time.

Between 1998 and 2005, both the balanced and imbalanced workers registered increased contracted and necessary time at the expense of committed and free time. Considered in terms of minutes per day between 1998 and 2005, both the balanced and imbalanced registered increased contracted time, 13 and 22 minutes, respectively, and decreased committed time, 7 and 17 minutes, respectively. During the same period, the time allocated to necessary time increased and the allocation to free time declined for both balance groups. The time allocation of the imbalanced to committed time declined over twice as much as did that of the balanced. The reverse held for free time, where the balanced allocation for free time fell over twice as much as the imbalanced allocation did. Balanced workers reallocated twice as much time to necessary activities. In short, lack of balance reflects increased productive activity and diminished free time for leisure and recreational activities. These gains and losses in time allocation among contracted, committed, necessary, and free time are remarkable and present an interesting avenue for further exploration.

Balance and Event Location

The data indicate that in 1998, balanced workers had significantly more of their events at home than imbalanced workers did. The difference, however, is very small. Over half of all events occurred at home, 55.55% for the balanced workers and 54.65% for the imbalanced (Table 8-5). In contrast, the imbalanced engaged in significantly more events at the workplace in 1998. For 2005, the difference in time spent at home and work between the balanced and imbalanced failed to be significant. While there are other statistically significant differences in terms of social space, the practical differences are all very small.

The share of events at home in 2005 increased for both the balanced and the imbalanced groups. This, coupled with the increased proportion of events alone, is consistent with Putnam's (1995) discussion on bowling alone. In the GSS, both the respondents reporting balanced and imbalanced lives had a larger share of events carried out at work and as a car driver, accompanied by a decline in the share of events by both groups as car passengers. With the increase of events at home and at work, there were fewer events in other locations.

Balance and Social Circle

Studies suggest that people need time with others and have more illness and shorter lives if they are excessively alone (Harvey & Taylor, 2000, House, 2001). One theorized dimension of life balance involves having "rewarding and self-affirming relationships with others" (Matuska & Christiansen, 2008, p. 11). Yet significantly more events engaged in by respondents reporting imbalanced lives are experienced alone or with children living at home (see Table 8-5). Significantly fewer events are spent with one's spouse and other household members. In terms of time allocation, compared to those reporting balanced lives, respondents reporting imbalanced lived spend significantly more time alone (391 minutes vs. 374 minutes), with household children (101 vs. 83), with nonhousehold persons in the company of others (229 vs. 201) and nonhousehold persons only (338 vs. 323; Table 8-6). Nonhousehold persons include contacts at work. These data indicate an objective basis for concern over lack of time spent with friends and family by

Table 8-4

COMPONENTS OF ACTIVITY CONTEXT BY YEAR AND BALANCE, WORKING POPULATION, CANADA

	1998		2005	
	BALANCED %	IMBALANCED %	BALANCED %	IMBALANCED %
Social Space (Location)				
Respondent's home	**55.55**	54.65	57.36	56.91
Work place	11.36	**12.55**	11.42	**11.86**
Someone else's home	**2.68**	2.44	2.08	**2.22**
Other neighborhood	**9.79**	9.35	**8.28**	7.72
Car (driver)	14.21	**14.82**	14.79	**15.36**
Car (passenger)	**2.88**	2.21	**2.54**	2.33
Walk	2.56	**2.76**	2.12	1.99
Bus and subway	0.72	**0.98**	1.05	**1.20**
Bicycle	0.14	0.12	0.16	0.16
Other	0.12	0.12	0.20	0.25
	100.00	100.00	100.00	100.00
Social Circle (Contact)				
Alone	55.95	**56.64**	58.31	**59.45**
Spouse	**15.86**	15.07	**23.13**	21.21
Children of the home	10.72	**13.89**	12.75	**16.6**
Parent(s)/in-laws in household	**1.64**	0.83	**2.29**	1.50
Other members in household	3.52	2.92	**3.61**	2.90
Child(ren) of respondent <15 out of home	0.32	0.29	0.59	0.67
Child(ren) of respondent >15 out of home	0.36	0.40	**0.64**	0.51
Parent(s)/in-laws not in household	**1.1**	0.73	1.41	1.34
Other family members	**1.98**	1.69	**2.72**	2.28
Friends	**7.62**	5.63	**7.20**	6.35
Others living out	11.99	**12.72**	11.36	11.23
	111.06*	110.81*	124.01*	124.04*
Temporal Space				
Morning	30.3	29.6	29.3	28.9
Afternoon	31.2	29.2	30.3	27.7
Evening	29.2	**31.8**	30.2	**32.5**
Night	9.2	9.4	10.2	**10.9**
	100.0	100.0	100.0	100.0
Duration				
Short	33.3	33.2	25.4	**26.2**
Medium	39.1	39.5	41.7	42.0
Long	27.6	27.3	**32.9**	31.8
	100.0	100.0	100.0	100.0

Note. For each significant pair, the higher value is **bolded**.
Data derived from Statistics Canada (1998) and Statistics Canada (2005).
*Greater than 100 because one can be with multiple others.

Table 8-5

TIME ALLOCATION TO ACTIVITIES, BY BALANCE, WORKING POPULATION CANADA, 1998 AND 2005 (MINUTES/DAY)

	1998		*2005*	
	BALANCED	*IMBALANCED*	*BALANCED*	*IMBALANCED*
Paid work	295.6	**349.6**	308.4	**369.7**
Travel: To/from paid work	28.3	**34.6**	31.2	**40.2**
Activities related to paid work	3.1	2.9	2.3	**3.1**
Education & related activities	23.5	20.2	**21.7**	16.1
Contracted	*350.6*	***407.4***	*363.7*	***429.0***
Cooking and washing up	38.3	37.3	32.7	32.7
Housekeeping	31.4	**36.3**	31.4	32.3
Maintenance and repair	9.6	10.3	12.6	11.5
Other household work	19.8	18.7	21.1	20.1
Shopping for goods & service	42.9	46.4	40.3	37.4
Childcare	24.3	**31.5**	21.1	**28.8**
Civic and voluntary activity	16.9	18.7	16.7	18.7
Committed	*183.1*	***199.2***	*175.9*	*181.6*
Night sleep/essential sleep	**472.8**	460.2	**490.1**	469.6
Meals (excluding restaurant)	**60.7**	57.7	58.9	52.4
Other personal activities	66.1	62.6	67.1	66.2
Necessary	***599.6***	*580.5*	***616.1***	*588.2*
Restaurant meals	19.2	17.8	16.2	15.7
Socializing in homes	**74.3**	60.9	66.4	61.1
Other socializing	**19.9**	15.7	14.7	11.5
Watching television	**107.3**	85.3	103.0	83.4
Reading books, newspapers	**19.2**	16.3	15.1	12.5
Other passive leisure	**4.4**	3.0	2.4	1.7
Sports, movies, & other	11.7	9.4	10.2	9.4
Active sports	**29.1**	23.0	27.8	22.5
Other active leisure	21.5	21.4	**28.2**	23.2
Free	***306.5***	*252.8*	***284.0***	*241.0*
Total	1440	1440	1440	1440

Note. For each significant pair, the larger category is bolded. Column totals reflect rounding.

Data derived from Statistics Canada (1998; 2005).

the imbalanced workers as indicated in Table 8-5. Stress appears to be exacerbated by time spent with household children and nonhousehold persons other than friends. Both are emblematic of work. Time with children is associated with child care and nonhousehold persons other than family or friends are predominantly work-based associations. Highly stressed individuals spend over an hour and a half (104 minutes) more time with such individuals. Most of this time is spent primarily at the expense of time with spouse, friends, and personal care. Distinct differences in the social circle between balanced and imbalanced individuals reflect forces giving rise to the problem of balance.

Balance and Social Space

The 2005 GSS provided a more detailed classification of generic locations than did previous GSS time-use studies, so the activity-setting components analysis is based only on the 2005 data. Not surprisingly, more of imbalanced workers' time is spent in work-related locations. Respondents reporting imbalanced lives spend 52 minutes more at the workplace and 50 minutes less at home. The respondents who are balanced spend more time at home (906 minutes vs. 856 minutes), someone else's home, restaurant/bar, place of worship, grocery store, other store/mall, school, outdoors away from home, library, other place, car as a passenger, and walking. While imbalanced respondents spend more time at work (338 minutes vs. 286 minutes), car as a driver, bus (includes street cars), subway/train (includes commute), and other locations (Table 8-7).

Time allocated to social spaces by workers identified with high and low stress are shown in Table 8-7. The significant relationships for stress parallel those for balance. The greater the time spent at home, the lower the stress, and greater the time spent at work, the higher the stress. There is a 68-minute difference at home compared with a 74-minute difference at the workplace. The only other difference is more time spent in the car as driver.

Balance and Time

The timing of events over the day (temporal space) and their duration can be expected to affect overall behavior and perceptions of it. If the distribution of events was totally random—independent of time of day and events were of roughly equal duration—a quarter of the daily events would start each quarter of the day. But this is not the case. Most significantly, only about 10% of events start between midnight and 6:00 a.m. because this time is occupied by sleeping events started before midnight. Expectations are that longer events generate fewer events, and shorter events generate more of them.

The reality is that there is a significant difference in the proportion of events started in the evening between respondents reporting balanced lives and respondents reporting imbalanced lives. Imbalanced individuals tend to have more events in the evening and night (see Table 8-5). They also registered significantly shorter events (15 min or less) and fewer long events (60 minutes or more) in 2005. These findings suggest that for individuals reporting imbalanced lives some activities may be crowded out of the normal daytime period. It can also be observed that for all workers there was a rather large decline in the share of short-duration events and total events that occur in the evening and night between 1998 and 2005. The extent, nature, and implications of these observations warrant further study.

Balance and Children

Segmentation indicated the importance of children as a factor strongly related to imbalance. With balance as the dependent variable, the first break variable was age, followed by time crunch, and then being with a household child under age 15. The next break was on marital status. The later showed married respondents had a below-average probability of experiencing imbalanced lives and an above-average probability of reporting imbalance, in decreasing order among the

Table 8-6

BALANCE, STRESS AND SOCIAL CONTACT, WORKING POPULATION, CANADA 2005

	BALANCED MIN/DAY	IMBALANCED MIN/DAY	LOW STRESS MIN/DAY	HIGH STRESS MIN/DAY
Alone	373.8	**391.3**	377.3	**382.9**
Spouse/partner	**184.8**	163.3	**199.5**	178.2
Household children <15	83.2	**101.2**	80.4	**126.3**
Parent/in-laws living in household	**16.8**	11.2	**18.9**	16.3
Other household members	**26.9**	20.8	28.1	**28.5**
Respondents nonhousehold children <15	4.7	**5.0**	5.3	**7.3**
Respondents nonhousehold children 15+	**5.6**	3.6	**7.3**	4.3
Parent/in-laws nonhousehold	**13.4**	12.7	13.1	**14.5**
Other family members nonhousehold	**29.7**	25.3	**35.5**	29.9
Friends nonhousehold	**87.1**	76.4	**94.1**	71.9
Other persons nonhousehold	201.1	**229.1**	151.7	**192.2**
Personal care	**0.4**	0.2	**0.5**	0.3
Household members only	**537.5**	517.8	**549.1**	527.1
Nonhousehold persons only	0.0	0.0	0.2	0.0

Note. For each significant pair, the larger category is **bolded**.

Data derived from Statistics Canada (2005).

---

separated, living common law, and the respondents who were divorced. This finding is consistent with the findings that single parents are the most time poor (Harvey & Mukhopadhyay, 2007).

Time spent engaged with children in the home, more than any other contextual dimension, differentiates balanced and imbalanced workers. The differences are 3.2% in 1998 (10.72 and 13.89) for the balanced and imbalanced, respectively, and 3.9% (12.7 and 16.6), respectively, in 2005 (see Table 8-4). The difference stands out against the great similarity of engagement by the two groups otherwise.

Balance and Stress

Balancing time use is similar to a juggler who has to keep several balls in the air. A successful juggler keeps all the balls in the air, and an unsuccessful one drops a ball occasionally. Similarly, people who work may successfully keep all their balls in the air (balance), or they may be unable to manage all the balls (imbalanced). The difference may be manifest in different stress levels. As will be observed below, stress and a sense of balance are closely and inversely related.

Segmentation analysis suggests that balance and stress go hand in hand. Three of the top five segmenting variables were stress related. Such a finding in essence highlights the definition of balance with which we started—that balance occurs in the absence of "grief, stress, or negative

Table 8-7

TIME ALLOCATION: SOCIAL SPACE, BALANCE AND STRESS, WORKING POPULATION, CANADA 2005

	BALANCED MIN/DAY	IMBALANCED MIN/DAY	LOW STRESS MIN/DAY	HIGH STRESS MIN/DAY
Home	**906.4**	856.2	**988.9**	921.2
Workplace	286.4	**338.4**	190.6	**265.4**
Someone else's home	**47.4**	46.9	**50.3**	48.7
Restaurant/bar	**16.6**	16.1	**16.3**	15.0
Place of worship	**2.8**	2.4	**3.1**	2.4
Grocery store	**6.8**	6.6	7.6	**8.2**
Other store/mall	**15.8**	13.7	17.1	**17.7**
School	**13.4**	8.5	**24.8**	22.2
Outdoors away from home	**16.9**	16.7	**18.6**	15.3
Library	**0.3**	0.2	**0.5**	0.5
Other place	**47.2**	44.5	**48.3**	41.1
Car as the driver	54.5	**63.4**	46.0	**54.1**
Car as a passenger	**10.2**	9.4	**12.1**	11.1
Walking	**4.1**	4.0	**4.9**	4.6
Bus (includes street cars)	5.1	**6.4**	5.4	**6.9**
Subway/train (includes commute)	2.6	3.2	2.2	**2.6**
Other	3.5	3.5	3.3	3.1
Total	1440	1440	1440	1440

Note. For each significant pair, the larger category is **bolded**.

Data derived from Statistics Canada (2005).

impact" (HRSDC, 2008, p. 1). Beyond stress, *feelings* about family time and work appear more prominent in distinguishing between the balanced and imbalanced than objective characteristics such as demographics and time allocations.

That the degree of satisfaction with work and family life balance is inextricably related to the experience and feelings of stress is immediately obvious in Table 8-3. In both 1998 and 2005, the top two segmenting variables were "time crunch" and "stated stress," with three additional stress or rush-related variables. It is notable that between 1998 and 2005, balance-related concerns appeared to have taken a slight shift from family driven toward work driven. In 2005, "feelings about main activity" and "constantly under stress" moved ahead of "time with family and friends" and "spending of nonwork/family time." Satisfaction with life as a whole ranked seventh in each year. Of the remaining variables, 1998 had one variable unique to it, "feelings about finances." "Hours worked the last 7 days" emerged in the 2005 data set, but was not present in 1998. Also present in 2005 was a willingness to change work hours by giving up hours for less pay. Such changes reflect an improved employment environment.

Time demand, both in terms of duration and scheduling, varies among the life roles people have. As the number of roles expands, it can be expected that time becomes more fragmented, and timing will create organizational problems as one tries to schedule work time, family time, social and community time, and personal time. Excessive or conflicting roles can create considerable stress, reducing both health and one's sense of happiness or life satisfaction. In contrast, individuals are likely to experience role balance if they have "a set of equally positive commitments to all their typical roles" (Marks & MacDermid, 1996, p. 421).

Balance and Happiness

Both the 1998 and 2005 GSS contained a question concerning perceived happiness, which can be used to shed light on the relationship between balance and well-being (Figure 8-2). Balance and happiness are clearly connected. In both 1998 and 2005, individuals who indicated they were unhappy were more than twice as likely to feel their work and family life were out of balance. Looked at in another way, in both years, 1998 and 2005, over three-quarters (75.9% and 78.7%, respectively) of happy individuals claimed they had a balanced work–family life. In contrast for the same years, half or less, (46.2% and 50.7%) of the unhappy indicated such balance.

Balance, Age, and Gender

Is the perception of balance affected by age and gender? The degree of satisfaction with work-home balance varies with both age and gender. There is a clear nonlinear relationship between age and balance, with younger and older individuals registering higher levels of satisfaction than individuals in the 25 to 44 year age group. Table 8-8 presents the findings related to single years of age (grouped by CHAID), gender, and balance from the 1998 Statistics Canada data set. Similar age data were not available for 2005.

The age groupings in Table 8-8 were calculated by CHAID in relation to the dependent variable balance. They do not conform to the standard 10-year groupings typically used, because the groupings were specifically determined in relation to stated balance. It is also notable that the age groupings are different for men and women. The age group 29–48 for men is broken into two groups for women: 29–42 and 42–48. Also, in the actual analysis, all six groups were used for men, while two sets of combined groups, the youngest and oldest groups, were combined for women. These groupings indicate a higher level of imbalance for women in the two groups. Women ages 42-48 registered the highest level (35.7%) of work–home imbalance. The second highest level (29.3% and 29.6% for men and women respectively) was for the 29-48 year age group for men, but for the 29–42 year age group for women. Relative to men, women register a higher ratio of imbalanced work-home life, for each age group (see Table 8-8).

Gender affects balance in two ways. First, at all ages women experience lower levels of perceived satisfaction than men. Second, the age structure of satisfaction with balance differs between men and women. There was no difference in balance across ages 29 to 48 for men, who registered 29.3% imbalanced. For women aged 29 to 42, the imbalanced rate was comparable to that of men, 29.6%. However, for women 42–48, the rate jumped to 36.7%—the highest rate recorded. There is a need for greater understanding of the age-gender dynamics relating to balance. The similarities and differences can generate both positive and negative effects in terms of understanding and support between partners. If both are experiencing the same level of imbalance, they may be able to understand how the other feels. On the other hand, a difference may cause misunderstanding.

Another aspect of balance relates to temporal scheduling of activities in relation to social times (work, store, daycare hours) and time with others. Finding mutual time together requires coordination in time and space (Larson & Zemke, 2003). Individuals moving through stages of the life course can face challenges in achieving coordinated daily schedules (Larson & Zemke, 2003). Temporal scheduling may serve to bring partners together or keep them apart and becomes increasingly complex as the schedules of other household members are taken into account (Larson and

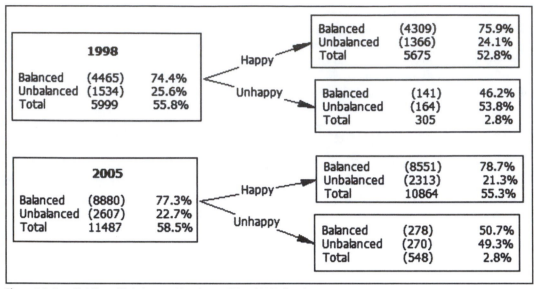

Figure 8-2. Stated job/home life balance and happiness, 1998 and 2005, Canada.

Zemke, 2003). Yet scheduling common time is important, since family closeness has been found to be enhanced by togetherness in both household and leisure activities (Garhammer, 1995).

DISCUSSION

Events form the foundation of time-use studies. Captured as diary entries, events show at any given time not only what individuals are doing but where they are and who they are with. The latter may be as important for life balance as what they are doing. Balance and time use must be viewed in terms of activities in context. People considering their life balanced between job and home, relative to those feeling imbalanced, engage in more events at home and someone else's home, and with household members and friends, and fewer events at work and alone. Individuals feeling imbalanced engage in more events alone, with household children, at work, and driving a car. They also engage in relatively more daily events in the evening, as work crowds out other events during the day. The daily time allocation of balanced and imbalanced workers across social space and social circle follows pretty well the pattern exhibited by the event data. Imbalanced workers spend about an hour more per day on work or commuting and spend relatively less time on virtually all other events. Imbalanced workers spend more time alone and with nonhousehold persons, the major share of whom are work colleagues. Hence, the picture painted by the time-use context data provides objective reasons for the feelings of individuals with respect to their sense of balance.

As individuals invest their time in one area such as contracted time, other areas have less time due to the "zero sum property of time" (Robinson, 1999, p. 55). Workers with balance allocated significantly more time to necessary and free time activities, while imbalanced workers allocated more to contracted and committed activities. The heavier time allocation to productive (contracted and committed) activities lead to a significant shortage of time allocated to virtually all free-time activities. More problematic, due to health considerations, was the smaller amount of necessary time, primarily sleep, registered by workers feeling imbalanced. Over the period from 1998 to 2005, contracted and necessary time increased (particularly sleep), while committed and free time decreased for both balanced and unbalanced workers. These changes are consistent with the improved employment environment in 2005. The net effect was an increase in productive time and decrease in free time.

Table 8-8

WORK/HOME LIFE BALANCE BY GENDER AND AGE, WORKING POPULATION, CANADA 1998

AGE GROUP	BALANCE	IMBALANCED	AGE GROUP	BALANCE	IMBALANCED
Men	%	%	*Women*	%	%
15–22	87.7	12.3	15–22,	77	23
22–29	75.6	24.4	22–29	77	23
29–48	70.7	29.3	29–42	70.4	29.6
48–55	77.4	22.6	42–48	64.3	35.7
55–62	85.5	14.5	48–55	75.8	24.2
62–80	95.4	4.6	55–62	86.0	14.0
Total	75.6	24.4	62–80	86.0	14.0
			Total	73.2	26.8

Note. Data derived from Statistics Canada (1998)

Compared with balanced workers, not only did imbalanced workers show more stress, they also were considerably more likely to be unhappy. Between 1998 and 2005, however, there was a decline in imbalanced workers and in the share of imbalanced workers who were unhappy. Does lack of balance arise from one or more areas getting crowded out as individuals fail to properly adjust priorities and time use as they move through life's course?

These findings have provided insights into how time use differs relative to individuals' evaluations of their life balance and how people feel regarding their time use. Earlier studies have shown that a person's gender, age, presence or absence of a spouse, or age of children have an impact on his or her time use. This chapter has examined objective and subjective contextual variables with a focus on balance that can provide further insights into time use across the life course. The probability of imbalance is highest between ages 25–54 years, peaking in the range of ages 25–44 year, the period of career and family building. This data coincides with our previous work that showed age 55 years as a turning point at which contracted work starts to diminish relative to other activities.

Particularly noteworthy is the increased sense of imbalance between 1998 and 2005 by individuals older than age 55 years whose probability of imbalance increased relative to those younger than age 55 years whose probability decreased.

It was noted that there is an unsettled question as to whether, over time, there has been an increase in work time or an increase in leisure time or little change in either. The answer ultimately depends on the population referent. For some population groups, work is increasing, for others leisure or necessary time is increasing.

We suggest that two forces are major contributors to one's sense of balance. One force is the diminished time at home and with one's spouse combined with the increased time spent with children, on work travel, and at the workplace. These conditions enhance stress and are a prime predictor of feelings of imbalance between one's job and home life. Secondly, there is reason to believe that the sense of imbalance is due to complexity generated by role responsibility. It is reasonable to assume that the greater the complexity of one's role, the individual has a greater number of transitions that, according to Michelson (1985), tend to generate stress. The presence of children in particular was a major contributor to the sense of imbalance. The time demands their presence imposes are both chronic and acute. Chronically, children add a greater number of recurring transitions that can be planned in which people are coming, going, and interacting. Acutely, unexpected events happen and they seem to happen more often when children are around, interrupting tasks and creating unplanned transitions.

CONCLUSIONS

The findings presented in this chapter indicate that the majority of time use is similar between respondents who perceived balance and those who perceived imbalance. The key differences include more time allocated to activities such as work, commuting to work, being at the workplace, and caring for children. However, as revealed by segmentation analysis, these factors do not appear to directly generate the sense of imbalance. Rather, the shift from perceived balance between work and home to perceived imbalance appears to be driven by subjective forces relating to stress and the lack of time for family and friends.

Research indicates that time use may have a weekly rhythm affecting how people perceive the days of the week and their time expenditure in relation to balance or imbalance (Zuzanek & Smale, 1999) . This study showed a relationship between starting times over the day and perceived balance. Our previous work, that of others, and the work here suggests a long-cycle rhythm in terms of the life course in which demands and responsibilities shift. The concept of balance and imbalance needs further exploration in relation to daily and weekly life course patterns of individuals who are working, not working, with children, and without children, and how such patterns relate to personal stress and happiness. The question of when these time shifts occur, and how they affect perceptions of balance, needs to be explored within the context of the various roles a person acquires across their life course.

REFERENCES

Andrews, F. M., & Morgan, J. N. (1971). *Multiple classification analysis: A report on a computer program for multiple regression using categorical predictors.* Ann Arbor: Survey Research Center, University of Michigan.

Apps, P., & Rees, R. (2005). Gender, time use, and public policy over the life cycle. *Oxford Review of Economic Policy, 21*(3), 439-461.

Bittman, M., & Wajcman, J. (2000). The rush hour: The character of leisure time and gender equity. *Social Forces, 79,* 165-189.

Bureau of Labor Statistics (2008). *American time use study.* Retrieved on May 25, 2008, from http://www.bls.gov/tus/.

Christiansen, C., & Matuska, K. (2006). Lifestyle balance: A review of concepts and research. *Journal of Occupational Science, 13,* 49-61.

Crawford, D. W., Godbey, G., & Crouter, A. C. (1986). The stability of leisure preferences. *Journal of Leisure Research, 18,* 96-115.

Elliot, D. H., Harvey, A .S., & McDonald, W. S. (1984). *Where does the day go? Time use of labour force aged Canadians.* Ottawa, ON: Employment and Immigration Canada.

Fast, J., & Frederick, J. (1998). *The time of our lives: Juggling work and leisure over the life cycle.* Catalogue no. 89-584-MIE, No. 4, Ottawa, ON: Statistics Canada.

Fast, J., & Frederick, J. (2004). *Days of our lives: Time use and transitions over the life course.* Catalogue no. 89-584-MIE2003004. Ottawa, ON: Statistics Canada.

Garhammer, M. (1995). Changes in work hours in Germany: The resulting impact on everyday life. *Time Sociology, 4,* 167-203.

Gershuny, J. (1999). *Changing times.* Oxford: Oxford Press.

Harvey, A. S., & Mukhopadhyay, A. K. (2007). When twenty-four hours is not enough: Time poverty of working parents. *Social Indicators Research. 82,* 57-77.

Harvey A. S., & Pentland, W. (2004). What do people do? In C. H. Christiansen & E. A. Townsend (Eds., pp. 63–90), *Introduction to occupation.* Upper Saddle River, NJ: Prentice Hall.

Harvey, A. S., & Singleton, J. F. (1989). Activity patterns across the lifespan. *Canadian Journal on Aging, 8,* 268–285.

Harvey, A. S., & Singleton, J. F. (1995). Stages of lifecycle and time spent in activities. *Journal of Occupational Science: Australia, 2,* 3-12.

Harvey, A. S., & Taylor, E. M. (2000). Activity settings and travel behavior: A social contact perspective. *Transportation, 27,* 53-73.

House, J. S. (2001) Understanding social factors and inequalities in health: 20th century progress and 21st century prospects. *Journal of Health and Social Behavior, 43*(June), 125–142.

Human Resources and Social Development Canada. (2008). *Work/life balance and new workplace challenges—Frequently asked questions for individuals.* Retrieved May 25, 2008, http://www.hrsdc.gc.ca/en/lp/spila/wlb/faq/01individuals.shtml#1

Larson, E. A., & Zemke, R. (2003). Shaping the temporal patterns of our lives: Social coordination of occupation. *Journal of Occupational Science, 10,* 80–89.

Matuska, K., & Christiansen, C. (2008). A proposed model of lifestyle balance. *Journal of Occupational Science, 15,* 9–19.

Marks, S. R., & MacDermid, S. M. (1996). Multiple roles and the self: A theory of role balance. *Journal of Marriage & Family, 58,* 417–432.

Michelson, W. (1985). *From sun to sun: Daily obligations and community structure in the lives of employed women and their families.* Totowa, NJ: Rowman & Allanheld.

Putnam, R. (1995). Bowling alone: America's declining social capital. *Journal of Democracy, 6,* 65–78.

Robinson, J. P., & Godbey, G. (1997). *Time for life.* University Park, PA: Pennsylvania State University Press.

Robinson, J. P. (1999). The time diary method structure and uses. In W. E. Pentland, A. S. Harvey, M. P. Lawton, & M. A. McColl (Eds.), *Time use research in the social sciences.* New York: Kluwer Academic/Plenum.

Schor, J. (1993). *The overworked Americans.* New York: Basic Books.

Shaw, S. (1985). The meaning of leisure in everyday life. *Leisure Sciences, 7,* 1-24.

Statistics Canada. (1998). *General social survey, cycle 12—Time use survey user's guide.* Ottawa, ON: Statistics Canada. Retrieved April 21, 2008, from http://www.statcan.gc.ca/bsolc/olc-cel/olc-cel?lang=eng&catno=12M0012G

Statistics Canada. (2005). *General social survey , cycle 19—Time use survey user's guide.* Ottawa, ON: Statistics Canada. Retrieved February 4, 2008, from http://www.statcan.gc.ca/bsolc/olc-cel/olc-cel?lang=eng&catno=12M0019X

Stone, L., & Harvey, A. S. (2000). Gender differences in transitions to total-work retirement. In V. W. Marshal, W. R. Heinz, H. Kruger, & A. Verma (Eds.), *Restructuring work and the life course.* Toronto: University of Toronto Press.

Szalai, A. (1972). *The use of time: Daily activities of urban and suburban populations in twelve countries.* Mouton: The Hague.

Zick, C. D., & McCullough J. L. (2004). Trends in married couples' time use: Evidence from 1977–78 and 1987–88. *Sex Roles, 24,* 459-487.

Zuzanek, J., & Box, S. J. (1988). Life course and the daily lives of older adults in Canada. In K. Altegrott (Ed.), *Daily life in later life.* Newbury Park: Sage.

Zuzanek, J., & Mannell, R. (1998). Life-cycle squeeze, time pressure, daily stress and leisure participation: A Canadian perspective. *Society and Leisure, 21,* 513–544.

Zuzanek, J., & Smale, B. J. A. (1999). Life-cycle and across the week allocation of time to daily activities. In W. E. Pentland, A. S. Harvey, M. P. Lawton, & M. A. McColl (Eds.), *Time use research in the social sciences* (pp. 127–153). New York: Kluwer Academic/Plenum.

Aspects of Daily Occupations That Promote Life Balance Among Women in Sweden

LENA-KARIN ERLANDSSON AND CARITA HÅKANSSON

INTRODUCTION

What constitutes a balanced, healthy, everyday life is a question increasingly present in popular science and everyday discussions in many of today's societies. In part, this is because perceived stress and stress-related disorders are growing (World Health Organization [WHO], 2001) and in Sweden stress has been recognized as a public health problem, especially among women (Socialstyrelsen, 2005). Despite this, there is no consensus about what is required by the individual or which conditions are needed in everyday life to achieve a healthy balance in life. In this chapter, we discuss the concept of *balance* from an occupational perspective. The term *occupation*, as used in this chapter, can be defined as "the ordinary and familiar things that people do every day" (American Occupational Therapy Association, 1995, p. 1015). Our focus is the daily occupations of Swedish women of working age, and we will explore the concept of balance considering the patterns of daily occupations. First, we will discuss and analyze the *structural* aspect, that is, occupational balance in women's patterns of daily occupations. Second, we will describe the *experiential* aspects reported by healthy women and by women with stress-related disorders in their patterns. Finally, we will show how these aspects are related to women's overall health and well-being.

Based on the theoretical framework of the Value and Meaning in Occupations Model (ValMO; Persson, Erlandsson, Eklund, & Iwarsson, 2001), we assume that experiences in everyday life are shaped by the individual's previous experiences in life as well as their conceptions about the future. Women evaluate their everyday experiences in a context that includes reflection on their earlier experiences in life and images of their future. We conclude with a presentation of occupational risk factors and suggestions for promoting healthy balanced everyday lives for women of working age.

PERSPECTIVES ON BALANCE

The concept of *balance* can be viewed in various ways. In ordinary terms, people often assume balance to be a state of equilibrium and, consequently, things that have equal proportions are considered to be well-balanced. From an occupational perspective, however, it is difficult to apply

K. Matuska & C. Christiansen (Eds.)
Life balance: Multidisciplinary theories and research (pp 115–130)
© 2009 SLACK Incorporated and AOTA Press

this kind of reasoning. There is little logic in expecting the time spent in different occupations, such as working, cleaning the house, going to the movies, filling the car with gas, getting dressed, and walking the dog, to take up an equal amount of an individual's time during a day, a week, or even a lifetime. The things we do occupy different proportions of our time. Thus, when it comes to everyday time use and occupations, balance seems to be about something other than a state of equilibrium. Another assumption is that balance or imbalance is related to what you are doing and how you experience your occupations rather than the proportion of time spent doing certain things.

The micro-, meso-, and macro-perspectives in the ValMO model (Persson et al., 2001) can be useful when investigating balance in daily occupations. According to the model, each occupation consists of a series of actions. Balance in this micro-perspective is of less importance because the stress resulting from a single action is easily compensated for by better conditions in later tasks.

The meso-perspective is more important and refers to occupations performed over days, weeks, and months. This perspective is made up of so-called *patterns of daily occupations* defined as all the occupations, including sleep that an individual performs during a 24-hour period, including the temporal and internal relationships among the occupations (Erlandsson, 2003). In these patterns, some occupations dominate in terms of time and awareness, while others are performed without any conscious thought. For example, having to give a talk at an important meeting might dominate your day in terms of awareness and effort, while having a cup of coffee between this meeting and the next may pass without any consideration at all. In patterns of daily occupations, some occupations can also be performed simultaneously (Davies, 1990), such as helping children with homework while cooking dinner, or may be enfolded (Bateson, 1996), such as, ironing and watching television at the same time.

Other researchers have offered various definitions of balance in the patterns of daily occupations. For example, it has been stated that occupational balance can mean variation in work, household chores, and recreation (e.g., Christiansen, 1996; Farnworth, 2003) or a balance between active occupations and sleep (e.g., Leufstadius, Erlandsson, & Eklund, 2006). However, these examples fail to consider personal experience or meaning in daily occupations. According to the ValMO model, each performance of an occupation is unique, giving a unique experience on every single occasion (Persson et al., 2001), and studies have shown that this subjective-experience component is related to health and well-being (Christiansen, 2000; Law, Steinwender, & Leclair, 1998; Wilcock et al., 1997). In the ValMO model (Persson et al., 2001), the lifestyle balance model (Matuska & Christiansen, 2008), and the model of lifestyle performance (Velde & Fidler, 2002), it is assumed that the experience of occupational balance depends on the individual's perception of a pleasurable combination of daily occupations in the daily pattern. Furthermore, Håkansson, Dahlin-Ivanoff, and Sonn (2006) have shown that a variation among experiences of obligation, enjoyment, and rest is an important prerequisite of occupational balance. Thus, in investigating balance in patterns of daily occupations, it may be important not only to consider the time spent in different occupations and the temporal relationships between different occupations but also to take into consideration the unique experiences of carrying out those occupations. Furthermore, the ValMO model suggests that experiences in the meso-perspective add up to form experiences of meaning in the macro-perspective (Persson et al., 2001). The macro-perspective is the total of all patterns of daily occupations performed in an individual's lifetime. Having a balanced life in this perspective would mean living, and having lived, a life—so far—that contains a combination of occupations corresponding to the individual's needs and desires in different stages of life.

Occupational repertoires, that is, the range of occupations performed daily, are influenced by age, gender, and culture. Thus the occupational repertoires of toddlers, teenagers, and senior citizens differ considerably. In Sweden, working women report being responsible for most of the daily household chores, whereas men reported having the main responsibility for the car, home maintenance, and household finances (Berntsson, Lundberg, & Krantz, 2006). Women of working age typically spend 77.7 hours each week in paid and unpaid work, while men spend 71.1 hours each week (Berntsson et al., 2006). Another illustration is the study by Håkansson and Ahlborg (2008). They found that absence of stress at work was the strongest predictor of good self-rated health among men in a general population. The strongest predictors of good self-rated health among women, however, were absence of stress in the patterns of daily occupations and, aside from having energy for paid work, having energy left to pursue unpaid work (e.g., household chores) and leisure activities.

Consequently, a balanced female repertoire may be slightly different from that of a male. According to several researchers, the prevailing explanation of increased ill health among women in the working population is their high total workload, including both paid and unpaid work (e.g., Lundberg & Frankenhaeuser, 1999; Orth-Gomér, 2003). For example, working women with children are constantly striving to achieve a balance between the demands of their job and the demands related to caring for children, home, and family (Elvin-Nowak, 1998). There are examples of other studies indicating that the specific situation of working mothers, in terms of paid and unpaid work, causes symptoms that could affect their health and well-being (e.g., Hallman, 2003; Johansson, Hamberg, Westmans, & Lindgren, 1999).

Self-rated health appears to be connected with engaging in certain occupations in time, as well as the experience of engaging in these occupations. Therefore, the focus in this chapter is on women of working age and their patterns of daily occupations, that is, what they do and how they experience it. Finally, we will suggest aspects promoting balance in daily occupations that in turn may lead to life balance.

WOMEN'S PATTERNS OF DAILY OCCUPATIONS

Most people who work or study have a balanced variation in the type of everyday occupations they perform. However, it may still be difficult to find the time to perform them all in a satisfying way and to experience balance. This is especially true for working mothers who have to juggle the challenges of a job, child care, and housework. For these women, balance would not simply be a matter of spending equal amounts of time in paid or unpaid work but in making all their daily occupations fit into 24 hours. A feeling of balance may instead be equated with being in control and feeling temporal harmony in their everyday tasks. It can be assumed that minor daily stressors result from the complexity of juggling multiple demands on time, dealing with interruptions and changes in occupations, and having too many things to do in a limited amount of time. For example, multiple interruptions and a feeling of lack of time may cause a feeling of imbalance and gradually lead to ill health. On the other hand, having a balanced repertoire of occupations that fit the time available, where occupations can be carried out without interruptions and are thus experienced positively by the doer, would be related to better health and well-being. To confirm these assumptions, the experience of everyday life must first be operationalized to describe and analyze the complexities and time limitations that women report.

The easiest way to analyze occupations is to map them on a *linear time* scale, assuming that occupations take place one after another and can be identified, scheduled, and quantified. This linear perspective is appealing, but reality is much more complicated. The conflict between what is actually being performed and what is measurable is striking. The starting and ending points of single occupations can be difficult to identify, some occupations may be being performed simultaneously or may be enfolded, and, in addition, occupations shape the experience of time (Zemke & Clark, 1996). Time flies when you are deeply engaged in an occupation, and you lose perception of how much time has passed. Likewise, an occupation may be experienced as lasting forever if it is difficult or unpleasant. Taking the subway to work every day may not be regarded as especially time consuming, except when a problem occurs. Even if the delay is only 10 minutes, it may seem like hours before the problem is fixed, and the train finally moves again. Furthermore, women's time has been characterized as cyclic (Davies, 1990), in that many of their chores keep coming back and are never really finished.

Another term used in describing women's time use is process time. *Process time* is the opposite of linear time, in which one thing is done after another. Process time means a constant readiness to respond to the needs of others (Hirdman, 1999), irrespective of one's own intentions, as well as having to wait for others. For example, caring for infants and toddlers or family members who are sick can hardly be planned for or scheduled. Thus, being in process time may result in instability in the flow of regular daily occupations.

In an attempt to describe working mothers' daily patterns of occupations, Erlandsson and Eklund (2001) applied four different methods of data collection to one woman's everyday occupations. The methods were a 24-hour diary, direct observation, video documentation, and an experience sampling method. All the data obtained from the diary, observation, video, and experience sampling were transformed into time and occupation logs describing what was performed and at what time. For each set of data, the notes concerning doing and time were arranged chronologically and the principles of latent content analysis (Sommer & Sommer, 1997) were applied. Category development was inductive in the sense that no previously formulated aspects were used, except for the formulated objective of determining the elements of a pattern of daily occupations. In the first step of analysis, single occupations were identified. In the second step, the actions that were the building blocks of each occupation were identified. Lastly, bearing in mind the pattern of occupations as a whole, the final analysis centered on how occupations were ordered in relation to each other.

The analysis revealed that the building blocks of a pattern of daily occupations consisted of a mixture of actions, performed in integrated or separate sequences, in turn forming occupations (Erlandsson & Eklund, 2001). Thus, the flow of actions created a complex fabric of several actions related to continuously performed occupations. Furthermore, the same occupation (e.g., cooking dinner) on different occasions was made up of different action sequences. In one case, the woman in the study was constantly interrupted by her children, dogs, and husband while cooking dinner. In another situation the woman was preparing the same dish but was able to concentrate on the cooking without being disturbed.

The analysis revealed that the pattern of daily occupations was dominated, in time and awareness, by a few *main occupations*. Intertwined with the main occupations were *hidden occupations* (e.g., emptying the dishwasher, making the bed). The hidden occupations belonged to the rhythm of the daily pattern but were performed between the main occupations and with apparently less attention from the performer. A third category of occupations was identified and called *unexpected occupations*. Such occupations were unforeseen in the pattern of daily occupations and interrupted the ongoing rhythm of main and hidden occupations. The three categories made up the weft in the daily fabric of occupations, forming unique patterns in time from day to day.

Time-Geographic Perspective on Women's Everyday Life

Viewing everyday experiences as a pattern of occupations organized in time is well established within the time-geographic methodology. One of the basic assumptions of time-geography is that everything takes place somewhere and that it takes time for everything to happen (Ellegård, 1999). In time-geography this is often illustrated as three related vectors in a diagram, one vector for time, one for the activity, and one for the place where the activity takes place. The time-geography method has its origin in Sweden and was developed by Hägerstrand (1978). It is usually applied in community planning and studies of women, but the idea of visually illustrating people's activities in relation to time can also be found in connection with health care. Adolph Meyer, a physician and a founder of occupational therapy, suggested that health-care professionals should fill out life charts for their patients because he believed that life events detected in this way could be of importance for a variety of physical illnesses (Cohen, Kessler, & Gordon, 1995). Life charts included notations of significant life events and the dates that they occurred in the life history of a patient. A life chart was made by interviewing the patient about crucial events in his or her life and marking these events on a timeline from birth until present time. Applied in an occupational perspective, Meyer's life charts may be viewed as reflecting the individual's occupational patterns from a lifecourse perspective. However, research has shown that it may not be the major traumatic and stressful events in a life that cause illness (e.g., Thoits, 1983). Instead, attention is being turned toward the cumulative effects of long-term, minor daily stressors on people's health (Eckenrode & Bolger, 1995). Thus, in the patterns of daily occupations, minor daily stressors, such as interruptions and time pressure, may result in experiencing imbalance and constitute a risk of ill health.

Furthermore, the complexity of the pattern of daily occupations revealed in the detailed description of one woman's day mentioned above serves as an illustration of the time-geography concept called the *packing dilemma* (Friberg, 1993). This means that the single occupations are not stressors in themselves, but packing them all into the frame of everyday life may lead to stress. The packing dilemma could be an occupational risk factor causing ill health. This leads to the question of whether it is possible to detect a limit for the number of occupations that can be crammed in before ill-health ensues.

Comparing Levels of Complexity in Women's Patterns of Daily Occupations

Time-use studies using identified behavior patterns to determine the characteristics of certain groups of people have been published previously (Farnworth, 2003; Stone, 1972). However, time-use studies do not consider the temporal relationships between single occupations. A process for characterizing patterns of daily occupations in terms of time-and-occupation graphs has been developed for studies of working women's patterns of daily occupations (Erlandsson, Rögnvaldsson, & Eklund, 2004). These graphs were found to be useful for comparing similarities and differences between actual patterns of daily occupations and those thought to constitute a healthy, balanced pattern of daily occupations.

One hundred working, cohabitant mothers with at least one child of preschool age were interviewed (Erlandsson et al., 2004) by means of *yesterday diaries* (Pentland, Harvey, Lawton, & McColl, 1999); that is, they reported what they did the day before. The women were encouraged to be as detailed as possible when recounting their activities of the previous day, which spanned from getting up in the morning to falling asleep at night. In addition, the women rated the day according to how well it represents their everyday type of day, from 1, meaning *not at all*, to a rating 5, meaning *absolutely*. On average, women gave these days a rating of 4.5. Thus the collected days data were considered representative examples from the women's everyday life. The women's descriptions were analyzed and their reported occupations were categorized. The three categories used to illustrate the pattern of daily occupations in graphs were main, hidden, and unexpected occupations. A fourth category, sleep, was used to indicate nonawake occupation time.

The time-and-occupation graphs, illustrating patterns of daily occupations, were further analyzed by means of a process based on visual inspection. The process is called *recognition of similarities* (ROS; Erlandsson et al., 2004). Each woman's pattern was compared, in pairs randomly sampled by a computer, with all the other women's patterns (in all 4,950 comparisons) to identify similarities and within groups, similar patterns. This resulted in three distinct subgroups of patterns of daily occupations being discerned among the 100 patterns: 12 of typically low complexity, 23 of typically medium complexity, and 24 of typically high complexity. The remaining 41 women's patterns were considered atypical and did not fit into any of the typical groups. Using the Mann–Whitney U Test (Mann & Whitney, 1947), it was determined that the group of women with heterogeneous patterns did not have a statistically significant difference from the groups of women with typical patterns, according to health, well-being, or lifestyle variables (Erlandsson & Eklund, 2006).

The women whose daily patterns of occupations were categorized as being of low complexity reported that their time was dominated by a few main occupations that were seldom or never interrupted by unexpected or hidden occupations (Figure 9-1).

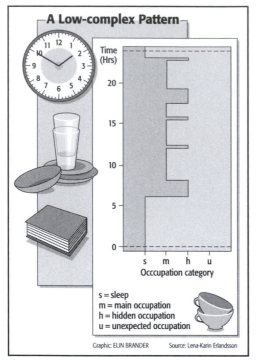

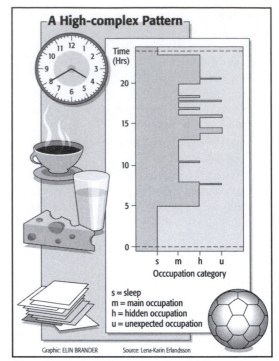

Figure 9-1. A typical low–complex pattern of daily occupations.

Figure 9-2. A typical high–complex pattern of daily occupations.

Among the women classified as having moderately complex patterns of daily occupations, some were disturbed during sleeping hours and had unexpected occupations in their daily patterns. The women whose patterns of daily occupations were characterized as highly complex reported both hidden and unexpected occupations and frequent interruptions of main and hidden occupations (Figure 9-2).

Thus far, we have shown how women's occupations can be described as main, hidden, and unexpected. We have also presented a method for characterizing working mothers' everyday situations according to the complexity of their patterns of daily occupations, based on their reported yesterday diaries. These are, however, measurements from an observer's perspective giving information on the visualized patterns. The actual experiences of the women are not elucidated.

Empirical results such as those reported by Håkansson et al. (2006) show that patterns of daily occupations can be experienced as balanced or imbalanced. The variation in the complexity of patterns of daily occupations (Erlandsson et al., 2004) described earlier confirms this assumption. It is probably particularly important to integrate paid work with additional occupations. Other studies have shown that work is a central part of women's daily patterns of occupations when they experience good health (Håkansson et al., 2003; 2005).

It can be concluded that patterns of daily occupations are unique to each individual, no matter how the occupations are categorized, and occupational balance seems to be an important consideration in a healthy, balanced, everyday life. Besides this structural aspect, experiential aspects are of great importance for a healthy balanced life and are discussed in the following section.

WOMEN'S EXPERIENCES REGARDING PATTERNS OF DAILY OCCUPATIONS

Studies of the relationships between occupation and health usually focus on categories of occupations or a single daily occupation, (e.g., drinking tea) (Hannam, 1997). One exception is a qualitative study in which Piskûr, Kinebanian, and Josephsson (2002) explored Slovenians' patterns of daily occupations. The findings of this study indicated that health was closely related to occupational balance, meaning, and control. Both men and women were studied together and the researchers did not show how women in particular experienced their patterns of daily occupations.

Women, however, were the focus of a qualitative study (Håkansson et al., 2006) in which women's patterns of daily occupations and well-being were explored. The women were of working age and had completed the first phase of recovery from a stress-related disorder. These women were chosen for the study because it was hypothesized that they would have gained valuable insight during their process of recovery. The findings were based on discussions with 19 women in five focus groups.

A combination of occupational balance, manageability, control, and meaning in relation to patterns of daily occupations seemed to be a prerequisite for the women's well-being. Furthermore, the findings showed that the women's occupational self-image influenced their daily occupations, which in turn influenced the women's well-being. The term *occupational self-image* was defined as the image of the self in relation to occupation (Håkansson et al., 2006). The occupations of everyday life seem to be the primary means through which people are able to communicate their image of their occupational selves to themselves and others. People use occupations to achieve a sense of being the person they want to be.

Experiences of Control and Manageability

Håkansson et al. (2006) found that the women in their study had developed different strategies to control occupational choices and to increase manageability in relation to patterns of daily occupations. *Manageability* means perceiving that the demands of daily occupations do not exceed the personal and contextual resources the individual can mobilize (Lazarus & Folkman, 1984). Control includes opportunities for reflection and the freedom to choose which occupations to pursue (Velde & Fidler, 2002). Furthermore, being able to influence or control one's situation results in a positive feeling (Townsend, 2007; Schultz & Schkade, 1992; Yerxa, 1998). However, control and manageability also depend on opportunities and obstacles provided by the context, which makes it impossible for people to control all the circumstances that affect their lives (Townsend, 2007). The strategies the women used included allowing themselves to be completely present, changing their level of ambition, prioritizing reciprocal relationships, getting a grasp of the structure of everyday life, and demanding that others respect their choices and the time needed to complete their chosen occupations. These strategies helped the women use their own values, needs, and resources to determine in which occupations they engaged (Håkansson et al., 2006).

In allowing themselves to be fully present, the women became focused and aware of the present, relaxed, rather than worrying whether this was the right thing to do or planning for or worrying about the next activity. Changing their level of ambition meant that they questioned their degree of responsibility in paid work, unpaid work, and relationships, and reduced it. Examples of this were ignoring some things, not worrying about appearances, leaving things half done, delaying things that had to be done, and still believing that things would be alright. Other examples included listening to other people without taking on their problems and only doing things for other people within certain limits. The third strategy they used was to leave one-sided relationships and prioritize reciprocal relationships. *Reciprocal relationships* are satisfying and stimulating social relationships in which both partners give and take. Another strategy was to get a grasp of the structure of everyday life. One way to do this was to write down, for example, in a diary, not only what they planned to do and whom they planned to meet, but also things they wanted to do as well as things they had to do, and to consider whether these were in accordance with their values, needs, and resources (Håkansson et al., 2006). Thus, it appears that two important considerations about whether the women's experiences in patterns of daily occupations constituted a healthy, balanced lifestyle were a (1) sense of control between the different occupations and (2) a sense of manageability in relation to all of them.

Experiences of Meaning

Scholars have found that when people engage in an occupation, it is more than just doing. Occupations are associated with meaning or value. Meaningful or valued occupations are characterized by how people understand or make sense of their experiences, and are uniquely individual and contextual. Occupations in everyday life are experienced as meaningful if they correlate with the individual's value orientation, that is, if they are experienced as good, important, and valuable to the individual (Hasselkus & Rosa, 1997).

Such experiences of value can be related to the results of a qualitative study among women with stress-related disorders (Håkansson et al., 2006). In this study, when experiences interpreted as being related to cultural meaning dominated the women's occupational choices—that is, the occupations they engaged in were mainly experienced as important or meaningful to others—they reported stress. However, when their personal interests dominated their occupational choices, and they experienced the occupations as personally meaningful, they reported greater well-being. Their personally meaningful occupations—for example, reciprocal relationships—were described as important, valuable, and intrinsically gratifying. That is, the women experienced pleasure, enjoyment, satisfaction, and self-improvement.

The occupations experienced as personally meaningful also included occupations in which they achieved a satisfying concrete result—for example, when they created something with their hands. Furthermore, for the women to experience an occupation as personally meaningful, it had to challenge their limits, be something that they were good at doing, or improve their performance. Personally meaningful or valued occupations were also experienced as sources of energy or restoration. The experiences in single occupations added up to experiences of meaning in the patterns of daily occupations (Persson et al., 2001). To achieve a healthy balanced life, it appears to be important that the patterns of daily occupations are experienced as meaningful.

Experiences of Hassles and Uplifts

Women's experiences in their patterns of daily occupations were also the subject of further investigation in the study of 100 working mothers presented earlier in this chapter. The concept of *hassles,* defined as perceived difficulties and irritations, and its opposite, *uplifts,* which denote pleasant experiences (Kanner, Coyne, Schaefer, & Lazarus, 1981), were used to detect positive and negative experiences in patterns of daily occupations. A self-report instrument called Targeted Hassles and Uplifts (THU; Erlandsson & Eklund, 2003a) was developed to reflect the occurrence of negative and positive experiences in everyday life. The participants formulated the target issues themselves and the process of filling out the instrument involved four steps. First, each woman was asked to write, on a blank sheet of paper, statements describing things that hassled her in everyday life. Second, she was requested to mark the five most annoying things, and third, to order these from 1 to 5, where 1 denoted the phenomenon she felt occurred most often in her everyday life. Lastly, each item was rated regarding the degree of hassle from *not at all* to *worst possible*. The same procedure was employed for uplifting occasions, although the scale was changed to include ratings from *not at all* to *the best that can happen*. The statements of hassles and uplifts were analyzed using content analysis.

The hassles reported by the women reflected their responsibility for home and children in combination with feelings of lack of time and difficult assignments at work. The women experienced hassles primarily in their social context, that is, their family and workmates, and they considered worries about their children to be one of the most irritating and disturbing hassles. Examples of hassles reported by the women were their children refusing to get dressed in the mornings, their husbands not helping with household chores, and interruptions by colleagues at work. The women also felt hassled by feeling responsible for the household, that is, having to plan for, shop for, and prepare dinner; clean the house; and do the laundry (Erlandsson & Eklund, 2003a). In contrast to men, women have been found to experience high levels of stress as a result of the complex interactions between paid work and circumstances related to their home and family situation (Lundberg, 1996). Men are usually stressed by conditions at their workplace. Furthermore, women have been described as more emotionally focused, and their level of stress thus increases in response to negative cultural pressures. Factors affecting women's experience of stress are often cumulative, for example, worries about sick children and household chores are added to problems at work (Stroud, Salovey, & Epel, 2002). Furthermore, the hassles experienced by working mothers were concerned with daily chores, lack of time, or events that caused delays and the upset of schedules (Erlandsson & Eklund, 2003a). In a way, the hassles described by these 100 women illustrate the need for strategies to maintain control and manageability, such as those reported by the women with stress-related disorders (Håkansson et al., 2006).

In analyzing the uplifting experiences in the women's patterns of daily occupations, it became evident that it is not the occupation itself that makes a difference. The experience of the occupation rather depends on the circumstances, that is, the experience of the specific sequence of actions when performed in a specific social and physical environment. The results showed that several occupations could be perceived as both hassling and uplifting. For example, both their physical environment, such as their home and place of work, and their daily occupations, such as cooking dinner or reading bedtime stories to children, generated hassles and uplifts. The women also reported aspects of work as being both hassling and uplifting. In other words, uplifts may be occupations and situations in women's patterns of daily occupations allowing for balance, manageability, and meaning.

FACTORS AFFECTING IMBALANCE IN WOMEN'S PATTERNS OF DAILY OCCUPATIONS AND ILL HEALTH

Humans need balance between different occupations, including variation in occupational categories as well as their duration (Wilcock, 2006). However, imbalance is always dependent on an individual's capacity, resources, interests, and responsibilities. In this section we will describe the factors we have found among women that might constitute risks of experiencing or developing imbalance and thus ill health. We found two main relationships between women's ill health and their pattern of daily occupations. First, the structure in patterns of daily occupations may affect self-rated poor health. The structure refers to how the daily occupations are organized in time. Second, women's ill health may depend on the amount of meaning, control, and manageability they have in their patterns of daily occupations.

Structure of Women's Patterns of Daily Occupations

Earlier we presented the ROS process as a method for categorizing women's patterns of daily occupations according to complexity (Erlandsson et al., 2004). This revealed three groups of women, who differed according to the complexity of their patterns. Erlandsson and Eklund (2006) formulated a hypothesis that a balanced, and therefore healthy, pattern of daily occupations, is where the occupations are organized with no or few interruptions and reasonably filled with varied occupations. They used nonparametric tests to compare groups exhibiting different levels of complexity in their pattern of daily occupations, and the Jonckheer–Terpstra test to see if an increasing level of complexity in patterns of daily occupations would lead to lower ratings of health and well-being. A linear trend was found with respect to self-rated health, indicating that an increasing level of complexity implied a lower rating of health (Erlandsson & Eklund, 2006). The working mothers who had a highly complex pattern of daily occupations reported a lower level of health than did mothers with a lower level of complexity. Thus, there seems to be a relationship between everyday patterns with frequent interruptions and changes in type of occupation and subjective health. This relationship applies specifically to working, cohabitant women with children of preschool age, but may be an illustration of a more general aspect of occupational imbalance and a risk factor for ill health.

The study of women with stress-related disorders (Håkansson et al., 2006) illuminated experiences that could be interpreted as reflecting the same phenomenon. These women experienced occupational imbalance when one or two occupations, mostly paid work and other obligations, dominated their patterns of daily occupations and took most of their time and energy. These women had no time or energy left for enjoyable occupations and rest, and reported feelings of stress and overload in the patterns of daily occupations. After a considerable time, these feelings of stress also correlated with long-term sick leave.

There are, however, additional illustrations of occupational structure affecting the experiences of health and well-being of the women in the previously described studies. For example, time limitations in the patterns of daily occupations were found to be one of the major themes among the working mothers' hassles, including lack of time, time pressure, and inflexibility (Erlandsson & Eklund, 2003a). Such time limitations might result in an additional occupational risk of ill health, namely occupational disruption or deprivation (Wilcock, 2006). In other words, certain circumstances may prevent the women from doing and enjoying things that they want to do. In addition, the perceived demands from the social and cultural environment could lead to denial of the women's own values or needs. Both were shown in the study of women with stress-related disorders (Håkansson et al., 2006), with the consequence that these women had no time or energy for enjoyable occupations and no time to rest.

A constant feeling of having too little time may result in passivity (Robinson & Godbey, 1997). For example, one may increase time spent watching television to escape from the pressures of daily life. This may be especially true in the case of women who feel that their freedom to choose what they want to do is restricted. Following this reasoning, women who experience time pressure would also be at risk of occupational imbalance, because of the risk of taking on too many passive or low-activity occupations.

Having imbalanced patterns of daily occupations with a structure that does not allow for reflection and variation in occupations may lead to a decrease in perceived meaning in everyday life. This phenomenon can be illustrated by the women with stress-related disorders, who felt their everyday lives were filled mostly with duties and obligations, which lead to an experience of stress and ill health (Håkansson et al., 2006). These women's descriptions indicated high complexity in their patterns because they felt they had to assume a high level of responsibility to ensure everything ran smoothly, both at work and at home. They also felt that they were responsible for the whole family, including parents, children, and grandchildren, as well as friends and colleagues. Consequently, they experienced no feelings of pleasure or enjoyment and no feelings of social belonging, but rather feelings of being exploited. They also felt they had no meaningful challenges or the opportunity to improve their skills and their daily occupations had no meaning or value.

Lack of Strategies to Manage and Control

It is unknown whether the stability reflected in the patterns of daily occupations of working mothers who reported low levels of complexity is the result of conscious strategies to control and manage their patterns of daily occupations or is the consequence of other circumstances.

However, strategies to manage and control seem to be useful because control appeared to be a crucial factor determining the extent to which the studied women experienced occupation-related hassles, and, in turn, how they rated their health and well-being (Erlandsson & Eklund, 2003b). The less control the women reported, the greater they perceived the severity of their hassles. Lack of control and manageability, that is not being able to decide what to do and how much time and energy to spend on different occupations, was also an important factor that influenced the feeling of ill health among women with stress-related disorders (Håkansson et al., 2006). The reason for this, according to the women, was their difficulty in saying no and setting limits on the spoken and unspoken demands due to feelings of guilt and fear of hurting someone's feelings.

An overall experience of lack of control and manageability is central to feeling stress, and a lack of control in the working environment has been found to constitute a risk of developing ill health. The demand/control model (Karasek & Theorell, 1990) is frequently mentioned in this context: Demands at work lead to feeling stress, whereas a feeling of being in control provides a buffer to stress. Similar to the demand/control model, those among the 100 working mothers who rated their sense of control as low typically had a low level of self-rated health (Erlandsson & Eklund, 2003b). Among women with stress-related disorders a lack of strategies to control and manage the every-day occupations lead to feelings of stress and ill-health (Håkansson et al., 2006). In these studies, no discrimination was made between control in relation to work and other occupations, but it has been shown elsewhere that women and men with low control either at work or at home may have an increased risk of developing depression and anxiety (Griffin, Fuhrer, Stansfeld, & Marmot, 2002).

An *internal locus of control* means that the individual can control the problems that occur in everyday situations (Theorell, 2003). An *external locus of control* means that the individual regards the possibility solving problems as being out of his or her hands. Applied to women's patterns of daily occupations, experiencing an internal locus of control would mean better ability to cope with complex and unstable patterns, while an external locus of control would lead to a higher risk of not being able to cope with the complexity of the pattern of daily occupations. The women with stress-related disorders allowed other people's demands to determine how they used their time and energy (Håkansson et al., 2006). Allowing this can also be seen as a form of external locus of control, although it controlled what the women actually did, not how they were allowed to handle it. We can thus conclude that not being able to control the choice of occupations and not having the ability to manage time and energy in daily occupations seem to be risk factors for poorer health in women.

Finally, the adequacy of the above-described findings among women was tested in another study by investigating whether a combination of occupational imbalance and lack of control, manageability, and meaning in women's patterns of daily occupations was related to perceived stress. Håkansson, Lissner, Björkelund, and Sonn (2009) surveyed 500 women of working age in a general Swedish population. The survey included questions on occupational experiences in the women's patterns of daily occupations, and, among other things, perceived stress. The findings confirmed previous findings. It was found that a combination of different experiences in women's patterns of daily occupations can be seen as risk factors for ill health and feelings of stress and overload. The results showed perceived stress was associated with a decreased ability to manage their daily occupations as well with occupational imbalance (Håkansson, et al., 2009).

BALANCE ASPECTS IN WOMEN'S PATTERNS OF DAILY OCCUPATIONS

As there are risk factors for imbalance, there are aspects that are important for maintaining or regaining balance in patterns of daily occupations. Such aspects may lead to improved health and well-being. In our studies we have uncovered several occupational aspects that seem to promote balance and health. These aspects are assembled in Table 9-1.

One successful strategy for experiencing control in the pattern of everyday occupations is a deliberate effort not to include too many occupations in one's schedule. The results presented by Erlandsson and Eklund (2006) indicated that such a strategy could also promote health because the women who had patterns of daily occupations that were classified as typically low complexity were found to have statistically significantly higher self-rated health.

Another means of experiencing control is to exercise occupational choices. The women with stress-related disorders emphasized how important it was that their values and needs guided their occupational choices. Furthermore, it was important for them to ensure that they had sufficient resources for both chosen and obligatory occupations (Håkansson et al., 2006).

It appears that the question of whether women's dual workload causes occupational balance or imbalance is related to personal and environmental conditions, not to the actual occupations performed. Achieving occupational balance is a question of fitting all types of occupations to the personal and contextual resources the individual is able to mobilize (Håkansson et al., 2009). Moreover, it is also important to have variation in the pattern of daily occupations and to do things that give energy and help the individual regain energy to maintain occupational balance. Enjoyable and recreational occupations as well as sleep are important ways of gaining energy (Håkansson et al., 2006). Thus, when personal choices and variation in the pattern of occupations can be accommodated by the personal and contextual resources of the individual, he or she is much more likely to experience meaning as well as balance in the pattern of daily occupations.

Women's experiences of health and well-being seem to be dependent on a combination of and the interaction among experiences of balance, meaning, and manageability in the patterns of daily occupations (Håkansson et al., 2009). However, if women do not have the ability to choose in which occupations to engage, it is unlikely that they will experience balance or meaning in their patterns of daily occupations. We therefore suggest that occupational balance, occupational meaning, manageability, choice, and control result in life balance and well-being. This is in line with the conclusions presented by Kielhofner (2002) and Backman (2004). They were of the opinion that the experience of balance reflects a dynamic interdependence between different occupations (occupational balance), and the occupations' relationship to an individual's internal values, interests, and goals (i.e., meaning, choice, and control), and to the external demands of the context (i.e., manageability). Matuska and Christiansen (2008) propose defining a *balanced lifestyle* as "a satisfying pattern of daily occupations that is healthful, meaningful, and sustainable to an individual within the context of his or her current life circumstances" (p. 9). The "satisfying pattern" in their model corresponds to "occupational balance" in ours. For this pattern to be sustainable for an individual within the context of his or her current life circumstances means that the opportunities and means for meeting needs vary according to the resources available within his or her given environments, and which corresponds to manageability in our model.

CONCLUSIONS

The studies presented in this chapter underline an additional aspect that is important for achieving balance in patterns of daily occupations, and that is the impact of the physical and social environment. Stress can be interpreted as the experience that emerges when an individual fails to adapt to environmental demands in his or her daily occupations. Environment may affect the level of complexity in women's patterns of daily occupations in that more input from the environment may result in unexpected occupations and more complex and unstable patterns of daily occupations. However, in the studies of working mothers, environmental aspects such as housing, number of children, and working hours could not be shown to have any impact on the level of complexity in their patterns of daily occupations (Erlandsson & Eklund, 2006). The social environment, however, did affect the complexity indirectly because having more children constituted a risk of experiencing more hassles (Erlandsson & Eklund, 2003b), which was, in turn being interpreted as having a more complex pattern of occupations. It seems likely that the social

Table 9-1

ASPECTS OF DAILY OCCUPATIONS PROMOTING LIFE BALANCE AMONG SWEDISH WOMEN OF WORKING AGE

STRUCTURAL FACTORS		EXPERIENCE FACTORS	
OCCUPATIONAL BALANCE	MEANING	CONTROL	MANAGEABILITY
Lower complexity (i.e., not too many occupations squeezed into the time frame)[1]	Perceived meaning in patterns of daily occupations[3,4]	Subjective experience of control[5]	Having the ability to mobilize personal and contextual resources to meet the demands[3,4]
Occupations accomplished with fewer interruptions[1,2]		Having the ability to choose[3,4]	
A variety and right amount of occupations[3,4]			

[1]Erlandsson & Eklund (2006).
[2]Erlandsson & Håkansson (2008).
[3]Håkansson, et al. (2006).
[4]Håkansson, et al. (2008b).
[5]Erlandsson & Eklund (2003b).

context, such as family members and colleagues, affects the individual's experience of balance.

In this chapter, we have shown that having life balance would mean living a life that contains a combination of occupations corresponding to the individual's needs, values, and resources at different stages in life. We have further shown that life balance seems, to a great extent, to be a matter of a combination of the organization or structure of the patterns of daily occupations and the subjective experiences derived from them. The studies presented in this chapter underline an additional aspect too, and that is the impact of the environment.

Finally, we would like to comment on the fact that this chapter on the patterns of daily occupations and life balance is based on studies on women of working age and it presents a gender-specific perspective. Knowledge about the structures of men's patterns of daily occupations and the way in which they experience such patterns is also important. However, in reflecting on the urban societies of today, it can be assumed that men's and women's patterns of daily occupations are becoming more and more alike. At least in Sweden, various strategies are being implemented by both the government and private industry to stimulate gender equality in terms of shared parental leave and support for women in higher managerial positions and on company boards. Such efforts will hopefully result in men and women having more similar conditions at work and at home. At the same time, the tempo and complexity of working life is increasing. Although there may now be fewer differences in the way men and women use their time and experience their patterns of daily occupations, today's society itself may constitute a general risk for people to experience imbalance.

REFERENCES

American Occupational Therapy Association. (1995). Occupation [Position paper]. *American Journal of Occupational Therapy, 49,* 1015–1018.

Backman, C. L. (2004). Occupational balance: Exploring the relationships among daily occupations and their influence on well-being. *Canadian Journal of Occupational Therapy, 71,* 202–209.

Bateson, C. (1996). Enfolded activity and the concept of occupation. In R. Zemke & F. Clark (Eds.), *Occupational science: The evolving discipline* (pp. 5–11). Philadelphia: F. A. Davis.

Berntsson, L., Lundberg, U., & Krantz, G. (2006). Gender differences in work–home interplay and symptom perception among Swedish white-collar employees. *Journal of Epidemiology and Community Health, 60,* 1070–1076.

Christiansen, C. (1996). Three perspectives on balance in occupation. In R. Zemke & F. Clark (Eds.), *Occupational science: The evolving discipline.* (pp. 431–451). Philadelphia: F. A. Davis.

Christiansen, C. (2000). Identity, personal projects, and happiness: Self-construction in everyday action. *Journal of Occupational Science, 7,* 98–107.

Cohen, S., Kessler, R., & Gordon, L. U. (1995). *Measuring stress: A guide for health and social scientists.* New York: Oxford University Press.

Davies, K. (1990). *Women, time, and the weaving of the strands of everyday life.* Aldershot, UK: Avebury.

Eckenrode, J., & Bolger, N. (1995). Daily and within-day event measurements. In S. Cohen, R. Kessler, & L. U. Gordon (Eds.), *Measuring stress: A guide for health and social scientists* (pp. 80–101). New York: Oxford University Press.

Ellegård, K. (1999). A time-geographical approach to the study of everyday life of individuals—A challenge of complexity. *GeoJournal, 48,* 167–175.

Elvin-Nowak, Y. (1998). *Flexibilitetens baksida: Om balans, kontroll och skuld i yrkesarbetande mödrars vardagsliv* [The flipside of flexibility: On balance, control and guilt in the everyday lives of employed mothers]. Report No. 101; Sweden: Stockholm University, Department of Psychology.

Erlandsson, L.-K. (2003). *101 Women's pattern of daily occupations. Characteristics and relationships to health and well-being.* Department of Clinical Neuroscience, Division of Occupational Therapy, Lund University.

Erlandsson, L.-K., & Eklund, M. (2001). Describing patterns of daily occupations—A methodological study comparing data from four different methods. *Scandinavian Journal of Occupational Therapy, 8,* 31–39.

Erlandsson, L.-K., & Eklund, M. (2003a). Women's experiences of hassles and uplifts in their everyday patterns of occupations. *Occupational Therapy International, 10,* 95–114.

Erlandsson, L.-K., & Eklund, M. (2003b). The relationships of hassles and uplifts to experience of health in working women. *Women and Health, 38,* 19–37.

Erlandsson, L.-K., & Eklund, M. (2006). Levels of complexity in patterns of daily occupations in relation to women's well-being. *Journal of Occupational Science, 13,* 27–36.

Erlandsson, L.-K., & Håkansson, C. (2009). Women's perceived frequency of disturbing interruptions and its relationship to self-rated health and satisfaction with life as a whole. Manuscript submitted for publication.

Erlandsson, L.-K., Rögnvaldsson, T., & Eklund, M. (2004). Recognition of similarities (ROS): A methodological approach to analysing and characterising patterns of daily occupations. *Journal of Occupational Science, 11,* 3–13.

Farnworth, L. (2003). Time use, tempo, and temporality: Occupational therapy's core business or someone else's business. *Australian Occupational Therapy Journal, 50,* 116–126.

Friberg, T. (1993). *Everyday life: Women's adaptive strategies in time and space.* Stockholm: Byggforskningsrådet.

Griffin, J. M., Fuhrer, R., Stansfeld, S., & Marmot, M. (2002). The importance of low control at work and home on depression and anxiety: Do these effects vary by gender and social class? *Social Science and Medicine, 54,* 783–798.

Hallman, T. (2003). *Gender perspectives on psychosocial risk factors: Conditions governing women's lives in relation to stress and coronary heart disease.* Thesis, Karolinska Institutet, Department of Clinical Neuroscience, Stockholm.

Hannam, D. (1997). More than a cup of tea: Meaning construction in an everyday occupation. *Journal of Occupational Science, 4,* 69–74.

Hasselkus, B. R., & Rosa, S. A. (1997). Meaning and occupation. In C. Christiansen & C. Baum. (Eds.), *Occupational therapy: Enabling function and well-being.* Thorofare, NJ: SLACK Incorporated.

Hirdman, Y. (1999). Om hantid och hontid: En modern historia [About male-time and female-time: A modern history]. *Folkets Historia, 3–4,* 62–129.

Håkansson, C., & Ahlborg, G. (2008). *Manageability, balance, and meaning in the activities of everyday life—Predictors of good self-rated health and balanced work attendance among women and men.* Unpublished manuscript, Lund University, Lund, Sweden.

Håkansson, C., Dahlin-Ivanoff, S., & Sonn, U. (2006). Achieving balance in everyday life. *Journal of Occupational Science, 13,* 74–82.

Håkansson. C., Eklund, M., Lidfeldt, J., Nerbrand, C., Samsioe, G., & Nilsson, P. M. (2005). Well-being and occupational roles among middle-aged women. *Work, 24,* 341–351.

Håkansson, C., Svartvik, L., Lidfeldt, J., Nerbrand, C., Samsioe, G., Schersten, B., et al. (2003). Self-rated health in middle-aged women—Associations with sense of coherence, socioeconomic, and health-related factors. *Scandinavian Journal of Occupational Therapy, 10,* 99–106.

Håkansson, C., Dahlin-Ivanoff, S., & Sonn, U. (2006). Achieving balance in everyday life. *Journal of Occupational Science, 13,* 74–82.

Håkansson, C., Lissner, L., Björkelund, C., & Sonn, U. (2009). Engagement in patterns of daily occupations and perceived health among women of working age. *Scandinavian Journal of Occupational Therapy, 16,* 1–8.

Hägerstrand, T. (1978). Survival and arena: On the life history of individuals in relation to their geographic environment. In T. Carlstein, D. Parkes, & N. Thrift (Eds.), *Human activity and time geography: Timing space and spacing time* (Vol. 2; pp. 122–145). New York: John Wiley & Sons.

Johansson, E., Hamberg, K., Westmans, G., & Lindgren, G. (1999). The meanings of pain: An exploration of women's description of symptoms. *Social Science and Medicine, 48,* 1791–1802.

Kanner, A., Coyne, J., Schaefer, C., & Lazarus, R. (1981). Comparison of two models of stress measurement: Daily hassles and uplifts versus major life events. *Journal of Behaviour Medicine, 4,* 1–39.

Karasek, R. A., & Theorell, T. (1990). *Healthy work: Stress, productivity, and reconstruction of working life.* New York: Basic Books.

Kielhofner, G. (2002). *A model of human occupation: Theory and application* (3rd ed.). Baltimore: Williams & Wilkins.

Law, M., Steinwender, S., & Leclair, L. (1998). Occupation, health, and well-being. *Canadian Journal of Occupational Therapy, 65,* 81–91.

Lazarus, R. S., & Folkman, S. (1984). *Stress, appraisal, and coping.* New York: Springer.

Leufstadius, C., Erlandsson, L.-K., & Eklund, M. (2006). Time use and daily rhythm in people with persistent mental illness. *Occupational Therapy International, 13,* 123–141.

Lundberg, U. (1996). Influences of paid and unpaid work on psychophysiological stress responses of men and women. *Journal of Occupational Health Psychology, 1,* 117–130.

Lundberg, U., & Frankenhaeuser, M. (1999). Stress and workload of men and women in high-ranking positions. *Journal of Occupational Health Psychology, 4,* 142–151.

Mann, H. B., & Whitney, D. R. (1947). On a test of whether one of two random variables is stochastically larger than the other. *Annals of Mathematical Statistics, 18,* 50–60.

Matuska, K. M., & Christiansen, C. H. (2008). A proposed model of lifestyle balance. *Journal of Occupational Science, 15,* 9–19.

Orth-Gomér, K. (2003). Kvinnors stress, sociala miljö och hälsa i ett livsperspektiv [Women's stress, social environment and health from a life perspective]. In T. Theorell (Ed.), *Psykosocial Miljö och Stress* (pp. 163–174). Lund, Sweden: Studentlitteratur.

Pentland, W., Harvey, A., Lawton, P., & McColl, A., (1999). *Time use research in the social sciences.* New York: Kluwer Academic.

Persson, D., Erlandsson, L.-K., Eklund, M., & Iwarsson, S. (2001). Value dimensions, meaning, and complexity in human occupation—A tentative structure for analysis. *Scandinavian Journal of Occupational Therapy, 8,* 7–18.

Piskûr, B., Kinebanian, A., & Josephsson, S. (2002). Occupation and well-being: A study of some Slovenian people's experiences of engagement in occupation in relation to well-being. *Scandinavian Journal of Occupational Therapy, 9,* 63–70.

Robinson, J., & Godbey, G. (1997). *Time for life. The surprising ways Americans use their time.* University Park, PA: The Pennsylvania State University Press.

Schultz, S., & Schkade, J. K. (1992). Occupational adaptation: Toward a holistic approach for contemporary practice, part 2. *American Journal of Occupational Therapy, 46,* 829–837.

Socialstyrelsen. (2005) *Folkhälsorapport 2005.* [Public health report 2005]. Stockholm: Socialstyrelsen; 2005.

Sommer, B., & Sommer, R. (1997). *A practical guide to behavioural research: Tools and techniques* (4th ed.). New York: Oxford University Press.

Stone, P. J. (1972). The analysis of time-budget data. In A. Szalai (Ed.), *The use of time: Daily activities of urban and suburban populations in twelve countries* (pp. 89–112). Hague, The Netherlands: Mouton & Co.

Stroud, L., Salovey, P., & Epel, E. (2002). Sex differences in stress responses: Social rejection versus achievement stress. *Biological Psychiatry, 52,* 318–327.

Theorell, T. (2003). *Psykosocial Miljö och Stress.* [Psychosocial environment and stress]. Lund, Sweden: Studentlitteratur.

Thoits, P. A. (1983). Dimensions of life events that influence psychological distress: An evaluation and synthesis of the literature. In H. Kaplan (Ed.), *Psychological stress: Trends in theory and research* (pp. 33–103). New York: Academic Press.

Townsend, E. (Ed.). (2007). *Enabling occupation: An occupational therapy perspective*. Ottawa: Canadian Association of Occupational Therapists.

WHO. (2001). *The World Health Report 2001: Mental health: New understanding. New hope*. World Health Organization: Geneva.

Wilcock, A. A. (2006). *An occupational perspective of health* (2nd ed.). Thorofare, NJ: SLACK Incorporated.

Wilcock, A. A., Chelin, M., Hall, M., Hamley, N., Morrison, B., Scrivener, L., et al. (1997). The relationship between occupational balance and health: A pilot study. *Occupational Therapy International, 4,* 17–30.

Velde, P. V., &, Fidler, G. S. (2002). *Lifestyle performance: A model for engaging the power of occupation*. Thorofare: SLACK Incorporated.

Yerxa, E. J. (1998). Occupation: the keystone of a curriculum for a self-defined profession. *American Journal of Occupational Therapy, 52,* 365–372.

Zemke, R., & Clark, F. (1996). *Occupational science: The evolving discipline*. Philadelphia: F. A. Davis.

SECTION III

Conceptualizing Life Balance

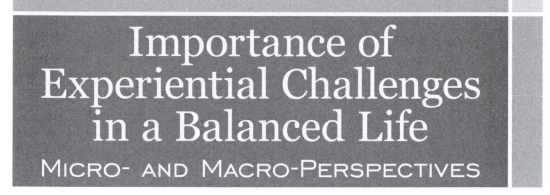

Importance of Experiential Challenges in a Balanced Life

MICRO- AND MACRO-PERSPECTIVES

DENNIS PERSSON AND HANS JONSSON

INTRODUCTION

This chapter focuses on aspects of life balance that concern the distribution of experiences that are generated by the occupations people have chosen as building blocks for their everyday life. We present the phenomenon of *flow* as a state with only a peripheral awareness of time or self due to the total focus and absorption in a doing process that is fundamentally engaging and enjoyable. The development of methodology to measure and analyze this experience are briefly presented, with a main focus on a so called eight-channel model that is based on reports on balance or imbalance between *challenges* and *skills* within occupations. Although this model captures the experiential optimization of single occupations, it fails to capture the bigger picture of the balance or imbalance of occupational dimensions in everyday life.

Therefore, the authors explore an alternative or complementary way to categorize the such data, using the eight-channel classification as a starting point. A Model of Experiential Balance condenses balanced and imbalanced experiences of challenges and skills into three dimensions: (1) *flowing*, (2) *exacting*, and (3) *calming* experiences.

Using this model, the authors present a secondary analysis of four different data sets from the United States, Italy, and Sweden, which are discussed from a health-promotion perspective. The authors discuss the importance of meaning and risk-taking for well-being, provide examples from the authors' additional research on retirement transition and everyday life strategies of people with long-term pain, and present a macro-perspective in which the importance of applying the notion of experiential balance in a global context is highlighted from ethical, political, and environmental viewpoints..

LIFE BALANCE AND EXPERIENCES

The notion of life as something that has to be balanced to be good is historically present within both Western and Eastern thinking. In ancient Greek philosophy, the balance of a good life was permeated by an ethical aspect. Plato saw real happiness or pleasure coming from the use of reason in everyday actions to reach a balance between passion and desires, pushing you in the direction of living a "just" life (Elias, 2008). If such a balance exists, there is no need to act unjustly, as

K. Matuska & C. Christiansen (Eds.)
Life balance: Multidisciplinary theories and research (pp 133–148)
© 2009 SLACK Incorporated and AOTA Press

one would be able to control passions and desires to receive proper rewards. Aristotle, on the other hand, argued that the ultimate human good is happiness—a good that is final and self-sufficient, irreplaceable by any other virtue such as honor, pleasure, and reason (Elias, 2008). In Eastern philosophy, the notion of balance is put in a universal context, such as the Taoist idea of *yin* and *yang* embodying the harmony of opposites in which nothing is completely yin or completely yang, although each contains the seed for its opposite and thereby represents a dynamic combination of opposites that keeps the world spinning and striving toward a state of balance in all aspects of life (Kaptchuk, 2000).

Action can be viewed as one of the most basic ways of expression for human beings, enabling the fulfillment of their fundamental needs, be it passion and desire or happiness. In this chapter *action* is referred to as *occupation*, defined as "the ordinary and familiar things that people do every day" (American Occupational Therapy Association, 1995, p. 1015). It may, in fact, even be appropriate to label humans as "occupational beings" (Zemke & Clark, 1996). The individually unique manner in which people choose and perform their occupations will greatly influence whether they experience balance or imbalance in their everyday lives. One of the most widely cited philosophical beliefs in occupational therapy literature is that a balance of occupations is beneficial to health and well-being (Christiansen, 1996). In the field of occupational therapy, balance was initially considered to be distribution of different categories of doing. For example, Meyer (1922/1977) in the early 20th century said that one must balance what he called the "big four"—work, play, rest, and sleep—to stay healthy. He argued, "Our conception of man is that of an organism that maintains and balances itself in the world of reality and actuality by being in active life and active use" (p. 641). However, life balance recently has been described in terms of more complex dimensions than the quantification of the four instrumental parameters of work, play, sleep, and rest (see Christiansen & Matuska, 2006). One example of a recent notion drawing on this complexity is Persson, Erlandsson, Eklund, and Iwarsson's (2001) Value, Meaning, and Occupations Model (ValMO), which emphasizes that a proper understanding of occupational content and balance has to be understood from the interplay between macro-, meso-, and micro-perspectives and the experiential and motivational dimensions of concrete, symbolic, and self-reward occupational values. In other words, what we choose to do every day is influenced by who we are as individuals, what the opportunities are in the environment, and the value we ascribe to certain experiences.

Thus, the experience of the everyday things we do, or *occupational performance* (Nelson, 1988; 1996), seems to be a fundamental motivation for what we choose to do. The memory of the experiences remains after the actual occupation is finished and influences us to do the same thing again if the experience was pleasurable, or alternatively, to stop it if it was not pleasurable. Thus it seems reasonable that the experience of an occupation has a fundamental impact on how the individual's occupational repertoire is constructed and ultimately on his or her sense of quality and well-being in life as a whole. We would expect, then, that if someone creates a lifestyle with a mix of occupations that gives him or her optimal experiences, that is, being perceived as pleasurable or meaningful, then he or she will most likely also report a sense of well-being or satisfaction with life. However, that might be too simplistic, considering the fact that people cannot be sure that what they experience as pleasurable or meaningful now will remain so in different contexts and at different times.

People in postindustrial societies have more lifestyle choices than ever yet do not experience the valuable and balanced everyday life they would like (Persson & Erlandsson, 2002). Warberg and Larsson (2005) believe this is a consequence of many small, unconscious choices people make under the influence of "the spirit of our time," which they consider to be an implicit but massively powerful influential phenomenon surrounding us. This social phenomenon is so powerful that the dominant culture dictates what we should think, do, and hold as important. The choices people make may not actually reflect their own values or what is really important to them.

As it turns out, doing things that reflect Western norms and values may lead to a sense of imbalance. This was partly illustrated in a validation study conducted using an instrument measuring occupational value (OV), based on the ValMO model (Persson et al., 2001). In this study, it was found that people were doing things that were within the Western cultural norms and expected from family and others in the social environment yet were no longer congruent with the values in their lives (Eklund, Erlandsson, Persson, & Hagell, 2007). The experiential aspects behind individuals' go-with-the-spirit-of-our-time might result in negative consequences and imbalances that they are not even aware of, because the dominant, sociocultural environment masks their own values and influences their choices.

OPTIMAL EXPERIENCE

The problem with discussing balance as a function of time spent in various occupational categories (e.g., work, sleep, leisure) is that people categorize their occupations very differently. For example, what might be considered work for one person could be perceived as leisure for another. Furthermore, individuals may perceive the same occupation differently at different times. For example, cooking for the family after a long day at work may be experienced differently than cooking with friends at a social gathering. Therefore, instead of examining balance by considering engagement in different occupational categories, it seems more effective and valid to examine the *experience* of engaging in occupations, regardless of how they are categorized. This experiential perspective has been highlighted as the intrinsic anatomy of optimal human experience, or *flow* (Csikszentmihalyi, 1990; Csikszentmihalyi & Larsen, 1987).

When flow theory was introduced about 30 years ago, it served as a theoretical model for understanding optimal experiences in human behavior. Starting from interviews of people having different creative or "free" occupations, Csikszentmihalyi and colleagues (1975) developed a model of flow based on how the interviewees experienced the relationship between the challenge of the occupation and their skill in doing it. *Flow* is described as an experience during which the doer has only a peripheral awareness of time or self due to his or her total focus and absorption in a doing process that is fundamentally engaging and enjoyable (Csikszentmihalyi, 1975, 1990). Flow theory became an alternative to the predominant psychoanalytical explanations of that time by focusing on the dynamic interaction between the person's skills and the challenge of an occupation. In the original version of the model, flow could be expected to occur when the challenges of a certain occupation were in balance with the doer's skills in that occupation.

To understand the experience of engaging in occupations, Csikszentmihalyi and Larson (1987) developed the experience sampling method (ESM), a procedure in which a programmed signaling device, usually a wristwatch, was worn by the informant for about a week. Every time the device beeped, the subjects filled out a 30-item questionnaire concerning the experience of the occupation being performed at the time. The items were mostly rated on a scale of 7 or 9 grades, with a few open questions. A crucial set of items concerned the rating of perceived challenges and skills related to each reported occupation.

They originally conceptualized a three-channel model (Figure 10-1) containing flow, anxiety and boredom, but revised this when they determined that four different variations of challenges and skills would be more useful when performing a certain statistical calculation of these items. Thus, a four-channel model, adding also *apathy*, became the new way of operationalizing the phenomenon of flow (see Figure 10-1).

Csikszentmihalyi and Larson (1987) used the individual average of the balanced challenge and skill scores for each occupation as the denominator in a ratio. A *flow experience* occurred if the balance for the experience was above the individual average; an *apathetic experience* occurred if it was below the individual average. This procedure revealed that different individuals required different levels of balanced challenge/skills ratios to reach a state of flow, so that one person might

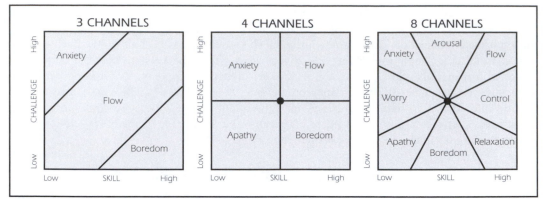

Figure 10-1. Three models of flow mirroring the development of the theory.

need only a lower score (e.g., 4) to reach the optimal experience level of flow, while another person needs 8 or 9 to reach this level. With this new method, it also became possible to compare groups of individuals with different levels of averages.

When Csikszentmihalyi, together with some Italian colleagues, increased the four channels in the model to eight channels (see Figure 10-1; Massimini, Csikszentmihalyi, & Carli, 1987), reports of experiences became even more differentiated. New cross-cultural studies were conducted, as well as studies on different traumatized or unhealthy groups (Farnworth, Mostert, Harrison, & Worrell, 1996; Persson, Eklund, & Isacsson, 1999).

Today, flow theory has become established and accepted in a variety of fields in the human sciences. Examples include creativity research (Csikszentmihalyi, 1997a; Feldman, Csikszentmihalyi, & Gardner, 1994) and positive psychology and happiness research (Csikszentmihalyi & Hunter, 2003; Seligman & Csikszentmihalyi, 2000). In occupational therapy literature and research, flow theory has been found to be an important therapeutic agent (e.g., Christiansen & Baum, 2004; Wright, 2004) and occupational therapy research projects have been carried out using the concept of flow as the theoretical base (Gerhardsson & Jonsson, 1996; Jacobs, 1994; Persson et al., 1999; Wright, Sadlo, & Stew, 2006, 2007). In the emerging field of occupational science, flow theory was identified as an important concept from the outset (Yerxa et al., 1990), and the use of ESM has been highlighted as an important method for developing knowledge on occupation (Carlson & Clark, 1991; Farnworth et al., 1996).

Thus, the concept of flow has heavily contributed to knowledge of the dynamic relationship between health and occupation, as people in general seem to benefit from flow experiences for satisfaction in their everyday occupations. However, it is reasonable to assume that more flow does not always lead to more satisfaction or health. While it is clear that there is a positive relationship between flow and satisfaction, there is reasonably a point where skill demands are at the limit of one's capacity and thus start to transform into a burden. Being at the maximum of your skill with a small amount of time for relaxation to recharge your batteries might in time lead to consequences, including symptoms of stress. Although they are performing rewarding activities, people within this overload situation say that eventually they "hit a wall." We thought that this negative aspect of flow was not sufficiently addressed in the literature, and furthermore, the concepts used in the theory seemed to imply that flow is the only valuable experience in human occupation.

This assumption is especially obvious in the four-channel model, which identifies only one positive experience—flow—and three negative experiences: boredom, apathy, and anxiety (see Figure 10-1). Not much was said about other possible positive aspects. Although flow experiences contribute to well-being, it is possible and reasonable that flow can sometimes have adverse consequences and show signs of being addictive. For example, people working with information technology at the beginning of the 1990s were so seduced by its novelty and possibilities that they became thoroughly absorbed by their experiences at the computer and in a short time developed symptoms of chronic fatigue, at that time known as the "yuppie disease" (Ware & Kleinman, 1992). A highly questionable means of experiencing flow was presented in a study of Japanese motorcycle gangs riding blindfolded against red traffic lights (Sato, 1988). Thus, we thought that when individuals organize their consciousness to experience flow, it is possible to do it in ways that stifle other important everyday tasks and experiences, leading to illness or practices that are destructive, dangerous, and even lethal. This highlights the concept of *occupational balance* or rather, balance between experiences in occupations, as was introduced in the beginning of this chapter. We raise the question about the need to balance the experience of high-challenge occupations with the experience of low-challenge occupations and wonder if occasional boredom might be necessary for being able to have highlights in flow.

TOWARD A MODEL OF EXPERIENTIAL BALANCE

The eight-channel model has been used mainly to map and discuss the importance of flow experiences, and further discussions of the ESM data tend to focus on concepts such as happiness (e.g., Seligman & Csikszentmihalyi, 2000), self-determination (e.g., Csikszentmihalyi & Hunter, 2003; Moneta, 2004), and social context (e.g., Kennedy & Vecitis, 2004). However, the eight-channel model, focusing the balance/imbalance between two items within a single occupation and fragmentized into eight different channels, captures the experiential optimization of that single occupation yet fails to capture the bigger picture of balance/imbalance among the occupational dimensions of everyday life as a whole. Thus, to be able to deal with the question of balance in this comprehensive respect, it seemed wise to begin with condensing the number of channels to get a more manageable starting point.

With that rationale, a condensed model was developed that grouped the eight channels into three dimensions of daily experiences in occupation (Jonsson & Persson, 2006). The first dimension, combining channels 2 and 3 (flow and control) describes highly or moderately challenging experiences matched with high skills. This dimension is called *high matched experiences* (HME). The second dimension, combining channels 1, 7, and 8 (arousal, worry, and anxiety) represents high challenge that cannot be matched with high skills. This dimension is called *high not matched experiences* (HNME). Finally, channels 4, 5, and 6 (relaxation, boredom, and apathy) are combined to form the third dimension, low to moderate challenge, called *low-challenge experiences* (LCE). The aggregated dimensions are illustrated in Figure 10-2, together with possible positive and negative attributes to each of the three dimensions.

In the second step, we used less technical terms for the three dimensions: *exacting, flowing,* and *calming*. These experiences are illustrated in a model (Figure 10-3) that also stresses the three-way dynamics and interdependent relationship between the dimensions (Jonsson & Persson, 2006).

ILLUSTRATION OF EXPERIENTIAL BALANCE

With our experiential model in place, we turned to four different data sets using the eight-channel model with participants from the United States, Italy, and Sweden (Jonsson & Persson, 2006). The Italian data set ($n = 47$) included adolescents between ages 16 and 18 in Milan (Massimini & Carli, 1988). One data set (sample) from the United States ($n = 75$) consisted of adolescents between ages 14 and 17 (Massimini, Carli, Delle Fave, & Massimini, 1988). A second data set from the United States was 19 women with HIV/AIDS living in the community (Kennedy & Vecitis, 2004). The Swedish dataset ($n = 18$) was collected in a mixed sample of adult men and woman (Persson, 2001; Persson et al., 1999).

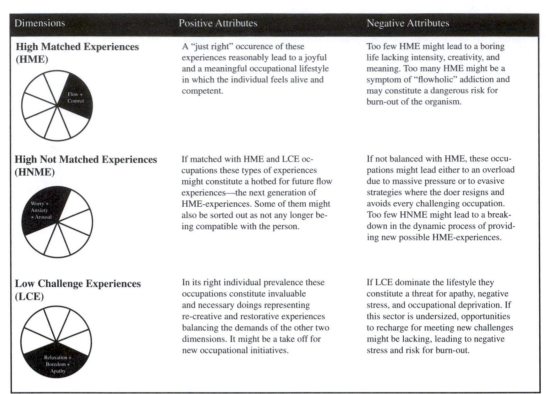

Dimensions	Positive Attributes	Negative Attributes
High Matched Experiences (HME)	A "just right" occurence of these experiences reasonably lead to a joyful and a meaningful occupational lifestyle in which the individual feels alive and competent.	Too few HME might lead to a boring life lacking intensity, creativity, and meaning. Too many HME might be a symptom of "flowholic" addiction and may constitute a dangerous risk for burn-out of the organism.
High Not Matched Experiences (HNME)	If matched with HME and LCE occupations these types of experiences might constitute a hotbed for future flow experiences—the next generation of HME-experiences. Some of them might also be sorted out as not any longer being compatible with the person.	If not balanced with HME, these occupations might lead either to an overload due to massive pressure or to evasive strategies where the doer resigns and avoids every challenging occupation. Too few HNME might lead to a breakdown in the dynamic process of providing new possible HME-experiences.
Low Challenge Experiences (LCE)	In its right individual prevalence these occupations constitute invaluable and necessary doings representing re-creative and restorative experiences balancing the demands of the other two dimensions. It might be a take off for new occupational initiatives.	If LCE dominate the lifestyle they constitute a threat for apathy, negative stress, and occupational deprivation. If this sector is undersized, opportunities to recharge for meeting new challenges might be lacking, leading to negative stress and risk for burn-out.

Figure 10-2. Combined dimensions of the eight-channel model and its possible attributes.

In Figure 10-4, the four data sets are presented together, using the combined model. The similarities across the groups are very obvious. Barely half of the occupations in a week are experienced as low-challenging occupations that do not require maximum skills (calming). A good half of the occupations in a week are challenging and half of those can be matched with areas of high skill (flowing). One of every four occupations is experienced as being too challenging to be achieved with existing skills (exacting).

In addressing the balance or imbalance of experiences, it seems that people need to experience occupations that balance challenges with skills as well as occupations with challenges that are too high or too low in relation to skills. Challenging occupations can be intrinsically rewarding or self-rewarding (Csikszentmihalyi, 1975, 1997b), and when met by high skills, people experience flow and competence. But functioning at maximum skill levels requires significant energy, so

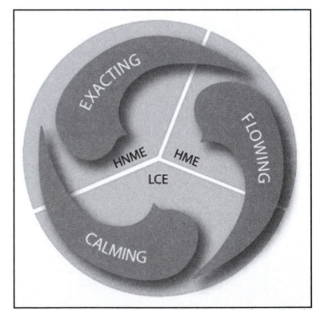

Figure 10-3. Trialectic model of experiential balance and its dynamic interdependent relationships among exacting, flowing, and calming dimensions.

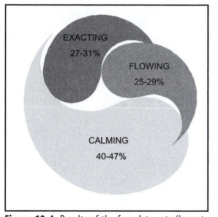

Figure 10-4. Results of the four data sets (lowest-highest) using the experiential model. *Note.* Each quality is dimensioned according to its average size.

people also need to have low-challenge occupations to relax and rest. Even being occasionally bored may have positive effects, as boredom can challenge initiative and creativity. Thus, in a balanced occupational life, relaxation, boredom, and apathy all need to be experienced, because they serve as sources of new energy and other positive emotional experiences.

Recreational occupations, such as sitting at the seaside watching the sun set on a gentle summer's evening, also referred to as *being* (Hammell, 2004; Wilcock, 1998), might, despite low levels of challenge, be as self-rewarding as being in flow (Persson et al., 2001). Further, Stigsdotter and Grahn (2002) found that relaxing in lush green surroundings had restorative impacts on people.

In challenging occupational experiences, people have sufficient skills to meet the demands of most occupations but occasionally face occupations that require more skills than they have at the time. In contrast to matched occupations, challenging occupations trigger individuals to continue to develop their skills in a dynamic process. These occupations may then become the next generation of flow experiences. In conclusion, we propose that the three dimensions in the combined model play complementary roles, and that having a balance between them is of great importance for people's experience of meaning and health in their overall occupational lifestyle.

ILLUSTRATION OF POSSIBLE IMBALANCE

Within the samples, individuals showed variations in their experiential patterns. We will present two case examples in the following shaded boxes from the Swedish study that indicated different forms of imbalance in their experiential pattern.

DYNAMICS AMONG THE EXPERIENTIAL DIMENSIONS IN THE MODEL

The analysis of the empirical material supports the condensed model, which collapses the eight experience channels into three dimensions, making it possible to analyze how these dimensions interact in a dynamic, everyday cycle and to determine whether a certain balance of experiences promotes health and well-being. All three dimensions and their relationships are important for achieving balance in occupational life; none of them are intrinsically positive or negative. The three dimensions have different relationships to each other and are needed within the total context of everyday experience. If any of these three dimensions is too dominating, an imbalance arises that in the long-term might risk developing into a destructive process—one that would lead to occupational deprivation or overload, with negative consequences on health and well-being.

It is reasonable to assume that calming experiences are needed to recharge people's batteries and for relaxation, but if they become dominant, experiences become too boring and depriving. Flowing experiences are a source of intrinsic rewards and feelings of competence, but if they are too dominant, experiences might become too energy demanding and even addictive, possibly leading to overload and social isolation. Exacting experiences are important and necessary sources of personal development that trigger new flow experiences as the dynamic process continues. During the actual experience, exacting experiences might initially arouse negative feelings of

ERIKA

Erika (not her real name)—experience-quality profile in Figure 10-5—was a 27-year-old cohabiting woman studying chemical engineering at a university who experienced a low level of challenge in at least half of her occupations. Erika's everyday life alternated between days with lectures at the university, which also seemed to contain most of her flowing experiences, and days when she studied at home. On days she studied at home, she also did household chores, took care of many domestic animals, cooked dinner, and watched TV with her partner. Of the challenging occupations that she experienced, a large majority were high skill, resulting in flowing experiences. On the other hand, she did not have many exacting occupations that were still too difficult for her. The exacting occupations that she did have were mostly on her days at home.

Seen from a dynamic and developmental perspective, this situation might be problematic for her future. Over time, she is likely to become more skilled and thus to no longer experience high levels of challenge. Furthermore, because she has so few exacting occupations, the likelihood of any of them developing into the next generation of

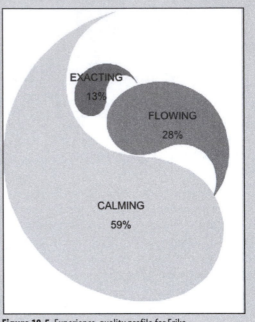

Figure 10-5. Experience-quality profile for Erika.
Note. Each quality is dimensioned according to its relative size.

balanced, highly challenging experiences is very small. Without these triggers, she is at risk of an expansion of calming experiences and, in the long run, might experience occupational deprivation.

JAN

Jan (not his real name)—experience-quality profile in Figure 10-6—was a 42-year-old university teacher living with his wife and son. In addition, he and his wife each have two more children from former relationships who occasionally live with them. Jan had over 40% of his experiential profile in challenging occupations. Compared with Erika, however, he has the opposite relationship between flowing and exacting occupations. Jan has experiences of high challenge in his occupational life, but in most cases his skills do not match the level of demand, resulting in exacting experiences. Having insufficient skills to satisfactorily perform demanding occupations can be very energy consuming without giving anything back in terms of intrinsic rewards and feelings of competence. If this imbalance continues, there might be a risk of burnout. A main part of Jan's exacting occupations were found within work, but he also had difficulties trying to solve problems within the family. From an individual perspective, one strategy would be to try to avoid challenging occupations or to shift experiences toward the calming dimension, with its inherent risk of occupational deprivation in the future. This would probably be a bad strategy, because none of his a-bit-too-challenging occupations from work or in the family are the kind he can ignore. A better alternative would probably be to continuously and stubbornly try to work on his tasks and, in time, increase his skills. In his work, he might try to get a slightly better fit between his capacities and his work tasks. Then these exacting experiences might develop into the next generation of flowing occupations and provide a better balance between the dimensions. As he has quite a lot of relaxed experiences, particularly at home, to back up these efforts, this could be possible.

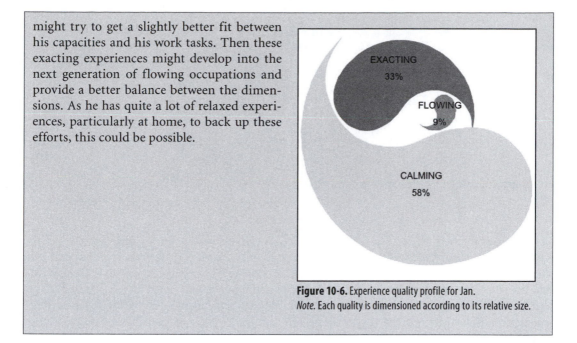

Figure 10-6. Experience quality profile for Jan.
Note. Each quality is dimensioned according to its relative size.

frustration and stress. Such feelings might be the price one has to pay to secure further development and creativity and to have flowing experiences in the future—advanced occupations that are eventually mastered, yet in the beginning are frustratingly difficult. If the exacting experiences are too dominant, experiences of negative stress, incompetence, and overload might arise.

The dynamic aspect of the model is of course very difficult to grasp by using the ESM method, which gives a frozen picture of the relationship among the qualities of experiences. Single occupations can travel through all dimensions in a back-and-forth process. An example of this is the different qualities of experience people have when beginning to learn a new computer program. At first, there are experiences of helplessness and anxiety, close to the limit of giving up (exacting). By overcoming these feelings, a mastery process begins, and individuals gradually experience a high level of skill and the ability to do advanced tasks with the program (flowing). With time and practice, the program becomes incorporated into day-to-day work and is no longer experienced as challenging (calming). Perhaps then, it is time for a new and more advanced program or for using it in a completely new way.

USING THE EXPERIENTIAL MODEL
TO UNDERSTAND EXPERIENCES OF IMBALANCE

In this section, using the experiential model as a theoretical tool with a longitudinal study of the retirement transition (conducted by the second author of this chapter) will demonstrate the experience of imbalance (Jonsson, Borell, & Sadlo, 2000; Jonsson, Josephsson, & Kielhofner, 2001a, 2001b). About 30 working participants were interviewed about their retirement process for 7 years (participants were 63–71 years of age). Several participants in this study expressed experiences of imbalance prior to retirement, and analysis revealed the following pattern. In the last years of work (typically after 60 years of age), participants felt that they did not have the same capacity to do as many things as they had previously done. This feeling that their general capacity to do things was shrinking was viewed by them as work taking increasing time and energy in their life. Participants expressed that earlier in their work career they had the strength to do

Figure 10-7. Using the experiential model to understand the process of going from one imbalance to another in the retirement transition.

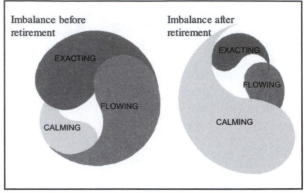

other things in the evening, but as they got older they used weekday evenings and parts of the weekend to rest and recharge their energy for next period of work. As one participant expressed in the interview, "It's going to be a tough year, this last one as I feel it now. And still, I am healthy. I haven't [used] any day[s] for sick-leave in the last year. But now I really feel that it will be nice to get out of work." Using the experiential model to frame this participant's comments, his experience can be seen as his general capacity shrinking without the demands of work lowering. In this case, exacting and flowing experiences expanded in the work setting, leaving little space for these types of experiences outside work and, consequently, the need to expand the calming experiences after work. With the experience of this type of imbalance, many participants were looking forward to retirement for greater rest and relaxation.

However, when several of these participants were interviewed about a year after retirement, another type of imbalance was expressed. One participant said, "I would very, very, very much like to have a small job. Not like in the old company, but some small job that I can manage. Like cutting the lawn or a hedge. Or go[ing] out with old people for a walk or shopping." In the analysis of the retirement process, comment indicated that the participant went from one type of imbalance before retirement to another kind of imbalance in retirement. Participants indicated the lack of demands and expectations that had provided more dynamics in their life. Another participant said, "You have had a fixed program all your life, and then suddenly you shall decide everything yourself. If you don't have anyone else that pulls the strings, you degenerate to be lazy." Another participant expressed the lack of challenges as, " Now I feel I must have something more to take a real bite in." Using the experiential model, these sentiments could be understood as a pattern in which calming experiences, with a lack of real exacting and flowing experiences, were dominant. This pattern—going from one imbalance to another in retirement—is illustrated in Figure 10-7.

Patterns of balance were also found in connection with engaging occupations in retirement, which provided flowing and exacting experiences in a dynamic relationship with calming experiences, allowing the participant to rest, relax, and recharge the batteries before more challenging occupations.

Cultural Images of Retirement

Cultural images in a society—toward retirement in Western societies, for example—can be seen as mirroring and shaping people's expectations and attitudes. Figure 10-8 provides two examples of typical cultural images of a contemporary view of retirement in a Western-European society.

From the experience of imbalance before retirement, it is understandable that an image of life in retirement might have many similarities to images of vacation—a sort of lifelong vacation. Cultural images of lifelong vacations as a pattern of occupational balance are quite common in

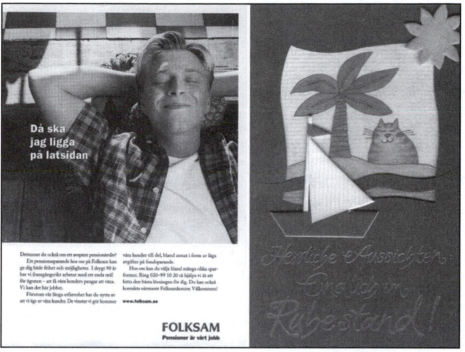

Figure 10-8. Two examples of contemporary cultural images of retirement. *To the left:* An advertisement of retirement funds from the Swedish Insurance company Folksam. The text in the picture says: "Then I'll really be on the lazy side." The text below the photo starts with: "Do you also dream about a relaxed retirement life?" (Photographer: Elisabeth Ohlson-Wallin reprinted with permission.) *To the right:* a German congratulation card. The text reads: Wonderful future views: Finally in retirement! (© Herlitz PBs Aktiengesellschaft, Berlin, Germany reprinted with permission.)

overworked Western societies. However, this dream of a nonchallenging life might be a nightmare if put into practice. In this chapter, we have argued that calming experiences are a necessary part of a balanced lifestyle pattern but are only one part of an interdependent dynamic relationship, where flowing experiences and exacting experiences are also necessary.

Long-Term Pain and Experiences of Flowing and Exacting Experiences

A study conducted by the first author of this chapter (Persson, 2001) showed that almost half of the experiences of people with long-term pain were flowing and exacting experiences. The people with long-term pain did not have particularly different distributions in and between the dimensions compared to the otherwise healthy or unhealthy cross-cultural groups. In fact, one strategy of these participants was to defy their pain to be able to experience the value in specifically meaningful occupations. This is thought provoking, as rehabilitation goals traditionally, on medical grounds, advise against defying pain! Following this line of thought, one can ask what is most important for a good life for these people: a life with the least pain and few peaks in flowing experiences or a life with more meaningful occupations but a higher amount of pain and exacting experiences? As proposed in our experiential model, a reasonable number of exacting and occasionally anxiety-generating experiences are natural in a meaningful and balanced lifestyle. The same goes for flowing and calming experiences.

Another study of motives for occupational performance among people with long-term pain in the Netherlands confirms the importance of taking certain risks to have flowing experiences

(Satink, Winding, & Jonsson, 2004). Participants expressed that they could choose between occupations "with or without pain." Sometimes they chose to do nothing in order to decrease the pain; at other times, they chose engaging activities even when they knew that it would cause more pain.

Health, Meaning, and Risk Taking

The above examples of people in retirement having too many calming, nondynamic occupational experiences and people with long-term pain defying their pain for meaningful experiences raises the question of the value of risk and risk taking in everyday life. A dynamic and creative life that is meaningful and healthy cannot be lived within rigid and secure routines and frames. One can argue that people defying their pain for short episodes of enjoyment is contradictory. The health of being able to experience as little pain as possible seems to oppose the health of participating in a dynamic, meaningful, yet risky daily life (with balance among calming, flowing, and exacting occupations). This conflict is accentuated in health care and rehabilitation that is solely biomedical, as this might lead to advising people to live a life within rigid restrictions, leaving out meaningful occupations or doing them in short fragmented doses. Such a health care paradigm does not recognize the perspective of experiential life balance. A multidimensional concept of health (Persson, 2001; World Health Organization [WHO], 1997) thereby seems warranted. This concept would consider meaningful experiences enabled through certain medical risks as a health-promoting factor that is occasionally as important as reducing risk in daily occupational behavior.

EXPERIENTIAL LIFE BALANCE CONSIDERED FROM A MACRO-PERSPECTIVE

"The true function of politics is not to make people richer, more secure, or powerful, but to let as many as possible enjoy an increasingly complex existence" (Csikszentmihalyi, 1990, p. 219).

The notion of daily life containing a balance of contrasting and complementing experiences generated by our everyday doings has hitherto been discussed only from the micro-perspective of the single individual's life. However, balance is required at many levels and in many aspects of our joint global life. Considering the increasing awareness of how lifestyles, particularly Western lifestyles, impact the use of global resources, causing climate changes and global economic injustice, there seems to be a reason for discussing the issue also from an ethical macro-perspective. Having access to flowing, calming, and exacting experiences and being able to balance these could be seen as a human right and expression of occupational justice on a higher organizational level (Kronenberg & Pollard, 2005; Townsend & Wilcock, 2004).

A majority of the world, in the so-called developing countries, lives under circumstances that contain occupational repertoires and patterns that are dominated by poverty, occupational deprivation, and lack of influence to improve their situation. On the other hand, people in industrialized Western countries use 10 times more global resources than their fellow humans in the developing world (Sanne, 2007). Still, it is questionable if people in industrialized countries are any happier (Csikszentmihalyi, 1999; Murray & Lopez, 1996). Welfare and happiness studies from an increasing number of nations show that the average happiness level increases along with the average income up to approximately 10,000 U.S. dollars (which corresponds to Sweden's average standard of living in the 1950s), then levels out (Donovan & Halpern, 2002; Sanne, 2007). Other studies have followed the average life satisfaction over time since the 1950s in the United States and since the 1970s in the United Kingdom. In both countries people's life satisfaction remains constant even as material wealth strongly increases (World Watch Institute, 2004).

People's happiness and well-being do not seem to need the political and ideological strivings toward an ever-increasing growth of economy, welfare, and consumption. For example, in 2003,

30% of the total sickness in Sweden was due to psychosocial ill health, and illnesses that seem to be stress related accounted for 80% of all sick leave (Statens Folkhälsoinstitut, 2004). Western culture presumes that time is money—that time should not be wasted, but used for something productive that preferably is worth money. With this idea comes an experience of lacking time, of time pressure. One probable effect of this hurried lifestyle is the drastic increase in psychosocial ill health seen in recent years. In America, there has been an increase in teen suicides, adult anxiety, and depression, as well as lifestyle and stress-related chronic health conditions (see, e.g., Stiles, 2005). Worldwide, major depressive episodes were shown to be one of the leading causes of disability-adjusted life years, overridden only by coronary disease (WHO, 2007). Another more paradoxical result of time pressure might be the drift toward passive and nonchallenging occupations. We know that without doubt the most common leisure occupation in Western societies, also expressed in this secondary data, is watching TV. The fact that people use so much of their free time to do something they don't think is challenging and requires no skills, is puzzling. Csikszentmihalyi (1990) discussed what he considers to be "deputy participation," which are all the things we do to mask the emptiness in our stressed and shallow lives. The problem is, he argues, that we do not use our own creativity and skills but spend lots of time, money, and energy on watching others perform sports and music and act in movies. The global entertainment industry, mostly based on Western consumption models, constantly increases its turnout because more and more people are filling their free time with passive entertainment.

Thus, experiential balance can be globally applied. The seemingly contradictory views of Plato, Aristotle, and the Taoists about balance now seem integrated here, in that we need to balance our own personal passions and desires in a harmonious way with our fellow humans for the healthy future of our planet. However, people must all realize how meaning, health, and balance issues on the individual micro-level connect to meaning, health, and balance issues on a global macro-level and the ethical dilemma that raises (Persson & Erlandsson, 2002).

Reaching individual balance in the Western world by overconsuming resources and negatively influencing global development causes serious threats to the planet's climate and a reasonable global balance of resources. With these issues becoming a top priority on the global agenda and heavily affecting individuals' lifestyles and patterns, it might be necessary to return to the well-known but seldom practiced wisdom that money (or consumption of resources) does not lead to a happier and richer life. This in itself is a challenge, but we have argued in this chapter that it takes awareness and then commitment and practice to create personally and globally balanced lives.

REFERENCES

American Occupational Therapy Association. (1995). Occupation [Position Paper]. *American Journal of Occupational Therapy, 49,* 1015–1018.

Carlson, M. E., & Clark, F. A. (1991). The search for useful methodologies in occupational science. *American Journal of Occupational Therapy, 45,* 235–241.

Christiansen, C. (1996). Three perspectives on balance in occupation. In R. Zemke & F. A. Clark (Eds.), *Occupational science: The evolving discipline* (pp. 431–451). Philadelphia: F. A. Davis.

Christiansen, C., & Baum, C. M. (Eds.) (2004). *Occupational therapy: Performance, participation, and well-being.* Thorofare, NJ: SLACK Incorporated.

Christiansen, C., & Matuska, K. (2006). Lifestyle balance: A review of concepts and research. *Journal of Occupational Science, 13,* 49–61.

Csikszentmihalyi, M. (1975). *Beyond boredom and anxiety: The experience of play in work and games.* San Francisco: Jossey-Bass.

Csikszentmihalyi, M. (1990). *Flow. The psychology of optimal experience.* New York: Harper & Row.

Csikszentmihalyi, M. (1997a). *Creativity: Flow and the psychology of discovery and invention.* New York: HarperCollins.

Csikszentmihalyi, M. (1997b). *Finding flow.* New York: HarperCollins.

Csikszentmihalyi, M. (1999). If we are so rich, why aren't we so happy? *American Psychologist, 54,* 821–827.

Csikszentmihalyi, M., & Hunter, J. (2003). Happiness in everyday life: The uses of experience sampling. *Journal of Happiness Studies, 4,* 185–199.

Csikszentmihalyi, M., & Larson, R. (1987). Validity and reliability of the experience-sampling method. *Journal of Nervous & Mental Disease, 175,* 526–536.

Donovan, N., & Halpern, D. (2002). *Life satisfaction: The state of knowledge and implications for government.* Retrieved on January 20, 2009, from the UK Prime Ministers Strategy Unit Web site : http://www.cabinetoffice.gov.uk/strategy/seminars/life_satisfaction.aspx

Eklund, M., Erlandsson, L.-K., Persson, D., & Hagell, P. (2007). *Rasch analysis of an instrument for measuring occupational value: Implications for theory and practice.* Manuscript submitted for publication.

Elias, M. (2008). *Introduction to the Greek philosophers.* Retrieved on April 4, 2008 from http//articles.directorym.com/Plato_vs_Aristotle-a639.html#68164

Farnworth, L., Mostert, E., Harrison, S., & Worrell, D. (1996). The experience sampling method: Its potential use in occupational therapy research. *Occupational Therapy International, 3,* 1–17.

Feldman, D. H., Csikszentmihalyi, M., & Gardner, H. (1994). *Changing the world: A framework for the study of creativity.* Westport CT: Greenwood Press.

Gerhardsson, C., & Jonsson, H. (1996). Experience of therapeutic occupations in schizophrenic subjects: Clinical observations organized in terms of the flow theory. *Scandinavian Journal of Occupational Therapy, 3,* 149–155.

Hammell, K. W. (2004). Dimensions of meaning in the occupations of daily life. *Canadian Journal of Occupational Therapy, 71,* 296–305.

Jacobs, K. (1994). Flow and the occupational therapy practitioner. *American Journal of Occupational Therapy, 48,* 989–996.

Jonsson, H., Borell, L., & Sadlo, G. (2000). Retirement: An occupational transition with consequences on temporality, rhythm and balance. *Journal of Occupational Science, 7,* 5–13.

Jonsson, H., Josephsson, S., & Kielhofner, G. (2001a). Narratives and experience in an occupational transition: A longitudinal study of the retirement process. *American Journal of Occupational Therapy, 55,* 424–432.

Jonsson, H., Josephsson, S., & Kielhofner, G. (2001b) Evolving narratives in the course of retirement. *American Journal of Occupational Therapy, 54,* 463–476.

Jonsson, H., & Persson, D. (2006). Towards an experiential model of occupational balance: An alternative perspective on flow theory analysis. *Journal of Occupational Science, 13,* 62–73.

Kaptchuk, T. J. (2000). *The web that has no weaver: Understanding Chinese medicine.* Taos, NM: Redwing Book Co.

Kennedy, B. L., & Vecitis, R. N. (2004). Context of the flow experience of women with HIV/AIDS. *OTJR: Occupation, Participation and Health, 24,* 83–91.

Kronenberg, F., & Pollard, N. (2005). Overcoming occupational apartheid: A preliminary exploration of the political nature of occupational therapy. In F. Kronenberg, S. Simo Algado, & N. Pollard (Eds.), *Occupational therapy without borders: Learning from the spirit of survivors* (pp. 58–86). Elsevier Limited.

Massimini, A., & Carli, M. (1988). Systematic assessment of flow in daily experience. In M. Csikszentmihalyi & I. S. Csikszentmihalyi (Eds.), *Optimal experience: Psychological studies of flow in consciousness* (pp. 266–287). Cambridge, UK: Cambridge University Press.

Massimini, A., Carli, M., Delle Fave, A., & Massimini, F. (1988). The quality of experience in the flow channels: Comparison of Italian and U.S. students. In M. Csikszentmihalyi & I. S. Csikszentmihalyi (Eds.), *Optimal experience: Psychological studies of flow in consciousness* (pp. 288–306). Cambridge, UK: Cambridge University Press.

Massimini, F., Csikszentmihalyi, M., & Carli, M. (1987). The monitoring of optimal experience: A tool for psychiatric rehabilitation. *Journal of Mental Disease, 175,* 545–549.

Meyer, A. (1977). The philosophy of occupational therapy. *American Journal of Occupational Therapy, 31,* 639–642. (Originally published 1922)

Moneta, G. B. (2004). The flow model of intrinsic motivation in Chinese: Cultural and personal moderators. *Journal of Happiness Studies, 5,* 181–217.

Murray, C. J. L., & Lopez, A. D. (1996). *The global burden of disease: A comprehensive assessment of mortality and disability from diseases, injuries, and risk factors in 1990 and projected to 2020.* Cambridge, MA: Harvard School of Public Health [on Behalf of the World Health Organization and the World Bank], 1996.

Nelson, D. L. (1988). Occupation: Form and performance. *American Journal of Occupational Therapy, 42,* 633–641.

Nelson, D. L. (1996). Therapeutic occupation: A definition. *American Journal of Occupational Therapy, 50,* 775–782.

Persson, D. (2001). *Aspects of meaning in everyday occupations and its relationships to health-related factors.* Unpublished doctoral thesis, Lund University, Lund, Sweden.

Persson, D., Eklund, M., & Isacsson, A. (1999). The experience of everyday occupations and its relation to sense of coherence—A methodological study. *Journal of Occupational Science, 6,* 13–26.

Persson, D., & Erlandsson, L.-K. (2002). Time to re-evaluate the machine society: Reasoning on postindustrial ethics from an occupational perspective. *Journal of Occupational Science, 9,* 93–99.

Persson, D., Erlandsson, L.-K., Eklund, M., & Iwarsson, S. (2001). Value dimensions, meaning and complexity in human occupations—A tentative structure for analysis. *Scandinavian Journal of Occupational Therapy 8,* 7–18.

Sanne, K. (2007). *Keynes barnbarn: En bättre framtid med arbete och välfärd.* [Keynes grandchildren: A better future with work and welfare]. Forskningsrådet Formas.

Satink, T., Winding, K., & Jonsson, H. (2004). Daily occupation with or without pain: Dilemmas in occupational performance. *Occupational Therapy Journal of Research, 24,* 144–150.

Sato, I. (1988). Bosozoku: Flow in Japanese motorcycle gangs. In M. Csikszentmihalyi & I. S. Csikszentmihalyi (Eds.), *Optimal experience: Psychological studies of flow in consciousness* (pp. 92–117). Cambridge, UK: Cambridge University Press.

Seligman, M. E. P., & Csikszentmihalyi, M. (2000). Positive psychology: An introduction. *American Psychologist, 55,* 5–14.

Statens Folkhälsoinstitut. (2004). *Levnadsvanor och hälsa—de första resultaten från den nationella folkhälsoenkäten Hälsa på lika villkor.* [Life conditions and health—The first results from the national public health survey Health on Equal Conditions]. R 2004:48. Retrieved (in Swedish) January 20, 2009, from: http://www.fhi.se/upload/ar2005/rapporter/r200448levnadsvanorhalsa0504.pdf

Stigsdotter, U., & Grahn, P. (2002). What makes a garden a healing garden? *Journal of Therapeutic Horticulture 13,* 60–69.

Stiles, P. (2005). *Is the American dream killing you? How the market rules our lives.* New York: Collins.

Townsend, E., & Wilcock, A. A. (2004). Occupational justice and client-centred practice: A dialogue-in-process. *Canadian Journal of Occupational Therapy, 71,* 75–87.

Warberg, F., &, Larsson, J. (2005). *Rik på riktigt: En värdefull vardag är möjlig* [Properly rich: A valuable everyday is possible]. Stockholm: Natur & Kultur.

Ware, N. C., & Kleinman, A. (1992). Culture and somatic experience: The social course of illness in neurasthenia and chronic fatigue syndrome. *Psychosomatic Medicine, 54,* 546–560.

Wilcock, A. A. (1998). *An occupational perspective on health.* Thorofare, NJ: SLACK Incorporated.

World Health Organization. (1997). The Jakarta declaration on leading health promotion into the 21st century. *Health Promotion International, 12,* 61–26.

World Health Organization. (2001). *Noncommunicable Diseases and Mental Health.* Retrieved January 20, 2009 from http//www.who.int/mip2001/files/2008/NCDDiseaseBurden.pdf

World Watch Institute. (2004). *State of the world 2004: Special focus—The consumer society.* London: Earthscan.

Wright, J. (2004). Occupation and flow. In M. Molineux (Ed.), *Occupation for occupational therapists* (pp. 66–77). Oxford, UK: Blackwell.

Wright, J. J., Sadlo, G., & Stew, G. (2006). Challenge-skills and mindfulness: An exploration of the conundrum of flow process. *OTJR: Occupation, Participation, and Health, 26,* 25–32.

Wright, J. J., Sadlo, G., & Stew, G. (2007). Further explorations into the conundrum of flow process. *Journal of Occupational Science, 14,* 136–144.

Yerxa, E. J., Clark, F., Frank, G., Jackson, J., Parham, D., Pierce, D., et al. (1990). An introduction to occupational science, a foundation for occupational therapy in the 21st century. *Occupational Therapy in Health Care, 6,* 1–17.

Zemke, R., & Clark, F. (Eds.). (1996). *Occupational science: The evolving discipline.* Philadelphia: F. A. Davis.

A Theoretical Model of Life Balance and Imbalance

Kathleen Matuska and Charles H. Christiansen

INTRODUCTION

A Web search using the term *lifestyle balance* produces 22 million hits, and a search for the term *life balance* produces roughly fourfold more. Clearly, the phrase has become commonly accepted, and people seem to accept the idea that living a balanced life is desirable and possible. A brief scan of the titles from the first 20 Web sites that appeared in the search showed that information and services are available that are intended to help people gain life balance, well-being, and more satisfying lives. The underlying assumptions gleaned from this search are that people can create optimal lives if they make the right choices about what they do in everyday living; that many people are not making the right choices and are therefore stressed, unhappy, or unhealthy; and that they could make improvements with the right information or service.

There seems to be an assumed understanding of what constitutes life balance and what influences it—such as stress, exercise, nutrition, relationships, adequate sleep, a positive attitude, or workplace satisfaction. For the most part, it seems that people have an intuitive sense about what a balanced life would be for them, and the popular press is full of examples and helpful hints to help them achieve whatever that is.

But do people ever actually achieve a balanced life? Does a balanced life mean a *better* life? And if that's possible, what does a balanced life look like? These are the same questions that all the authors in this book are asking and the very questions that started our quest to study the phenomenon.

Discovering the complexities of the questions ultimately led us to bring together multidisciplinary scholars, who have studied various related aspects of life balance for an International Life Balance conference held in Kingston, Ontario, in 2007. Many of the presentations at the conference are reflected in this book, and many of them helped us clarify our thinking about a life balance model we have been developing for several years.

In this chapter, we will describe a proposed a model of life balance that was created after reviewing and synthesizing multidisciplinary research related to the phenomenon of life balance (Christiansen & Matuska, 2006). This model, drawn from work in positive psychology, personality studies, studies of successful aging, studies of resilience, and the literature in occupational science, is a multifaceted way of explaining the recurring patterns of living that define and influence relationships, self-esteem, identity, meaning, purpose, and basic problem solving. In this model,

K. Matuska & C. Christiansen (Eds.)
Life balance: Multidisciplinary theories and research (pp 149–164)
© 2009 SLACK Incorporated and AOTA Press

balanced lives are viewed as resulting from experience, that is, coping with life's demands requires some basic skills in organizing time and managing personal and environmental resources—the kinds of lessons one would imagine being taught if everyone were required to take a course called Life Skills 101. In fact, given the widespread interest in life skills and the emerging demand for life coaching, offering such a course might be well received indeed.

The popular interest in creating balanced lives seems to come from a sense of lacking something; a feeling of imbalance; or a longing for a healthier, more satisfying life. That these feelings are also widespread is suggested in the emergence of terms in popular parlance such as *quality time, mental-health day, stress relief, getaway,* and *burnout.* These terms communicate feelings of imbalance, so it seems valuable to also explore the perceived life imbalance that seems to be driving people to consume information and services to change how they live their lives.

PROPOSED MODEL OF LIFE BALANCE

Our model describes life balance from the standpoint of how everyday patterns of activity meet essential human needs (Matuska & Christiansen, 2008). People can meet their needs through participation in different types of daily activities. For example, some people fulfill their social and relationship needs through friendships and participation in social groups, while others may meet these needs through interactions with family and partners. Thus, the model allows for variability in activity configurations based on individual differences and cultural and environmental influences.

We view life balance as the extent to which an individual's unique patterns of activities (in context) enable needs essential to resilience, well-being, and quality of life to be met. The focus on *activity patterns* and the combination of their perceived and actual states of balance (i.e., what people actually do relative to what they desire doing) differentiates this concept from other positive-state constructs such as happiness or satisfaction with life (Matuska & Christiansen, 2008). Our model asserts that life balance is best represented as a continuum of activity patterns over the life course, during which the individual will experience a variable range of satisfactory states. We view a balanced state as having a range, where activity patterns meet important needs, rather than a designated or precise point on a fulcrum. Instead of prescribing a static or ideal state of balance, our model suggests a dynamic interaction between the person's environment and his or her everyday patterns of activity that result in varying degrees of satisfaction and sustainability over time. Thus, the balance "range" is considered from the standpoint of how activities meet important needs and are congruent with a person's values and expectations at any particular point in time.

The model defines a *balanced lifestyle* as "a satisfying pattern of daily occupations that is healthful, meaningful, and sustainable to an individual within the context of his or her current life circumstances" (Matuska & Christiansen, 2008, p. 11). The term *satisfying* in this definition means congruence between actual participation in activities and desired participation in activities. This definition recognizes that individuals have different roles, role requirements, personalities, values, and interests and that these change over time. It also recognizes that the opportunities and means for meeting needs vary according to the resources available within given physical, social, and cultural environments. It is conceivable, then, that resource limitations can influence the extent to which a person is able to meet needs and participate in valued activities, thus constraining the opportunity to attain a lifestyle with a greater degree of balance.

Furthermore, we identified five dimensions of activities that meet essential needs for a life with greater balance. These dimensions represent a congruent array of daily activities that enable people to do the following:

(1) meet basic instrumental needs necessary for sustained biological health and physical safety; (2) have rewarding and self-affirming relationships with others; (3) feel engaged, challenged, and competent; (4) create meaning and a positive personal iden-

tity; (5) organize their time and energy in ways that enable them to meet important personal goals and renewal. (Matuska & Christiansen, 2008, p. 11)

The model indicates that to the extent people are able to engage consistently in overall patterns of activities that address these dimensions, they will perceive their lives as more satisfying, less stressful, and more meaningful, or *balanced*. The model also shows that lifestyles with greater balance contribute to psychological well-being and overall health, that is, people with greater balance will be less likely to become victims of illness, chronic disease, or depression. (For a more complete description and support for the model, see Matuska & Christiansen, 2008.)

LIFE IMBALANCE

Because we describe life balance as requiring activity patterns that meet important needs related to health, relationships, identity, challenge, and effective time use, then it is reasonable to assume that lifestyles without these attributes are more likely to result in imbalances, *because* their daily activity patterns would not be conducive to meeting these needs. Thus, we view life imbalances as characterized by patterns of daily activities that are perceived to be unsatisfactory to the individual and that (1) increase the risk for physical and mental health problems; (2) limit or compromise participation in valued relationships; (3) are incongruent with establishing or maintaining a satisfactory identity; (4) are felt to be mundane, uninteresting, or unchallenging; or (5) are not sufficiently organized, managed, or comprehensible to enable life meaning, self-renewal, or goal achievement.

People seem to know when their lives feel too stressful, too boring, too rushed, or too unfulfilling, but may not know how to improve those situations. Within the general population, life imbalance is often experienced as difficulty in meeting the demands of modern life because of perceived or actual time constraints. These constraints limit peoples' ability to meet important personal or social needs in a satisfactory or meaningful manner and lead to stress. People often adapt to these time-stress demands by seeking new strategies, such as attending time-management seminars, learning to multitask, taking working vacations, or making more drastic changes in lifestyle by downsizing living environments, changing jobs, or moving to the country (or even other countries). Time-coping strategies are also facilitated by digital technologies such as laptop computers, smart phones, personal digital assistants (PDAs), or use of the Internet for banking, shopping, social networking, or correspondence.

Life imbalances may lead to changed physical, cognitive, or emotional states, such as fatigue or drowsiness resulting from insufficient sleep or a nagging anxiety about the dearth of leisure or opportunities for meaningful socialization with family and friends. This last condition has given rise to the Western expression *quality time*, intended to mean time use that results in richer, more satisfying, and more meaningful social experiences, or in the broader sense, activities that are viewed as representing a higher quality of life.

Wilcock (1998) defines *imbalance* as a

> state that occurs because people's engagement in occupation fails to meet their unique physical, social, mental, or rest needs and allows insufficient time for their own occupational interests and growth as well as for the occupations each feels obliged to undertake in order to meet family, social, and community commitments" (p. 138).

Wilcock and others have proposed that opportunities for engagement in daily activities that enable fulfillment of essential needs are distinguishing features within a socially just society because these needs are so closely related to health and well-being (Townsend and Wilcock, 2004).

Thus, because leading more balance lives requires conditions not wholly under control of individuals, it would not be appropriate to suggest that individuals are accountable for all the situations that contribute to imbalances in their lives. Bickenbach and Glass (2009) write in Chapter

2 in this volume that the "concept of life balance [should] not become one more example [of a condition] that serves only to medicalize personal troubles that are reflections of broader social and cultural tensions" (p. 16).

The dynamic interaction between people and their environments suggests that both internal and external factors influence what people do every day. The internal factors relate to personality and unique individual differences that influence what activity patterns are chosen. For example, even though healthy relationships are associated with well-being (Achat et al., 1998) and an internal factor such as relational insecurity may drive a person to choose activities that are engaged in alone. Another example might be a person who feels the need to spend long hours at one or more jobs because of a personal ambition whose spousal and family relationships are strained as a result.

External factors from the environment influence what activities are chosen. Environments may encourage and support activity patterns through the availability and character of physical and social resources, what Gibson (1979) termed *affordances*, or possibilities for action. There are also advantages to having stable living environments, because consistent and recurring features, such as social conventions, customs, and rituals, can influence habits and routines that provide helpful rhythms to sustain satisfying activity patterns (Clark, 2000; Zerubavel, 1981). For example, having family and friends who are physically active and living in a community that has sidewalks, bike lanes, attractive parks, and recreational facilities is helpful for maintaining a physically active lifestyle. Alternately, other social and cultural environments may not offer such resources nor even place value on a particular activity such as exercise. For an individual to choose a regular exercise regime without environmental support would require different internal resources than what is required of individuals in supportive environments. In other words, as Westhorp (2003) observed, imbalance can be attributed to conditions in the larger community or society as well as to individual habits, routines, and skills.

When people are unable to participate in a variety of meaningful activities because of external constraints or conditions, their ability to lead balanced, healthy lifestyles is compromised. Wilcock (1998) uses the term *occupational deprivation* to describe a state in which people are unable to participate in meaningful activities for prolonged periods of time as a result of factors outside their control. Environmental factors that limit a person's ability to participate in meaningful activities can include social and geographic isolation, economic constraints, cultural differences, and sociopolitical conditions resulting in repression or conflict (Whiteford, 2004). Unemployment, retirement, disability, incarceration, and forced dislocation (including homelessness and refugeeism) are examples of such conditions of deprivation that place an individual at higher risk for life imbalance (Whiteford, 2004).

Chronic health conditions also influence what people are able to do and whether or not they can create a satisfactory balance of activities in their lives. In a phenomenological study of women with multiple sclerosis (MS), Matuska and Erickson (2008) found that the symptoms of MS had a profound influence on the women's perceived life balance. The women with MS expressed how managing their health needs became a major factor in their lives and how they needed to make daily adaptations to continue doing things that were important to them. Fatigue and other physical symptoms required that they adjust their aspirations and self-perceptions and how they nurtured important relationships and modify their hobbies and interests to stay as active as possible. Their disease often dictated what their activity options were in a given day.

Similarly, Kralik, Koch, Price, and Howard (2004) found that people who had arthritis learned about what they could or couldn't do through daily life experiences and as a result of trial-and-error learning. The self-management of their illness occurred through regular reconfiguration of their daily lives and reconstruction of their self-identity by exploring their personal limitations or boundaries. It is easy to imagine that trying to cope with the limitations of a mental or physical disease would add an increased challenge to living a balanced life. Additional reports have been published about people whose balance in life activities was constrained by health conditions.

For an account of work adjustments associated with mental health problems, see Crist, Davis, and Coffin, (2000); for the effects of cognitive problems associated with MS on life balance, see Shevil and Finlayson (2006); and for the challenges of managing everyday self-care for people with chronic obstructive pulmonary disease, see Cicutto, Brooks, and Henderson (2004).

People make choices about what they do, and some choices are better for meeting their needs than others. As discussed earlier, many factors can influence those choices, some more salient than others. In the following sections, we discuss specific conditions that indicate, contribute to, or result from imbalanced activity patterns that have negative consequences to health and well-being, often mediated through stress. These include workaholism, burnout, retirement, obesity, insomnia and sleep disorders, and circadian desynchronosis, or jet lag syndrome. This discussion is not intended to be a comprehensive or complete review but rather a sample of different states where there is evidence to support a link between activity patterns and health consequences with physical, psychological, or social implications.

WORKAHOLISM

Workaholism is a social term modeled after the term *alcoholism*, implying an addiction, but is not a generally accepted medical term. However, the term is widely accepted in the popular parlance to describe an addicted-to-work state. In fact, the 2005 General Social Survey in Canada revealed that one-third of employed Canadians ages 19 to 64 years identify themselves as *workaholics*. This group was not satisfied with their work–life balance and wished they could spend more time with their family and friends (Keown, 2007). The syndrome has become so commonly understood that there are now Workaholics Anonymous 12-step programs for people "identifying themselves as 'powerless over compulsive work, worry, or activity' including, but not limited to, workaholics" (Workaholics Anonymous, 2008, "definition" para. 1). The assumption underlying this state is that when too much time is spent at work, another area is neglected, such as the family or other important relationships. This phenomenon is sometimes described as *spillover*.

The scientific community is only now exploring workaholism, and researchers are calling for more empirical support for the syndrome and its effects. In a review of the available research on the topic, Piotrowski and Vodanovich (2006) concluded that workaholism is associated with an increase in perceived work–life conflict, high levels of family distress, and dissatisfaction in life. A workaholic has been described as someone who has all three of the following characteristics: (1) high work involvement, (2) high drive to work, and (3) low work enjoyment (Spence & Robbins, 1992). People who had the three characteristics of the workaholic profile were more likely to label themselves as workaholics, more likely to have acquaintances label them as workaholics, and more likely to have lower life satisfaction and higher work–life imbalance than people who had only one or two of the characteristics (Aziz & Zicker, 2006). People with workaholic profiles delegated responsibility less, were more likely to be perfectionists, perceived their experiences as more stressful, and had more health complaints than people without the profile (Spence & Robbins, 1992).

Workaholism has also been associated with social problems. Indeed, people who self-reported high work addiction also reported greater interference with social and intimate relationships (Robinson & Post, 1995). Living with a workaholic spouse has also been shown to be significantly related to marital disaffection and lower positive feeling toward spouses (Robinson, Carroll, & Flowers, 2001; Robinson, Flowers, & Ng, 2006). Moreover, workaholism also has been found to affect the entire family, with adult children having significantly more psychological problems and health complaints (Carroll & Robinson, 2000).

Interestingly, research has also shown that workaholics were aware of their problems and used relationships as a form of coping mechanism or stress buffer. McMillan, O'Driscoll, and Brady (2004) tested the proposition that workaholics deny their workaholism and experience greater disturbances in close relationships than do *non-workaholics*. Through workers' own self-ratings and partner or spouse ratings, they found that workaholics self-rated their level of workaholism similar to the ratings provided by their spouse or partner. They also found that satisfaction with their personal relationship (with their spouse or partner) was minimally affected by workaholism and that intimate relationships may act as stress buffers for workaholics. Clearly, the conflicting findings about the characteristics of workaholics and the social consequences of workaholism warrant further study into the syndrome and its defining characteristics.

Workaholism is most likely affected by broader sociocultural and economic influences, such as competitive job markets, stagnant wages and salaries, and higher costs of living, but surprising little attention is paid to this in the academic literature. Moreover, it seems unlikely that workaholism as it is defined here would be very prevalent in poor and developing nations. Many magazine and newspaper articles bemoan the blending of work and nonwork activities and blame technological advances (e.g., Erase-Blunt, 2001) for the ease of doing work tasks at home or on vacation. Other insidious factors that may be influencing the perceived incidence of workaholism stem from the employer, such as increased productivity demands, incentive systems for higher productivity, and a work culture that emphasizes job loyalty (Piotrowski & Vodanovich, 2006). The increased competition in the global marketplace, economic insecurity, and cultural value of consumerism may also influence perceived job insecurity, creating a sense of urgency in work that fuels the beginning stages of overwork.

Workaholism represents a form of life imbalance when the drive to work becomes a pattern of everyday activity that is no longer considered satisfactory and fails to meet an individual's needs. Preliminary evidence suggests workaholism may increase the risk for physical and mental health problems and may place a strain on valued relationships. Finally, if workaholism persists, many believe the final consequence is burnout (Schaufeli, Taris, & van Rhenen, 2008) a topic to which we now turn our attention.

BURNOUT

Is burnout an end-product of workaholism? Schaufeli, Taris, and van Rhenen (2008) investigated this question with 587 telecom managers to determine whether workaholism, burnout, and work engagement were actually different constructs or simply versions of the same thing. They concluded that the three constructs are different because they each retained unique patterns of relationships among five work-related variables. *Burnout* is a result of perceived imbalance in work or in other major responsibilities that presents as a psychological syndrome resulting from prolonged response to chronic interpersonal stressors. It is commonly described as a state of mental weariness, and the most widely used conceptualization originates from Maslach (1993), who described three major components of burnout: (1) *exhaustion,* (2) *cynicism,* and (3) *inefficiency.* The *exhaustion* component refers to feelings of being overextended and depleted of emotional and physical resources and is the strongest predictor of negative health outcomes (Schaufeli et al., 2008). The *cynicism* (or depersonalization) component represents the interpersonal dimension of burnout and refers to a negative, callous, or excessively detached response to various aspects of the job. The component of *inefficiency* (or reduced accomplishment) represents the self-evaluation dimension of burnout and refers to feelings of incompetence and a lack of achievement and productivity (Breso, Salanova, & Schaufeli, 2007; Maslach & Leiter, 2008). Burnout is often seen in high-stakes and high-stress jobs such as critical health care (Peterson et al., 2008) and disaster relief (Figley, 2002), where there is an intense emotional component.

Burnout is identified as a condition in the *International Classification of Diseases* (ICD-10; World Health Organization [WHO], 2007), under the category Z73, problems related to life management difficulty. Burnout can be considered a life imbalance because employment is no longer meeting important needs of competence and challenge or contributing to a satisfactory identity. Furthermore, people who are experiencing burnout may not find opportunities for renewal and experience reduced productivity, thus diminishing their self-esteem and overall affect. For example, significantly more self-reported depression, anxiety, sleep disturbance, memory impairment, and neck and back pain were reported by Swedish health-care workers who were burned out than workers who were not (Peterson et al., 2008). On the other hand, getting adequate sleep seems to be a buffer against the risk for long term burnout (Sonnenschein et al., 2008). One surprising finding was that burned out managers did not have higher stress consequences than healthy managers as measured by their allostatic load, which is an emerging index of the effects of cumulative stress consisting of 10 physiological indicators (Langelaan, Bakker, Schaufeli, van Rhenen, & van Doornen, 2007). The authors of this study concluded that the mediating physiological mechanisms between burnout and objective physical health have not yet been identified.

A common lay perception of other types of imbalance (such as obesity and workaholism) is that these represent an inability of the individual to self-manage behavior or lifestyle. In contrast, however, it is commonly perceived that burnout is less subject to personal control and that anyone may experience burnout if the work conditions are demanding enough. As it turns out, there is some evidence that certain work conditions are more predictive of burnout than others. Even though some evidence shows that workaholism can be a precursor to burnout (Schaufeli et al., 2008), the environmental presses from the job are the strongest predictors. The job characteristics that are predictors of burnout include a perceived imbalance of effort and reward (Uterbrink et al., 2007), work overload that is paired with poor resources (lack of social support from supervisor or coworkers), lack of job control (Schaufeli et al., 2008), and lack of perceived fairness (Maslach & Leiter, 2008).

Bullying is a form of unfairness in its extreme expression, and for Portuguese nurses it took the form of being expected to do tasks below their level of competence, having areas of responsibility removed or replaced with more trivial or unpleasant tasks, and being exposed to unmanageable levels of workload (Fleming, 2008). The bullied nurses had significantly higher levels of emotional exhaustion and lowered levels of mental health compared with nonbullied colleagues.

Evidence shows that the work environment contributes to employee burnout, but are there certain internal factors or personal characteristics that increase the risk for burnout? Research is limited on this question, except for the evidence linking the personal traits associated with workaholism to eventual burnout (Schaufeli et al., 2008). Most studies of burnout have emphasized work environments and their influence on employees rather than examining potential interactions between personal characteristics and the work environment and how this might serve to mediate consequences such as burnout. However, some research has been done on identifying the early warning signs of burnout.

Toward this end, Ericson-Lidman and Strandberg (2007) obtained narratives from coworkers of people who were on sick leave because of burnout and found that coworkers retrospectively recalled a multiplicity of signs in their work mates before they were burned out. They perceived that the people concerned were attempting to manage alone, showing self-sacrifice, struggling to achieve unattainable goals, becoming distanced and isolated, and showing signs of falling apart. Some of the signs preceding workmate's burnout may be difficult to interpret as signs of the condition, because they may be regarded as characteristics that are to some extent encouraged in the prevailing culture (Ericson-Lidman & Strandberg, 2007).

We surmise that it is likely that most people readily recognize when they are ready for change and, if conditions permit, often take corrective action to change their job circumstances to create more favorable circumstances for their well-being. Often, these changes take the form of new projects, new work locations, new jobs, or retirement. Retirement might be an antidote to burnout for some, but it can also represent a change in life circumstances and patterns that is less than satisfactory for others. The sudden change from one set of activities to another that often accompanies retirement has been the focus of increased study in recent years. Retirement is often regarded as the point at which people have more control over their lives and therefore a greater chance at obtaining the life balance they see as ideal. However, this does not always occur. (See for example, the discussion of retirees by Persson and Jonsson in Chapter 10 of this volume.) In the following section, we briefly review what other literature reveals about the changes in lifestyle that occur during retirement. In keeping with the present theme, we focus particularly on the imbalances that often result in the transition from work to retirement.

RETIREMENT

Employment offers people many benefits beyond a paycheck. It contributes to identity development, provides structure and routine, stimulates social interactions, and affords challenges and an opportunity to feel engaged and competent. Although these benefits may diminish over time, or with age, they are no longer available in the same way once retired. Many people put so much time and effort into their work that they have few interests or hobbies that will keep them stimulated when they retire. For white men in particular, the rates of depression, illness, and death increase fairly dramatically within 3 to 5 years after the person has retired (Chop, 1999). There is speculation and evidence that these consequences are related to the lack of need fulfillment, life purpose, and identity that can result from the dramatic lifestyle changes following retirement.

The first wave of baby boomers are starting to retire now, and it is predicted that, because of economic realities and changing attitudes toward work by people ages 60 years and older, most baby boomers will continue working at least part-time during their retirement years. In a study of people in this category, three-quarters specified needs other than financial as their most important reason for working after retirement (Jonsson & Andersson, 1999). According to an AARP (2006) survey of 60-year-olds, of those responding, 54% were still working, 37% specified they would work "until I drop," and 14% who were not currently working plan to go back to work in the next few years. This group of 60-year-olds was substantially satisfied with their lives, but 87% want to take better care of their physical health, 72% plan to spend more time on interests and hobbies, and 47% want to do more volunteering.

Typically, new patterns of work by retiring baby boomers involve mid-level jobs that are less demanding and stressful. This is because workers of retirement age desire less-demanding lifestyles. Retirement is viewed as a time when they should be able to engage in more leisure activities and enjoy life more. Studies have shown that certain types of leisure activities are more related to life satisfaction than others. Higher life satisfaction is associated with leisure activities that have the following characteristics: *self-determination* (feel in control of leisure behaviors), *competence* (leisure behaviors with competence feedback), and *challenge* (leisure experiences that stretch one's limits and provide novel stimuli). Of these, leisure activities that afford challenge seem to offer the most explanatory power relative to life satisfaction (Guinn, 1999).

Most people do not take up new activities after retirement but do more of the familiar activities. People who adapt most successfully to retirement are those who have to make the least changes (Jonsson, Josephsson, & Kielhofner, 2001). Although it is widely perceived that volunteering is a retirement activity that promotes satisfaction, Oakley found that volunteering was not, in itself, associated with life satisfaction (Oakley & Pratt, 1997).

Four personal characteristics seem to be linked to retirement satisfaction: (1) health, (2) income, (3) attitudes, and (4) preparedness for retirement (Sterns, Junkins, & Bayer, 1999). Positive attitude is important, but many retirees are still not ready for the changes that occur in their lifestyles. A realistic attitude seems to be more important (Sterns et al., 1999). People who plan for major life changes are more successful in dealing with them. Thus, those who plan for retirement seem to adjust more successfully (Sterns, Junkins, & Bayer, 1999).

Some additional insights into the factors related to successful adaption to retirement were provided through a study reported by Jonsson et al. (2001). In this qualitative longitudinal study, retirement-age workers were followed for 7 years and interviewed before and following retirement. Among other findings from this important study, retirees generally found that the transition from work to retirement was more complex and unpredictable than they imagined. A key factor related to adjustment seemed to involve the shift from external demands to internal motivation as an incentive for participation. Some workers found it difficult to create satisfying routines without external demands to help them structure their lives.

Another interesting finding related to the subjects' daily occupational rhythms and the surprising lack of free time. Subjects found that the time made available with the absence of paid work was quickly consumed if they were not mindful of allocating their time to obligatory activities such as housework, self-care, and shopping. Unless they specifically structured their day, casual plans for taking up new activities were often not realized.

The respondents also found that the meaning of some occupations changed when work was not there to provide a contrast. For example, going to the cabin, which was seen as a special event during the working years, became more ordinary. The authors concluded that the meaning of occupations changed in relation to the narrative or story line of the person's life. That is, the meanings of the activity were different in the context of a longer time frame, when the activities preceding and following a given leisure occupation changed. It is easy to imagine that a fishing trip wedged between months of demanding work is different than a fishing trip that it breaks periods of boredom or inactivity.

Another finding of the longitudinal study reported by Jonsson and colleagues (2001) was that retirement occupations characterized by keen interest and sustained involvement were related to greater life satisfaction. This characteristic or quality was described as a factor of engagement. The presence or absence of engaging occupations appeared to be the main determinant of whether participants were able to achieve positive life experiences as retirees. Those who had difficulty adjusting to retirement had no truly engaging occupations.

OBESITY

Obesity is a maladaption of wealth (from a global perspective) but also an indicator of life imbalance. Approximately 60% of American adults are obese (Ogden, Carroll, McDowell, & Flegal, 2007), and sedentary lifestyles have been directly linked to an increased risk of obesity (Jebb & Moore, 1999). This incidence has been at epidemic proportions for several years, but even more alarming is the increasing trend for childhood obesity, with one in six children or adolescents in the United States being obese (Baskin, Ard, Franklin, & Allison, 2005), with significant variation in incidence found among ethnic and socioeconomic groups (Crawford, Story, Wang, Richie, & Sabry, 2001). Childhood obesity not only carries with it increased health risks but significant risks for decreased self-esteem and elevated levels of loneliness, sadness, and nervousness (Strauss, 2000).

The generally understood cause of obesity is increased calorie consumption relative to decreased energy output. At an individual lifestyle level, changes in daily patterns of activity that increase energy output relative to calorie input will make a big impact on obesity. It is a relatively simple formula: If individuals change their regular patterns of activity to include more physical activity and less high-calorie snacking, they will reduce their weight and improve their health and well-being (Jebb & Moore, 1999). Yet if the principles for avoiding weight gain or losing excess pounds are so clear and simple, why is intensive pharmacological and behavioral therapy for weight loss only moderately effective at best (McTigue et al., 2003)? An entire medical system exists to address the problem, including invasive surgery, yet the problem still persists and grows.

Within the model of life balance proposed in this chapter, obesity provides an excellent example of how factors work in combination to promote or disturb healthy lifestyles. It is true that sedentary lifestyles contribute to obesity, but it is also true that sedentary lifestyles are often a product of social isolation, low self-esteem, and a self-identity that is viewed as unsatisfactory. It is often the case that obesity contributes to low self-esteem and identity dissatisfaction, which in turn reduces the tendency of some people to participate in the more active lifestyles that tend toward more rather than less social interaction.

One model applied to eating behavior, borrowed from studies of alcohol consumption, characterizes eating as responding to one or more of four primary motives: (1) to cope with negative feelings, (2) to be social, (3) to comply with others' expectations, and (4) to enhance pleasure (e.g., see Jackson, Cooper, Mintz, & Albino, 2003). There are obvious connections between these motives and the need-based activity categories in the life balance model, particularly those associated with self-identity and rewarding relationships with others.

While many studies focus on the relationship between sedentary activity, such as watching television, and obesity, even the prevalence of sedentary activity must be viewed in a larger context, such as the ability of the individual to manage time and organize individual activity toward productive pursuits. A study reported by Feldman, Barnett, Shrier, Rossignol, and Abenheim (2003) showed the prevalence of sedentary activity in adolescent subjects was not inversely related to physical activity but was, instead, related to time management and engagement in other productive activity, such as part-time employment. Clearly, a complete understanding of obesity and its relationship to lifestyle must encompass more than a determination of the physical activity and sedentary activity profiles of subjects.

However, environmental factors also contribute to the obesity epidemic in the United States. Environmental factors are largely ignored in the medical system, where, when it occurs, the focus is typically only on personal lifestyle change. The production and marketing of food that is more fully prepared, readily available, and highly promoted through competitive business strategies contributes to diets that have a higher fat and calorie content (Tillotson, 2004). In general, healthier foods with less fat content are usually more expensive, and thus less-healthy foods have become a major source of the American diet in lower socioeconomic groups. Although personal choice is still important for balanced eating, broader agricultural and economic policies and practices create an environment that makes it more difficult to make healthy choices. These factors, driven in part by a profit motive, must be acknowledged in any serious discussion of the obesity epidemic in the United States.

Poor food options driven by economic factors may partially explain why socioeconomically disadvantaged populations have a greater prevalence of obesity compared to white, economically advantaged populations (Ford & Dzewaltowski, 2008). Economic factors, such as cost and the proximity or availability of recreational facilities, also partially explain why there is a greater prevalence of obesity and lower activity levels among rural youth than urban youth (Joens-Matre et al., 2008).

Environments with lower-than-average neighborhood availability of healthful foods and higher than average availability of fast food restaurants, along with exposure to ethnically targeted food marketing may contribute to reliance on high-calorie foods and beverages. In addition, these foods may be socially and culturally valued. Attitudes about and environmental contexts for physical activity are also relevant. "Increasingly, it is acknowledged that individual behaviors and lifestyles (e.g., food choices, child feeding practices), are responsive to the ecological contexts in which they are practiced" (Kumanyika, 2008, p. 61).

The model of life balance presented in this chapter shows that multiple factors contribute to imbalance, and these are often interconnected, as we have related in this short discussion of obesity. Not mentioned above, however, has been the connection between obesity and sleep duration. While one might be tempted to conclude that these two factors are positively correlated (i.e., less sleep equals less obesity), studies show that the relationship is inverse. Less sleep tends to equate with higher levels of obesity (Chaput, Després, Bouchard, & Tremblay, 2007; Vioque, Torres, & Quiles, 2000). The central role of sleep as an indicator of life balance is a topic to which we turn in the following section.

INSOMNIA AND SLEEP DISORDERS

Sleep is an important and obligatory daily human occupation, and on average, normal healthy adults spend nearly one-third of their lives sleeping (Roehrs & Roth, 2004). Recent research has shown that sleep is vital for health and that sleep deficits are related to the emergence of many chronic diseases as well as to life expectancy (Chaput et al., 2007; Dew et al., 2003). Although sleep is not yet completely understood, empirical research over the past half-century has revealed the phases of normal sleep; the importance of rapid eye movement (REM) sleep; and clear associations between sleep quality and duration and immune function, overall health, and longevity (Dew et al., 2003). Sleep disorders include insomnia, fragmented sleep, sleep of limited duration, and sleep of poor quality (unrestful sleep).

It is generally accepted that there is clear a association between stress and sleep, and current theory postulates that an important purpose of sleep is to serve as a stress buffer, with normal sleep serving to provide resilience against the damaging health effects of everyday stressors (Mohr et al., 2003). Sleep disorders often follow significant traumatic events (Clum, Nishith, & Resick, 2001) and psychiatric disturbances, such as severe depression (Lustberg & Reynolds, 2000).

Because sleep is such a major and necessary daily occupation, its disturbance almost by definition constitutes an imbalance in time use and lifestyle. Further, the literature on sleep disorders shows that sleep quality is related to what people do during the day, their experiences of stress, and the manner in which they cope with stressful circumstances (Atkinson & Davenne, 2007; Landis et al., 2003). There is emerging evidence on the relationship among sleep disorders, daily lifestyle experiences, and health. This highlights the importance of sleep disorders as important manifestations of life imbalance.

CIRCADIAN DESYNCHRONOSIS: JET LAG SYNDROME

Some people experience insomnia because of *desynchronosis*, a condition where the body's internal clocks are not synchronized with the external environment. The study of chronobiology has provided scientists with a keen understanding of how hormones work to influence normal rest–activity cycles. These cycles are important for maintaining health and enabling the body to adjust to changes in the environment, such as day and night, and allowing people to be alert or to sleep when it is necessary for them to do so. Scientists have learned that light is an important regulator of our internal clocks and that regular activity helps to "reset the clocks" to enable entrainment, that is, to have the body's internal clocks synchronized with the external environment. These regular, time-adjusting activities are known as *zeitgebers*, and the importance of zeitgebers to entrainment and health is being better understood. Scientists have found some important biological reasons for maintaining a relatively consistent daily routine. When desynchronosis occurs, such as with travel across multiple time zones, the body's clocks are out of adjustment with the environment, and drowsiness or sleeplessness result when people should be respectively alert or resting. Most people know this condition by its popular label, "jet lag syndrome."

People whose work schedules require them to disregard their natural biological rhythms are at risk of disentrainment because their activity schedules cause them to be active when they would ordinarily be at rest. Airline workers, emergency personnel, and a host of other shift workers may be at greater risk for the deleterious effects of such disentrained activity patterns, which can include performance decrements and diminished safety, as well as insomnia, immune dysfunction, and increased risk for cancer and cardiac conditions (Boivin, Tremblay, & James, 2007; Boggild & Knuttson, 1999; Costa, Sartori, & Akerstedt, 2006; Haus & Smolensky, 2006). Shift work can be related to diminished sleep quality and quantity. In turn, diminished sleep duration and quality have been associated with affective disorders and higher rates of mortality (Dew et al.,

2003). Existing approaches to correcting desynchronosis are based on the current understanding of the reciprocal influences of human activity and internal timekeeping mechanisms and involve dietary, pharmacologic, and behavioral regimens, including exercise and lifestyle changes (Peate, 2007). Taken together, existing evidence on sleep disorders and desynchronosis suggest that these are important consequences of irregular activity patterns that should be considered in models of life balance.

CONCLUDING COMMENTS

In this chapter, we have presented a model of life balance based on a perspective of activity patterns within daily lives and over time. The model emphasizes that it is important that people engage regularly in activities that enable them to meet essential human needs for physical health, satisfactory social relationships, personal identity, and meaning. An added requirement is that people possess the skills and competencies necessary to manage time and personal resources effectively.

This model goes beyond traditional public health approaches that view lifestyle from the standpoint of human participation in specific behaviors that compromise health and safety, to a comprehensive view of time use that acknowledges the relationships among activities within the context of lives. We assert that comprehensive programs aimed at promoting health and achieving wellness must recognize the central role that psychological needs play in motivating behavior. They must also recognize the need to assist people to manage all facets of their lives to avoid patterns that lead to ineffective adaptation and the chronic health consequences that result.

We believe that beyond basic life skills, engagement in interesting and meaningful activities is a central part of a healthy lifestyle. When people are unable to manage their time and their competencies to enjoy feelings of personal productivity and worth, they experience stress, which is a central mediator between lifestyle, health, and longevity. We contend that recognition of the confluence of these activities in defining and explaining a continuum of healthful activity patterns is key to explaining the relationship between lifestyle and health and should be central to future population-based approaches toward preventing disease.

Although the life balance model presented in this chapter was formulated based on research about human flourishing and resilience, the unified model itself is largely untested and serves as a beginning point for additional study. Research supports the idea that meeting important needs is linked to positive physical and mental health outcomes, but additional research is needed to support linking the five need dimensions proposed in the model to consistent patterns of activity within lives. We contend that just as good nutrition requires careful attention to planning meals, healthy lifestyles require attention to planning activities that are need fulfilling.

Matuska and Erickson (2008) reported that the model has validity evidence when used to understand life balance for women who have MS. Their study supports the claim that the five need dimensions proposed in the model were important to the participants' sense of life balance. However, additional evidence of validity is needed before the model can be justified as a guide for intervention.

Furthermore, there is no evidence that a *balance* among the five need dimensions contained in the model is essential. It is possible that, as Maslow suggested in borrowing a concept from chemistry, some needs have stronger "valences" (or are more important to overall well-being) than others. Still unexplored is the possibility that some people might do very little to meet one or two of the five proposed needs outlined in the model, yet perceive their lives to be satisfactory or experience little stress. This is an important question for future research. We anticipate that differences in personality, temperament, and experience may provide for differences in the amount of activity required to fulfill needs in each area. In other words, we doubt that there is a "balanced life" regimen that works for everyone based on time allocation. However, we do believe that attention to planning regular activity that addresses the needs identified in the model will contribute to better resilience, greater satisfaction, and better long-term health.

We also acknowledge that some life activities can meet many needs simultaneously. For example, playing in a marching band or organized team sports may fulfill needs for simultaneously experiencing challenging, engaging activity; creating meaningful social relationships; building identity; and perhaps improving physical fitness. Indeed, it is the ability to find synergistic activities (i.e., those that simultaneously meet multiple needs) that seems so important to managing the time, energy, and other resources that are necessary for effectively balancing a life. Often, balancing lives requires improvisation.

This is one of the messages Mary Catherine Bateson, the renowned writer and anthropologist, wrote in her book *Composing a Life,* describing the ways through which her artist friends were able to meet multiple needs as they crafted their lives. She noted that the challenges and changes of the modern era have made the satisfactory "composition "of a life a more daunting task:

> Just as the design of a building or of a vase must be rethought as the scale has changed, so must he design of lives. Most of the most basic concepts we use to construct a sense of self or the design of a life have changed their meanings: Work. Home. Love. Commitment. (Bateson, 2001, p. 2)

We are convinced that living balanced lives requires role models, reflection, and improvisation. Together these represent the resource management or crafting competencies identified in the model, and described with such eloquence and insight by Bateson.

Additionally, an entire line of research is necessary to explore the assertion that the five need dimensions are universal. Although it is likely that different activities will be pursued to meet the needs across different cultures and environmental contexts, it is not clear that the needs identified in this model as being necessary for a balanced and resilient life are culturally universal. We assume that the model applies mainly to people living in developed Western nations because the idea of developing a coherent and satisfying personal identity might not apply or may differently apply in cultures where the individual gains identity through participation as part of a larger social collective (e.g., Japanese culture).

Our participation in conceptualizing and organizing the conference that led to this volume was based on the expectation that sharing diverse perspectives through an international and interdisciplinary group of social scientists would help us shape and refine this model, and we were not disappointed.

We keenly recognize that in order for the proposed model to evolve it will need a valid and reliable approach for measuring need-related activity participation, satisfaction, and life management skills. It then will require evidence that these skills, perceptions, and activities are collectively related to reduced stress and improved well-being. Most importantly, the model must result in a condition that is demonstrably different than other well-defined and measured positive states. This is a point that was clearly made by our colleague Kennon Sheldon in Chapter 6. That is, collectively our model must provide information that is different from existing concepts such as subjective well-being or life satisfaction.

Achieving this may make it necessary to identify specific types of activities that typically meet various needs. For example, playing competitive board games may reside in a category of activities that provide for challenge and socialization. Sketching, doing pottery, or singing might be activities that meet needs for creativity and self-expression. A good deal of research has been done on personality and activity preference, and work has also been done linking personality types and needs. What may be needed is additional work that links needs and activity preferences.

Otherwise, it may be necessary to devise a means for measuring time use while including certain qualitative dimensions, such as identity congruence, enjoyment, challenge, or meaning. Hybrid measurement approaches have been developed and validated in action psychology that can provide data that include individual perceptions (or qualitative information) as well as empirical observations that can be compared across groups, such as actual time use. An example of a successful and novel measurement approach of this type is Personal Projects Analysis, which was devised by Brian Little, who wrote the foreword to this volume (see Christiansen, Little, and Backman, 1998, for a description).

Clearly, there is much work to be done. In our view, however, it is less important that the model we propose endures or prevails than it is to draw attention to and encourage the work of social scientists on the important questions addressed in this volume. In the end, if society succeeds in answering the larger question of what characteristics are most likely to bring satisfaction, health, and well-being to people as they live their lives, an important advance that will benefit many people will have been accomplished.

REFERENCES

Achat, H., Kawachi, I., Levine, S., Berkey, C., Coakley, E., & Colditz, G. (1998). Social networks, stress, and health related quality of life. *Quality of Life Research, 7,* 735–750.

AARP (2006). *Lifestyles: Boomers turning 60.* Retrieved May 24, 2008, from http://www.aarp.org/research/family/lifestyles/boomers60.html

Atkinson, G., & Davenne, D. (2007). Relationships between sleep, physical activity and human health. *Physiology and Behavior, 90,* 229–235.

Aziz, S., & Zicker, M. J. (2006). A cluster analysis investigation of workaholism as a syndrome. *Journal of Occupational Health Psychology, 11,* 52–62.

Bateson, M. C. (2001). *Composing a life.* New York: Grove/Atlantic.

Baskin, M. L., Ard, J., Franklin, F., & Allison, D. B. (2005). Prevalence of obesity in the United States [electronic version]. *Obesity Reviews, 6,* 5–7.

Bickenbach, J. E., & Glass, T. (2009). Life balance: The meaning and the menace in a metaphor. In K. Matuska & C. Christiansen (Eds.), *Life balance: Multidisciplinary theories and research* (pp. 13–22). Bethesda, MD: AOTA Press/ SLACK Incorporated.

Boggild, H., & Knutsson, A. (1999). Shift work, risk factors and cardiovascular disease. *Scandinavian Journal of Work, Environment and Health, 25,* 85–99.

Boivin, D. B., Tremblay, G. M., & James, F. O. (2007). Working on atypical schedules. *Sleep Medicine, 8,* 578–589.

Breso, E., Salanova, M., & Schaufeli, W. B. (2007) In search of the "third dimension" of burnout: Efficacy or inefficacy? *Applied Psychology, 56,* 460–478.

Carroll, J. J., & Robinson, B. E. (2000). Depression and parentification among adults as related to parental workaholism and alcoholism. *Family Journal, 8,* 360–367.

Chaput, J. P., Després, J. P., Bouchard, C., & Tremblay, A. (2007). Short sleep duration is associated with reduced leptin levels and increased adiposity: Results from the Quebec family study. *Obesity, 15,* 253–261.

Chop, W. C. (1999). Demographic trends of an aging society. In W. C. Chop & R. H. Robnet (Eds.), *Gerontology for the healthcare professional* (pp. 1–16). Philadelphia: F. A. Davis.

Christiansen, C. H., Little, B. R., & Backman, C (1998). Personal projects: A useful approach to the study of occupation. *American Journal of Occupational Therapy 52,* 439–446.

Christiansen, C., & Matuska, K. (2006). Life balance: A review of concepts and research. *Journal of Occupational Science, 13,* 49–61.

Cicutto, L., Brooks, D., & Henderson, K. (2004). Self-care issues from the perspective of individuals with chronic obstructive pulmonary disease. *Patient Education and Counseling, 55,* 168–176.

Clark, F. A. (2000). The concepts of habit and routine: A preliminary theoretical synthesis. *Occupational Therapy Journal of Research, 20,* 123S–138S.

Clum, G. A., Nishith, P., & Resick, P. A. (2001). Trauma-related sleep disturbance and self-reported physical health symptoms in treatment-seeking female rape victims. *Journal of Nervous and Mental Disease, 189,* 618–622.

Costa, G., Sartori, S., & Akerstedt, T. (2006). Influence of flexibility and variability of working hours on health and well-being. *Chronobiology International, 23,* 1125–1137.

Crawford, M., Story, M., Wang, L., Ritchie, Z., & Sabry, Z. I. (2001). Ethnic issues in the epidemiology of childhood obesity [Electronic version]. *Pediatric Clinics of North America, 48,* 855–878.

Crist, P. H., Davis, C. G., & Coffin, P. S. (2000). The effects of employment and mental health status on the balance of work, play/leisure, self-care, and rest. *Occupational Therapy in Mental Health, 15,* 27–42.

Dew, M. A., Hoch, C. C., Buysse, D. J., Monk, T. H., Begley, A. E., Houck, P. R., et al. (2003). Healthy older adults' sleep predicts all-cause mortality at 4 to 19 years of follow-up. *Psychosomatic Medicine, 65,* 63–73.

Erase-Blunt, M. (2001). The busman's holiday. *HR Magazine, 46,* 76–80.

Ericson-Lidman, E., & Strandberg, G. (2007). Burnout: Coworkers' perceptions of signs preceding workmates' burnout. *Journal of Advanced Nursing, 60,* 199–208.

Feldman, D. E., Barnett, T., Shrier, I., Rossignol, M., & Abenhaim, L. (2003). Is physical activity differentially associated with different types of sedentary pursuits? *Archives of Pediatrics and Adolescent Medicine, 157,* 797–802.

Figley, C. (2002). *Treating compassion fatigue.* New York: Brunner-Routledge.

Fleming, M. S. (2008). Bullying, burnout, and mental health amongst Portuguese nurses [Electronic version]. *Issues in Mental Health Nursing, 29,* 411–426.

Ford, P. B., & Dzewaltowski, D. A. (2008). Disparities in obesity prevalence due to variation in the retail food environment: Three testable hypotheses. *Nutrition Reviews, 66,* 216–228.

Gibson, J. J. (1979). *The ecological approach to vision perception.* Boston: Houghton-Mifflin.

Guinn, B. (1999). Leisure behavior modification and the life satisfaction of retired persons. *Activities, Adaptation, and Aging, 23,* 13–20.

Haus, E., & Smolensky, M. (2006). Biological clocks and shift work: Circadian dysregulation and potential long-term effects. *Cancer Causes and Control, 17,* 489–500.

Jackson, B., Cooper, M. L., Mintz, L., & Albino, A. (2003). Motivations to eat: Scale development and validation. *Journal of Research in Personality, 37,* 297–318.

Jebb, S., & Moore, M. (1999). Contribution of a sedentary lifestyle and inactivity to the etiology of overweight and obesity: Current evidence and research issues: Roundtable Consensus Statement [Electronic version]. *Medicine and Science in Sports and Exercise, 31(Suppl 11),* S531–S534.

Joens-Matre, R. R., Welk, G. J., Calabro, M. A., Russell, D. W., Nicklay, E., & Hensley, L. D. (2008). Rural–urban differences in physical activity, physical fitness, and overweight prevalence of children. *Journal of Rural Health, 24,* 49–54.

Jonsson, H., & Andersson, L. (1999). Attitudes to work and retirement: Generalization or diversity. *Scandinavian Journal of Occupational Therapy, 6,* 29–35.

Jonsson, H., Josephsson, S., & Kielhofner, G. (2001). Narratives and experience in an occupational transition: A longitudinal study. *American Journal of Occupational Therapy, 55,* 424–432.

Keown, L. A. (2007). Time escapes me: Workaholics and time perception. (Canadian Social Trends, No. 83, May 15, 2007) *Statistics Canada, Catalogue #11-008,* 28–32.

Kralik, D., Koch, T., Price, K., & Howard, N. (2004). Chronic illness self-management: Taking action to create order. *Journal of Clinical Nursing, 13,* 2, 259-267.

Landis, C. A., Frey, C. A., Lentz, M. J., Rothermel, J., Buchwald, D., & Shaver, J. L. (2003). Self-reported sleep quality and fatigue correlates with actigraphy in midlife women with fibromyalgia. *Nursing Research, 52,* 140–147.

Langelaan, S., Bakker, A. B., Schaufeli, W. B., van Rhenen, W., & van Doornen, L. J. P. (2007). Is burnout related to allostatic load? *International Journal of Behavioral Medicine, 14,* 213–221.

Kumanyika, S. K. (2008). Environmental influences on childhood obesity: Ethnic and cultural influences in context. *Physiology and Behavior, 94,* 61–70.

Lustberg, L., & Reyolds, C. F. (2000). Depression and insomnia: Questions of cause and effect. *Sleep Medicine Reviews, 4,* 253–262.

Maslach, C. (1993). Burnout: A multidimensional perspective. In W. B. Schaufeli, C. Maslach, & T. Marek (Eds.), *Professional burnout: Recent developments in theory and research* (pp. 19–32). Washington, DC: Taylor & Francis.

Maslach, C., & Leiter M. P. (2008). Early predictors of job burnout and engagement. *Journal of Applied Psychology, 93,* 498–512.

Matuska, K., & Christiansen, C. (2008). A proposed model of life balance. *Journal of Occupational Science, 15,* 9–19.

Matuska, K., & Erickson, B. (2008). Life balance: How it is described and experienced by women with multiple sclerosis. *Journal of Occupational Science, 15,* 20–26.

McMillan, L. H. W., O'Driscoll, M. P., & Brady, E. C. (2004). The impact of workaholism on personal relationships. *British Journal of Guidance and Counselling, 32,* 171–186.

McTigue, K., Harris, R., Hemphill, B., Lux, L., Sutton, S., Bunton, A., et al. (2003). Screening and interventions for obesity in adults: Summary of the evidence for U.S. preventative services task force. *Annals of Internal Medicine, 139,* 933–949.

Mohr, D., Vedantham, K., Neylan, T., Metzler, T. J., Best, S., & Marmar, C. R. (2003). The mediating effects of sleep in the relationship between traumatic stress and health symptoms in urban police officers. *Psychosomatic Medicine, 65,* 485–489.

Oakley, C., & Pratt, J. (1997). Voluntary work in the lives of postretirement adults. *British Journal of Occupational Therapy, 60,* 273–276.

Ogden, C. L., Carroll, M. D., McDowell, M. A., & Flegal, K. M. (2007). *Obesity among adults in the United States: No change since 2003–2004* (NCNS Data Brief No. 1). Hyattsville, MD: National Center for Health Statistics.

Peate, I. (2007). Strategies for coping with shift work. *Nursing Standard, 22,* 42–45.

Peterson, U., Demerouti, E., Bergström, G., Samuelsson, M., Asberg, M., & Nygren, A. (2008). Burnout and physical and mental health among Swedish healthcare workers [Electronic version]. *Journal of Advanced Nursing, 62,* 84–95.

Piotrowski, C., & Vodanovich, S. J. (2006). The interface between workaholism and work–family conflict. *Organization Development Journal, 24,* 84–91.

Robinson, B. E., Carroll, J. J., & Flowers, C. (2001). Marital estrangement, positive affect, and locus of control among spouses of workaholics and spouses of nonworkaholics: A national study. *American Journal of Family Therapy, 29,* 397–410.

Robinson, B. E., Flowers, C., & Ng, K. (2006). The relationship between workaholism and marital disaffection: Husband's perspectives [Electronic version]. *Family Journal: Counseling and Therapy for Couples and Families, 14,* 213–220.

Robinson, B. E., & Post, P. (1995). Work addiction as a function of family of origin and its influence on current family functioning. *The Family Journal: Counseling and Therapy for Couples and Families, 3,* 200–206.

Roehrs, T., & Roth, T. (2004). Sleep disorders: An overview. *Clinical Cornerstone, 6,* S6–S16.

Schaufeli, W. B., Taris, T. W., & van Rhenen, W. (2008). Workaholism, burnout, and work engagement: Three of a kind or three different kinds of employee burnout? *Applied Psychology: An International Review, 57,* 173–203.

Shevil, E., & Finlayson, M. (2006). Perceptions of persons with multiple sclerosis on cognitive changes and their impact on daily life. *Disability and Rehabilitation, 28,* 779–788.

Sonnenschein, M., Sorbi, M. J., Verbraak, M. J., Schaufeli, W. B., Maas, C. J., & van Doornen, L. J. (2008). Influence of sleep on symptom improvement and return to work in clinical burnout [Electronic version]. *Scandinavian Journal of Work, Environment and Health, 34,* 23–32.

Spence, J., & Robbins, A. (1992) Workaholism: Definition, measurement, and preliminary results. *Journal of Personality Assessment, 58,* 160–178.

Sterns, H., Junkins, M. P., & Bayer, J. (1999). Work and retirement. In B. Bonder & M. Wagner (Eds.), *Functional performance in older adults* (2nd ed., pp. 179–195). Philadelphia: F. A. Davis.

Strauss, R. S. (2000). Childhood obesity and self esteem [Electronic version]. *Pediatrics, 105,* 1–5.

Tillotson, J. (2004). America's obesity: Conflicting public policies, industrial economic development, and unintended consequences. *Annual Reviews of Nutrition, 24,* 617–643.

Townsend, E., & Wilcock, A. (2004). Occupational justice. In C. Christiansen & E. Townsend (Eds.), *Introduction to occupation: The art and science of living* (pp. 243–273). Upper Saddle River, NJ: Pearson Education.

Uterbrink, T., Hack, A., Pfeifer, R., Buhl-Grießhaber, V., Müller, U., Wesche, H., et al. (2007). Burnout and effort–reward-imbalance in a sample of 949 German teachers [Electronic version]. *International Archives of Occupational and Environmental Health, 80,* 443–441.

Vioque, J., Torres, A., & Quiles, J. (2000). Time spent watching television, sleep duration and obesity in adults living in Valencia, Spain. *International Journal of Obesity and Related Metabolic Disorders, 24,* 1683–1688.

Westhorp, P. (2003). Exploring balance as a concept in occupational science. *Journal of Occupational Science, 10,* 99–106.

Wilcock, A. A. (1998). *An occupational perspective of health.* Thorofare, NJ: SLACK Incorporated.

Whiteford, G. (2004). When people can't participate: Occupational deprivation. In C. Christiansen & E. Townsend (Eds.), *Introduction to occupation: The art and science of living* (pp. 221–242). Upper Saddle River, NJ: Prentice-Hall.

Workaholics Anonymous. (2008). In *Wikipedia, the Free Encyclopedia.* Retrieved on May 6, 2008, from http://en.wikipedia.org/wiki/Workaholics_Anonymous

World Health Organization. (2007). *ICD-10: The ICD-10 Classification of Mental and Behavioural Disorders: Clinical Descriptions and Diagnostic Guidelines.* Geneva: Author.

Zerubavel, E. (1981). *Hidden rhythms, schedules and calendars in social life.* Chicago: The University of Chicago Press.

Another Perspective on Life Balance

LIVING IN INTEGRITY WITH VALUES

WENDY PENTLAND AND MARY ANN MCCOLL

INTRODUCTION

In this chapter, we offer an alternative perspective on life balance. We propose that the extent to which people perceive their life to be in balance derives from the extent to which they are living congruently with their personal values and strengths. We define this state as *occupational integrity*. The metaphor of *balance* obscures the fundamental characteristics and nature of this sought-after state. Instead of focusing on an idealistic and dualistic outcome (balance), we instead propose instead going deeper into the concept of *integrity* to understand the processes that may lead to what is colloquially referred to as a *balanced life*. Through clarifying and unpacking the concept of occupational integrity, approaches and strategies can become apparent for designing or redesigning and maintaining a life that feels balanced.

COMMON CONCEPTUALIZATIONS OF LIFE BALANCE

The notion of *life balance* has received considerable attention in the past few decades, particularly in the developed world. There is currently no single definition for the term; it seems generally agreed that whatever it is, it's a good thing if you can get it. A balanced life is commonly associated with feeling relaxed, happy, and free, with positive outcomes such as improved health and characteristics such as kindness, gentleness, compassion, creativity, innovation, reflection, and perspective (Danner & Snowdon, 2001; Diener, Suh, Lucas, & Smith, 1999; Fredrickson, 1998; Marks & Fleming, 1999; Maruta, Colligan, Malinchoc, & Offord, 2000; Peterson, Park, Seligman, 2005; Ryff, 1995; Segerstrom, Taylor, Kemeny, & Fahey, 1998; Selye, 1974; Sheldon & Niemiec, 2006; Stone, Neale, Cox, & Napoli, 1994). Although there seems universal agreement about the positive outcomes of a balanced life, what life balance actually means, how to go about it, and how we will know when we get there have not been well defined.

Notwithstanding the recorded thinking of the past 2,500 years from both Western and Eastern philosophers on what constitutes human happiness and well-being, life balance is a relatively recent term. Discussions of life balance have originated primarily in developed and industrialized societies, reflecting various features of these cultures:

K. Matuska & C. Christiansen (Eds.)
Life balance: Multidisciplinary theories and research (pp 165–180)
© 2009 SLACK Incorporated and AOTA Press

- Tremendous freedom of personal choice although perhaps not often fully acknowledged and exercised

- Escalating consumerism and valuing of material possessions, security, and luxury, leading in turn to increased valuing of money, growth and productivity and the consequent need to work harder, longer, and more productively

- Women entering the work force in greater numbers

- More households with all members either in school or the paid workforce (based on the Multinational Time-Use Study (MSTU) in Harvey & Pentland, 2010).

The terminology used to refer to life balance can vary, and meanings are often unclear or appear to overlap. The terms *work–life balance* and *work–family balance* are common in the corporate world and human resources literature. The underlying construct is a subjective perception of the extent to which time allocation successfully responds to workers' combination of personal, family, and workplace demands in the context of time pressure. Evidence of organizations attempting to address employee work–life balance may be seen in policies that support family leave or caregiver leave, on-site childcare services, flexible hours, and teleworking options. Although it is common for employers to have policies promoting work–family balance and work–life balance, the over-simplification of such a multifaceted concept of human behavior has been previously recognized (see Primeau, 1995). Despite this, workplace policies addressing work–life balance or work–family balance are becoming both increasingly politically correct and essential for attracting and retaining the best talent.

The term *life balance* appears in the media, popular press, everyday conversation, and scholarly literature. It is significant to note that the vast majority of those publicizing, speaking, and writing about life balance are of working age. This raises questions as to whether the concept of life balance is symptomatic of what is known to be a time- and role-intensive time of life, although indeed the true construct of what is being referred to is broader. The pervasiveness of the term life balance can lead to perceptions that although the term is not clearly defined, it is both important and universally understood.

Research is lacking on the meaning of life balance to different groups, such as children, youth, older people, and those in non-American cultures. Interviews conducted with six community-dwelling urban Canadians ages 80–88 years revealed that for them, the term *life balance* had virtually no meaning whatsoever. Although some had heard the term before, when asked to select a phrase that felt more relevant to what they were striving for, they suggested things like "keeping breathing," "contentment," and "peace." They talked about being able to do what was important to them, but because they had less and less energy and ability, they had become increasingly selective and prioritized where they devoted their time and attention. One couple raised the notion that, "with the importance you young people place on independence, success, and rushing around and being productive, you're going to find growing old a bit of an adjustment." They talked a lot about needing community and connection—one lived in a seniors' building that she described as a "vertical village"; others did their best to avoid isolation and found meaning in helping and supporting each other and the next generations (Pentland, 2007).

Life balance has been examined across various disciplines, almost always from the perspective of overt human behavior (what people actually do). Examples include the following:

- Allocation of time and energies to daily activities and activity patterns (Aas, 1982; Csikszentmihalyi & Larson, 1987; Hofferth, 2003; Monk et al., 1996; Pentland, Harvey, Lawton, & McColl, 1999); Statistics Canada, 2005; Zuzanek & Smale, 1997)

- Roles, role balance, and role conflict (Greenhaus, Collins, & Shaw 2002; Marks, 1977; Marks & MacDermid, 1996)

- Time pressure (Jonsson, Borell, & Sadlo, 2000; Zuzanek & Smale, 1997)

- Satisfaction of psychological needs (Sheldon & Niemiec, 2006)
- Life or personal projects (Little, 1983; Palys & Little, 1983)
- *Occupations*, which are defined as groups of activities and tasks of everyday life (Crist, Davis, & Coffin, 2000; Håkansson, Dahlin-Ivanoff, & Sonn, 2006; Jonsson, Josephson, & Kielhofner, 2001; Larsen & Zemke, 2003; Law, Steinwender, & Leclair, 1998; Meyer, 1922; Pentland, Harvey, Smith, & Walker, 1999; Wilcock et al., 1997).

Although we typically view balance as a blissful ideal state, when we look at people whose livelihood depends on balance, we see that it can be time consuming and demanding. To use a metaphor, one only needs to look closely at people who are balance experts (in the physical sense)—jugglers, tightrope walkers, unicycle riders, and gymnasts. They are very good at balancing, and they are unquestionably talented, courageous, and awe-inspiring. They are indeed balanced, but do they appear to be relaxed, open, spontaneous, free, creative, flourishing; are they having fun? In looking more closely at their faces, we see stress, inward focus, seriousness, and an apparent tuning out of their environment lest they become distracted. They also need spotters, ropes, and safety nets.

Balance represents dualistic thinking: One is either balanced or not. Once one has it, one will presumably be motivated to work hard to keep it. This can lead to becoming rigid and inflexible, overreactive, resistant, and suspicious of change of anything that might threaten that balance. It could lead us to want to avoid taking risks or trying new things as we desperately hold on to our balanced life.

The behavioral approach to understanding life balance is based on the assumption that there is a correct configuration of time, roles, activities, and projects that leads to balance and subsequently to well-being. This approach fails to take account of the underlying choices that lead to these configurations. From the perspective that people create their own reality and have tremendous choice in how they create their lives (Frankl, 1984; Jung, 1961; Buddhism, in Thurman, 2005), the metaphors and language used and the questions asked are powerful shapers of the choices people think they have, the choices they make, and hence their lives (Goldberg, 1997; Lakoff & Johnson, 1980). Questions such as, "How do I balance my life?" or "How can I get more balance in my life?" focus attention on how to reconfigure the same set of activities or roles into a perfect state, thereby entrenching thinking and leading people to seek the answer down a path of futility or of increasingly untenable and dissatisfying lifestyles.

We and our society have been asking questions like "How do I get more balance in my life?" for some time, and things do not seem to be getting much better. Marilee Goldberg (1997), who developed an approach to psychotherapy based on specific types of questions, observed that innovation and new thinking about how to design and do things begin with a new question or an old question asked in a different way. Albert Einstein similarly observed that our current problems cannot be solved by the same level of thinking or the same world view that created them. Perhaps then, the questions we are asking ourselves about how to lead a balanced life are leading us in the wrong direction.

REFRAMING LIFE BALANCE AS OCCUPATIONAL INTEGRITY

The concept that truly links the configuration of daily life (occupations) with well-being is not life balance but rather the extent to which a person lives in integrity with his or her personal values, strengths, and attributions of meaning. We propose that this concept be referred to as *occupational integrity*. Integrity has a number of definitions: (1) incorruptibility, (2) soundness, and (3) being whole, undivided, complete (Coulson, Carr, Hutchinson, & Eagle, 1962). It is the latter meaning to which we refer when we speak of living in occupational integrity. Living in

Figure 12-1. Model of occupational integrity.

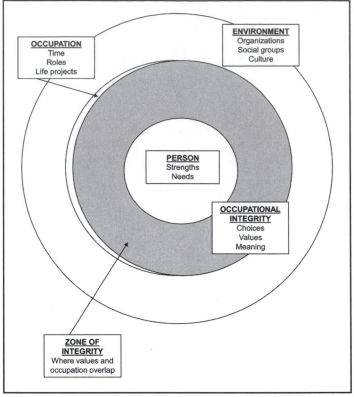

occupational integrity is integrating into one's occupational choices the values that matter most (Figure 12-1). The extent to which an individual can design an occupational life that is consistent with his or her values will be the extent to which he or she feels a sense of balance and well-being. Please refer to the shaded box containing the story that has circulated in recent years illustrates designing a life of occupational integrity.

Our sense of well-being derives from the extent to which we have designed a life that is congruent with our values; that is, in integrity with them. This is consistent with Westhorp's (2003) discussion of balance in occupational science and with work on happiness and subjective well-being (see Deiner & Seligman, 2002; Peterson et al., 2005; Seligman & Csikszentmihalyi, 2000). Seligman and Csikszentmihalyi (2000) argue that three elements are necessary for well-being: the "pleasant life," which depends on minimizing negative emotions and maximizing positive emotions; "engagement," which is generated when an individual finds opportunities to use his or her strengths in daily living; and "meaning," which involves an individual acting in congruity with his or her values, in service of a cause that is greater than the self

A MODEL OF OCCUPATIONAL INTEGRITY

We propose a conceptual model of occupational integrity as a way of thinking about life balance. The model is illustrated in Figure 12-1. The concepts in the model are to be understood as a system, in that they are interactive and in dynamic interrelationship. The essence of the model of occupational integrity is that the extent to which a person feels fulfillment and well-being lies in his or her ongoing ability to design and live a life that is in congruence with personal values. Such a life resolves the paradox between the human desire to be authentic in terms of his or her own values and strengths versus the demands and expectations of being in relationship with the

---

ILLUSTRATION OF A LIFE OF OCCUPATIONAL INTEGRITY

A professor of philosophy stood before his class and wordlessly picked up a large empty jar and proceeded to fill it with rocks about 2 inches in diameter. He then asked the students if the jar was full. They agreed that it was full. So the professor picked up a box of pebbles and poured them into the jar. He shook the jar lightly and the pebbles rolled into the open areas between the rocks. The professor again asked the students if the jar was full. They chuckled and agreed that it was indeed full this time. Next, the professor picked up a box of sand and poured it into the jar. The sand filled the remaining open areas of the jar.

"I want you to recognize that this jar signifies your life. The rocks are the truly important things, such as family, health, and relationships. The pebbles are the other things that matter in your life, such as work or school. The sand signifies the remaining small stuff and material possessions.

"If you put sand into the jar first, there is no room for the rocks or the pebbles. Similarly, if you spend all your time and energy on the small stuff, you will never have room for the things that are truly important. Take care of the rocks first—things that really matter. Set your priorities. The rest is just pebbles and sand."

(Author Unknown).

---

environment. This tension is continuous throughout life, resulting in ongoing iterations and negotiations between the self and the environment.

The model (Figure 12-1) consists of the person (made up of strengths and needs) and their environment (made up of organizations, culture and social groups). The person interacts with their environment through their occupations (in time use) and through roles and life projects. The person assembles their constellation of occupations by making choices based on personal meaning and values. The person does this within the context of the demands and expectations they perceive to come from the environment. In our model, people will feel "dis-ease" when their lifestyle is designed exclusively to meet either their own or the environment's values, needs, and demands. The optimal place for ease, fulfillment, and well-being is an occupational lifestyle that remains within the zone of integrity, that is, when we honor personal values, strengths, and sense of meaning and simultaneously live in relationship with our environment. Hence the individual's well-being will be predicted by the extent to which they have designed their occupational life within their zone of integrity.

Concepts and Definitions

This section offers definitions for each of the key concepts in the model: person, occupation, environment, and integrity. Further, it offers some theoretical background on several secondary concepts, such as strengths, life projects, and choices.

WELL-BEING

The ultimate goal of occupational integrity is *well-being*. Well-being is defined as a flourishing condition that derives from a life where there is congruence among the person's occupations and their values and meaning.

PERSON

According to the model, the *person* is made up of strengths and needs.

STRENGTHS

Strengths are defined according to the work in positive psychology by Seligman (2002; Peterson & Seligman, 2003; Seligman, Parks, & Steen, 2004). Positive psychology has identified 24 human strengths (Table 12-1) that will lead to more effective functioning and positive experiences in life. Strengths are qualities we desire for their own sake. People are seen as having a set of core strengths that can be used and developed to enhance mastery and happiness. The application of one's core strengths in service to something beyond the self is viewed as fundamental to finding meaning in life. Work in the field of positive psychology is ongoing with regards to distinguishing among strengths, talents, abilities, and skills. Presently Peterson and Seligman (2003) differentiate them as follows:

> Talents and abilities on the face of it seem more innate, more immutable, and less voluntary than strengths and virtues. There is a limit as to how much talent you can acquire. Talents are viewed as relative and automatic in that you either have a talent or you do not. Talents and abilities seem valued more for their tangible consequences (acclaim, wealth) than their own right. (p. 309)

NEEDS

In the occupational integrity model, the definition of *needs* is limited largely to requirements for survival and subsistence. When viewed in the context of Abraham Maslow's (1943) hierarchy of needs, the needs within this model would fall under the first four levels, *deficiency needs*. Maslow regarded deficiency needs as those the individual notices only when unmet and which once met do not typically result in motivating the individual further. Maslow defined the four levels of deficiency needs as physiological (e.g., breathing, food, water, sex, sleep), safety and security (e.g., structure, order, predictability), love and belonging (e.g., supportive family, friends, intimate relationships, identification with a group), and esteem (both from others and self).

OCCUPATION

Occupation is defined in the model as what people do; groups of activities and tasks to, for example, take care of themselves, enjoy themselves, or be productive (Canadian Association of Occupational Therapists [CAOT], 1997; Townsend & Polatajko, 2007). The constellation or pattern of a person's activities and tasks will be largely governed by their roles and life projects.

TIME USE

In this model, *time use* is the means through which humans exercise their occupations, life projects, and roles. There is an extensive literature on human time use, and national time-use studies have been conducted in virtually all eastern and western European countries since the early 1900s. Time use is complex in that just as a computer can multiprocess, a human also can. People engage in primary, secondary, and even tertiary activities, because they have multiple senses and generally use them concurrently. An individual can be watching soccer on TV, listening to the better play-by-play on the radio, minding children, and drinking a beer, all with friends. These activities—watching TV, listening to the radio, caring for children, drinking, and socializing—are concurrently engaged in. Unquestionably, it is the mix of activities and contexts that provide life with meaning and richness. Overlapping activities also are one way humans create efficiencies in time use, because time use is constrained by the amount of time available.

The concept of *time* dominates much of the existing literature on life balance. The model of occupational integrity shows time as an environmental constraint that the person has to reckon with in the process of reconciling their own authenticity with the expectations of the environment. It is our sense that when people report feeling their life is not balanced, they are often actually referring to this one aspect of trying to live in the zone of integrity. In this sense, it is possible

Table 12-1

24 HUMAN STRENGTHS

The 24 signature strengths delineated based on the work by Petersen & Seligman (2003):

1. **Creativity (originality, ingenuity):** Thinking of novel and productive ways to conceptualize and do things.

2. **Curiosity (interest, novelty-seeking, openness to experience):** Taking an interest in ongoing experiences for their own sake; exploring and discovering

3. **Open-mindedness (judgment, critical thinking):** Thinking things through and examining them from all sides; weighing all evidence fairly.

4. **Love of learning:** Mastering new skills, topics, and bodies of knowledge, whether on one's own or formally.

5. **Perspective (wisdom):** Being able to provide wise counsel to others; having ways of looking at the world that make sense to oneself and to other people

6. **Bravery (valor):** Not shrinking from threat, challenge, difficulty, or pain; acting on convictions even if unpopular.

7. **Persistence (perseverance, industriousness):** Finishing what one starts; persisting in a course of action in spite of obstacles.

8. **Integrity (authenticity, honesty):** Presenting oneself in a genuine way; taking responsibility for one's feeling and actions

9. **Vitality (zest, enthusiasm, vigor, energy):** Approaching life with excitement and energy; feeling alive and activated

10. **Love:** Valuing close relations with others, in particular when sharing and caring are reciprocated.

11. **Kindness (generosity, nurturance, care, compassion, altruistic love, niceness):** Doing favors and good deeds for others.

12. **Social intelligence (emotional intelligence, personal intelligence):** Being aware of the motives and feelings of other people and oneself.

13. **Citizenship (social responsibility, loyalty, teamwork):** Working well as a member of a group or team; being loyal to the group.

14. **Fairness:** Treating all people the same according to notions of fairness and justice; not letting personal feelings bias decisions about others.

15. **Leadership:** Encouraging a group of which one is a member to get things done and at the same time maintain good relations within the group.

16. **Forgiveness and mercy:** Forgiving those who have done wrong; accepting the shortcomings of others; giving people a second chance; not being vengeful

17. **Humility/Modesty:** Letting one's accomplishments speak for themselves; not regarding oneself as more special than one is.

18. **Prudence:** Being careful about one's choices; not taking undue risks; not saying or doing things that might later be regretted.

19. **Self-regulation (self-control):** Regulating what one feels and does; being disciplined; controlling one's appetites and emotions.

20. **Appreciation of beauty and excellence (awe, wonder, elevation):** Appreciating beauty, excellence, and/or skilled performance in various domains of life.

21. **Gratitude:** Being aware of and thankful for the good things that happen; taking time to express thanks.

22. **Hope (optimism, future-mindedness, future orientation):** Expecting the best in the future and working to achieve it.

23. **Humor (playfulness):** Liking to laugh, tease; bringing smiles to other people; seeing the light side.

24. **Spirituality (religiousness, faith, purpose):** Having coherent beliefs about the higher purpose, the meaning of life, and the meaning of the universe.

Note. Adapted from Petersen and Seligman (2003).

to live within the zone of integrity and feel time pressure, much as if you selected from a buffet of favorite foods, only to get back to your table and find you have put more on your plate than you can comfortably eat. The solution to this lies in reconciling and prioritizing what you do on the basis of personal values (awareness and what matters most), using choice, assertiveness (e.g., being able to say no), and living with the consequences of making choices that may let others down or incur disapproval from the environment.

ROLES

A *role* is defined as a pattern of behavior that a person performs in a particular situation. A role may evolve from certain rights and duties. Roles may be performed to meet personal needs and expectations, societal needs and expectations, or both (Kielhofner, 1985). Role has been defined as "a culturally defined pattern of occupation that reflects particular routines and habits" (CAOT, 1997, p. 182). Keep in mind that while roles may carry with them cultural expectations, the individual chooses how they will perform any given role. Roles do not necessarily imply a particular commitment of time. Roles may be temporary (e.g., airplane passenger, sporting event spectator, patient while having a mammogram) or of very long duration (e.g., child, parent, spouse). Any one occupation may be performed in a number of roles (e.g., skating for pleasure or skating as a professional athlete). Some roles are chosen, others may be ascribed, and still others lie somewhere between free choice and a sense of obligation.

LIFE PROJECTS

Life projects are defined in the model as a constellation of occupations aimed at a goal or personal project (Christiansen, Backman, Little, & Nguyen, 1988; Ellegard, 1993; Little, 1983). People may have any number of goals or personal projects they are pursuing at any time. Examples include learning to play the guitar, choosing a postsecondary education institution, buying a house, harvesting rice, changing the brake pads on the car, or raising a child. These projects influence the person's behavior and what they do with their time. Like roles, life projects and goals are also largely selected by individual choice, although the perceived power of environmental expectations may not always mean the person feels they have much choice. Research has shown that increased life satisfaction is associated with engagement in projects that the person has chosen, values, and feels they are competent to perform (Palys & Little, 1983).

ENVIRONMENT

The model shows environment as both distinct from and a function of the individual (Lee, 2002). The aspects captured in the model under the term *environment* (culture, organizations, and social groups) all exert their own values, demands, and expectations. Some common current Anglo-European environmental values are personal control over the environment, the importance of time, individualism, self-help, competition, future orientation, and goal orientation. Some common Eastern environmental values are collectivism, interrelationship, karma, and reciprocity. How cultural values and information evolve and are transmitted has been explored in various fields, including the sociocultural and sociopolitical literature (Dawkins, 1976).

The environmental demands and expectations experienced by the person may be real or simply perceived. Walter Lippmann, in his 1922 book *Public Opinion*, described the *pseudo-environment* as a mental image of the real environment that a person creates and then responds to as if it were reality. He proposed that we create our own mental image of the environment and then insert it between us and our environment because "the real environment is altogether too big, too complex, and too fleeting for our direct acquaintance... we are not equipped to deal with so much subtlety, so much variety, so many permutations and combinations... and although we have to act in that environment, we have to reconstruct it on a simpler model before we can manage with it" (p. 18). And that was in 1922, when the environment was arguably much simpler and where the fastest way to communicate at a distance was often Morse code! Research has shown the alarming extent to which people appear to get swept along and conform to environmental expectations and values, even when it undermines their health and well-being (Deiner & Seligman, 2004; Frank, 2004; Scitovsky, 1976; VanBoven & Gilovich, 2003).

While the values of the environment may differ from those of the individual, the individual is one part of the collective that makes up the environment and, as such, can theoretically influence its values. It is this ongoing possibility of reciprocal influence between the individual and the environment that makes social change possible (individual affects the environment) and can foster individual change (environment affects the individual).

The model of occupational integrity includes the notion that there are negative costs to the person over time of granting too much power and influence to environmental demands and expectations. This negative effect increases as the difference between the person's strengths and values and those of the environment do not fit. Evidence for these negative costs to both the individual and the environment appears in the burnout literature related to the workplace (Maslach, 2003). When a person, consciously or not, pays more attention to and is pulled too strongly by environmental demands or has internalized environmental values at the expense of his or her own authenticity, he or she may say things like "I have lost myself. I don't know what matters to me anymore." Then we lose track of who we are or sometimes never even stop to think about our own strengths, what is important to us, and what we value.

INTEGRITY

Occupational integrity is achieved through living in congruence with personal values, choices, and meaning.

VALUES

Values are defined as the things, beliefs, attitudes, and behaviors viewed as desirable and good by the individual (Dewey, 1972; Perry, 1968). They are the criteria we use for deciding what is worth doing and the goals and aspirations to which we will commit (Kielhofner, 1983; Rohan, 2000). Our values are what we stand for; they are the thumbprints of our souls. Values evolve beginning in childhood. Although they are essentially stable across the life course, personal values do shift and change both in character and priority as we proceed though various life stages and experiences in the environment (Johnson, 2002). Values are unique to each person. Life crises can precipitate heightened awareness of values. For example, disability or life-threatening illness may challenge one's ability to conform to environmental values like individualism and personal control and thus may result in a heightened clarity about personal values (Fuhrer, Rintala, Hart, Clearman, & Young., 1992; McColl, 2003; McColl, Bickenbach, Johnston, Nishihama, et al., 2000; McColl, Bickenbach, Johnston, Schumaker, et al., 2000).

Values are very powerful and can be the cause of wars. Their power and importance are well-recognized in the conflict literature, in that values-based conflicts are commonly regarded as unresolvable and best managed by acknowledging the differences and agreeing on superordinate goals (Lewicki, Saunders, & Minton, 2001; Moore, 1996). Yet many people have become disconnected from their values and certainly do not consciously plan their lives to honor them. Personal-values clarification is an ongoing process. It involves questioning, awareness, mindfulness, and self-observation. We can watch for our own values by noticing what brings us joy, when we feel at our best, what frustrates or deeply angers us, and what keeps showing up in our lives.

Values can be classified in terms of whether they are ultimate desires (often referred to as ends, terminal values, or inherent values) or values necessary to achieve those desires (means, instrumental values). Typically, when people are asked what they value, they initially identify *means values*. Examples of means values are money, family, health, nature, and teamwork. *Ends values* are typically deeper, more fundamental, and desired for their own sake (Riukas, 1998). To help people clarify their ends values, one can ask questions like "What about your family (i.e., means value) is important to you?" or "What do you have when you have that?" Examples of ends values are unconditional love and acceptance, beauty, independence, freedom, fairness and equality, safety, and security.

CHOICES

When individuals construct their lives, they exercise *choice*. What drives our choices about how we design our lives? How do we decide what occupations get our attention and time? According to Maslow (1943), safety and survival needs must be met before attention and time can be devoted to self-actualization. Adult human development includes learning to differentiate from the need to receive external approval toward becoming aware of and taking a stand for our own uniqueness, values, and beliefs (Laske, 1999). Similarly, it has been said that one of our life-development tasks is making choices that resolve the paradox between fully expressing our unique selves versus meeting the demands and expectations of being in relationship with others (Lippman, 1922; Mezirow, 2000). Part of this process of moving toward personal autonomy, and autonomous choice entails awareness and critical self-reflection about our own and others' assumptions and beliefs and the consequences of conforming with them. A *liberated person* has been described by Siegel (1990) as a person "free from unwarranted and undesirable control of unjustified beliefs, unsupportable attitudes, and paucity of ability which can prevent one from taking charge of her own life" (p. 58).

The Person–Environment–Occupation (PEO) model (Law et al., 1997) of human behavior illustrates the paradoxical nature of the choices between self-expression and embeddedness. In this model, a person's occupations are located at the intersection of the person and his or her environment. Often without realizing it, we are pulled more by the demands and expectations we perceive from those around us and our environment. People can lose track of who they are or sometimes never even stop to think about their own strengths, what is important to them, or what they value (Mezirow, 2000). We may have heard family members, colleagues, or perhaps even ourselves, when feeling stressed and unfulfilled or in crisis from illness saying "I feel like I have lost myself; my sense of who I am, and what matters to me." A critical first step to creatively resolve the paradox and live a life of occupational integrity is finding our self and understanding our own values and uniquenesses. The next step is taking stock of whose values we are living: ours or those of the world around us.

MEANING

It has been observed that, perhaps at least in the developed world, we have evolved lifestyles of such unprecedented comfort, safety, and control that we have reached the crest of a hill and do not quite know where to head next. One result is a growing focus on the search for *meaning* in life. Some pursue this search directly. Many others get uncomfortable and backfill their lives with busyness, stimulation, complexity, and change and create the need for more wealth, control, security, material acquisitions, and diversions. What do we mean by "meaning"? McColl (2003) suggests that there are three types of meaning: personal meaning, sociocultural meaning, and spiritual meaning.

- *Personal meaning* refers to attributions that an individual makes about events, people, or statements based on his or her own personal history. Events or ideas may have a unique psychological meaning for an individual based on his or her experience with similar events in the past.

- *Sociocultural meaning* refers to the shared meanings that members of a social or cultural group attribute to particular events or ideas. These shared beliefs are a product of the history of the group and are communicated to young or new members as they attain full membership in the culture or as part of their socialization. Often these shared meanings are so effectively transmitted that we do not even recognize them as assumptions that others might not hold. Religious beliefs were once like that, but to a large extent, have become less tenable as the scientific paradigm has become the dominant shared belief system in Western society.

■ *Spiritual meaning* refers to attributions that we make about events and ideas that are universal, on the basis of our shared history with the whole human race and with the larger universe or cosmos. For some, spiritual meaning is associated with the concept of a higher power and may conform to religions or faith traditions.

Meaning is typically not overtly expressed but through *symbols*. These symbols may be metaphors, stories, particular affiliations or preferences, idiosyncratic behaviors, or images. It is through exploring these symbols that individuals attain perspective on meaning and capture the meaning that is available in events or experiences. In pursuing occupational integrity for oneself or assisting a another, such as a client, to do the same, it becomes critical to recognize potential symbols and afford clients an opportunity to explore them and thereby mine the meaning or significance that may be available in particular occupations.

HOW THE MODEL WORKS

The model of occupational integrity shows how human beings interact with the environment through the medium of occupation or daily activity (Townsend & Polatajko, 2007). The model of occupational integrity is unique in that it *superimposes* another circle representing personal values, choices, and meaning (see Figure 12-1). This values–choices–meaning circle floats over the PEO interaction.

It is important to note that within the model of occupational integrity, time use is simply one dimension through which humans can honor or express or fail to honor their values. Examples of other dimensions might be intensity, focus, exclusivity, and depth of engagement. Understanding this concept is critical to avoiding the erroneous assumption that the amount of time spent honoring a value is an indication of the extent to which a person feels he or she living congruently with that value.

As illustrated in Figure 12-2a, occupational integrity is achieved when the person's occupational choices are congruently with their values choices and meaning as the person at the same time lives in harmonious relationship with their environment. The model shows that the greater or more aligned the overlap between the person's values–choices–meaning and their occupations (what they actually do in their life), the greater their perceived occupational integrity and fulfillment. As stated earlier, individuals will feel "dis-ease" when their lifestyle is designed to meet exclusively either their own (Figure 12-2b) or the environment's values (Figure 12-2c), needs, and demands. Rather, an individual's well-being, ease, and fulfillment comes from living in their zone of integrity, a lifestyle that honors their personal values, strengths, and sense of meaning that also allows living in relationship with one's environment.

In terms of the less-ideal ways in which values–choices–meaning and occupation may be aligned, Figure 12-3c represents a situation where a significant proportion of daily occupations activities fall outside of the zone of integrity in that they are aligned largely with the values, demands, and expectations of the organizations, culture, and social groups of the environment. As such, these occupations may fail to express the values of the individual; they may indicate a life where the individual feels they have had to design and make choices about their occupational behaviors (i.e., roles, life projects, time use) that are not honoring their own values but more meeting the needs of the environment. This may stem from feeling powerless to make choices or being unable to find or engage in activities that add meaning to life. These activities that fall outside of the zone of integrity not only do nothing to add to the sense of well-being, they may, in fact, detract from it by drawing the individual away from valued activities, leaving them feeling resentful, without purpose, or unfulfilled.

Another example of the way the model may express nonalignment between occupations and values–choices–meaning is shown in Figure 12-2b. In this example, the sum of daily occupations falls outside the zone of integrity because they have been exclusively chosen to meet the individual's personal values, strengths, and needs. Although the person may well be engaged in

Figure 12-2. Three options for occupational integrity.

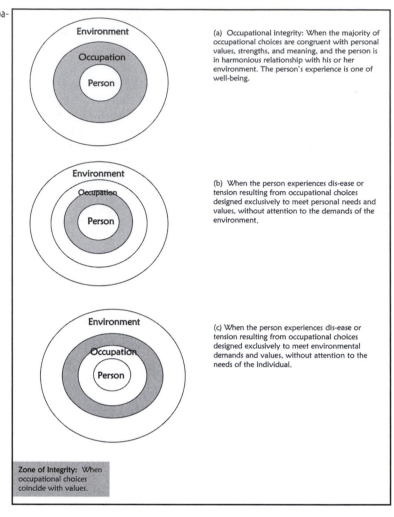

(a) Occupational integrity: When the majority of occupational choices are congruent with personal values, strengths, and meaning, and the person is in harmonious relationship with his or her environment. The person's experience is one of well-being.

(b) When the person experiences dis-ease or tension resulting from occupational choices designed exclusively to meet personal needs and values, without attention to the demands of the environment.

(c) When the person experiences dis-ease or tension resulting from occupational choices designed exclusively to meet environmental demands and values, without attention to the needs of the individual.

Zone of Integrity: When occupational choices coincide with values.

the environment (i.e., culture, organizations, social groups), the model postulates that by designing their occupations based on their own exclusive choices, meaning, and values, they are likely to ultimately experience reduced well-being or "dis-ease" resulting from conditions such as environmental resistance, conflict, isolation, disconnection, and feeling they are not making a difference. In its extreme, this may be thought of as a sort of alienation or disengagement and might occur to varying degrees in, for example, older persons or immigrants. It may also occur in the presence of a disability, either physical or mental, when the choice of activities is restricted by the disability, rendering the individual unable to choose those occupations that add meaning to life. These are just a few examples of different permutations of the model and its ability to reflect the relationship between activities and values that results in occupational integrity. In summary, a person's well-being is enhanced by their ability to recognize and use their own values and attributions of meaning (i.e., their zone of integrity) as the basis upon which they make choices about how they simultaneously design their life and live in relationship with their environment.

CONCLUSION

Throughout our lives we are caught in a paradox between being ourselves and being in relationship with others. We are individuals, with a strong need to express our unique selves fully in our life and work. At the same time, we face demands and expectations from relationships with others, membership in multiple systems, and being an inextricable part of the human community. Our creativity in resolving this paradox between self-expression and embeddedness has a powerful impact on our success, fulfillment, and well-being.

The resolution of this tension between the self and the environment is expressed as occupation—what we do, how we spend our time, and the choices we make. One of the ways that this paradox can be resolved is through occupational integrity. Occupational integrity is achieved when our choices of activities or occupations honor our values, while at the same time allowing us to live in relationship with our environment. The model shows that a life designed and lived with integrity is at the root of the sense of well-being that is often attributed to life balance. The zone of occupational integrity is where the paradox between the authentic self and the environment is resolved. The person has designed a life that allows him or her to be at once an authentic self while living successfully with the needs and expectations of his or her environment. The individual and the environment are in dynamic relationship, and the person is motivated and working at adjusting so that he or she can stay within this zone.

Despite innovations and coping strategies such as maximizing efficiency, multitasking, delegating, and replacing face-to-face and voice contact with technological substitutes, we all still only have 24 hours in the day and whatever number of years of life we manage to end up with. Typical conceptualizations of life balance show life balance as a correct configuration of time, roles, activities, and projects that leads to balance and subsequently to well-being. This configuration may allow for evaluation of whether there is balance or not but provides limited guidance on how to make improvements. By grounding the design of a lifestyle in personal values, meaning, and choices, the model of occupational integrity provides both a framework to evaluate lifestyle and a basis to make changes for improved well-being. The model offers a place for the individual to begin to reflect on and evaluate life choices, see and examine new options, and choose differently to enhance well-being.

REFERENCES

Aas, D. (1982). Designs for large scale time use studies of the 24 hour day. In Z. Staikov (Ed.). *It's about time; International research group on time budgets and social activities* (pp. 17-53). Sofia, Bulgaria: Institute of Sociology at the Bulgarian Academy of Sciences, Bulgarian Sociological Association..

Adler School of Professional Coaching. (2004). *Welcome to Adler School of Professional Coaching.* Retrieved September, 14, 2004, from http://www.adlercoach.com/

Canadian Association of Occupational Therapists. (1997). *Enabling occupation: An occupational therapy perspective.* Ottawa, ON: Author.

Christiansen, C., Backman, C., Little, B. R., & Nguyen, A. (1988). Occupations and well-being: A study of personal projects. *The American Journal of Occupational Therapy, 53,* 93–99.

Coulson, J., Carr, C. T., Hutchinson, L., & Eagle, D. (Eds). (1962). *Oxford Illustrated Dictionary* (p. 421). Oxford, UK: Oxford University Press.

Crist, P. H., Davis, C. G., & Coffin, P. S. (2000). The effects of employment and mental health status on the balance of work, play/leisure, self-care and rest. *Occupational Therapy in Mental Health, 15,* 27–39.

Csikszentmihalyi, M., & Larson, R. (1987). Validity and reliability of the experience-sampling method. *Journal of Nervous and Mental Disease, 175,* 526–536.

Danner, D., & Snowdon, D. (2001). Positive emotion in early life and longevity: Findings from the nun study. *Journal of Personality and Social Psychology, 80,* 804–813.

Dawkins, R. (1976). *The selfish gene.* New York: Oxford University Press.

Deiner, E., & Seligman, M. E. P. (2002). Very happy people. *Psychological Science, 13,* 81–84.

Deiner, E., & Seligman, M. E. P. (2004). Beyond money: Toward an economy of well-being. *Psychological Science in the Public Interest, 5,* 1–31.

Diener, E., Suh, E. M., Lucas, R. E., & Smith, H. L. (1999). Subjective well-being: Three decades of progress. *Psychological Bulletin, 125,* 276–302.

Dewey, J. (1972). *Theory of valuation.* Chicago: University of Chicago Press.

Ellegard, K. (1993). Activities in their everyday context: Using individual diary data to set forth the complex pattern of people's activities in their everyday life. In *Time use methodology: Toward consensus.* Rome: Italian National Statistical Institute.

Frank, R. H. (2004). How not to buy happiness. *Daedalus: Journal of the American Academy of Arts and Sciences, 133,* 69–79.

Frankl, V. (1984). *Man's search for meaning.* New York: Washington Square Press.

Fredrickson, B. (1998). What good are positive emotions? *Review of General Psychology, 2,* 200–319.

Fuhrer, M. J., Rintala, D. H., Hart, A. H., Clearman, R., & Young, M. E. (1992). Relationship of life satisfaction to impairment, disability, and handicap among persons with spinal cord injury living in the community. *Archives of Physical Medicine and Rehabilitation, 73,* 552–557.

Goldberg, M. (1997). *The art of the question: A guide to short-term question centred therapy.* New York: Wiley.

Greenhaus, J. Collins, R., & Shaw, L. (2002). The relations between work–family balance and quality of life. *Journal of Vocational Behavior, 63,* 510–531.

Håkansson, C., Dahlin-Ivanoff, S., & Sonn, U. (2006). Achieving balance in everyday life. *Journal of Occupational Science, 13,* 74–82.

Harvey, A. S., & Pentland, W. (2010). What do people do? In C. Christiansen & E. Townsend (Eds.), *Introduction to occupation: The art and science of living* (2nd ed., pp. 128–134). New York: Pearson.

Hofferth, S. L. (2003). The American family: Changes and challenges for the 21st century. In H. Wallace, G. Green, & K. Jaros (Eds.), *Health and welfare for families in the 21st century* (pp. 71–79). Sudbury, MA: Jones & Bartlett.

Johnson, R. E. (2002) A critical review of research on personal values, 1990–2000: Implications for pastoral counselors. *Dissertation Abstracts International, 62,* 5357B.

Jonsson, H., Josephson, S., & Kielhofner, G. (2001). Narratives and experience in an occupational transition: A longitudinal study. *American Journal of Occupational Therapy, 55,* 424–432.

Jonsson, H., Borell, L., & Sadlo, G. (2000). Retirement: An occupational transition with consequences on temporality, rhythm, and balance. *Journal of Occupational Science, 7,* 5–13.

Jung, C. G. (1961). *Memories, dreams and reflections.* New York: Vintage.

Kielhofner, G. (1983). *Health through occupation: Theory and practice in occupational therapy.* Philadelphia: F. A. Davis.

Kielhofner, G. (1985) *A model of human occupation.* Baltimore: Williams & Wilkins.

Lakoff G., & Johnson, M. (1980). *Metaphors we live by.* Chicago: University of Chicago Press.

Larsen, E. A., & Zemke, R. (2003). Shaping the temporal patterns of our lives: The social co-ordination of occupation. *Journal of Occupational Science, 10,* 80–89.

Laske, O. (1999). An integrated model of developmental coaching. *Consulting Psychology Journal, 51,* 139–159.

Law, M., Cooper, B. A., Strong, S., Stewart, D., Rigby, P., & Letts, L. (1997). Theoretical contexts for the practice of occupational therapy. In C. Christiansen & C. Baum (Eds.), *Occupational therapy: Enabling function and well-being* (2nd ed.). Thorofare, NJ: SLACK Incorporated.

Law, M., Steinwender, S., & Leclair, L. (1998). Occupation, health, and well-being. *Canadian Journal of Occupational Therapy, 65,* 81–90.

Lee, R. G. (2002). Ethics: A gestalt of values/The values of gestalt: A next step. *Gestalt Review, 6,* 27–51.

Lewicki, R. J., Saunders, M., & Minton, J. W. (2001). *Essentials of negotiation.* Boston: McGraw-Hill/Irwin.

Lippmann, W. (1922). *Public Opinion.* New York: Free Press.

Little, B. R. (1983). Personal projects: A rationale and method for investigation. *Environment and Behavior, 15,* 273–309.

Marks, S. R. (1977). Multiple roles and role strain: Some notes on human energy, time and commitment. *American Sociological Review, 39,* 567–568.

Marks, S. R., & MacDermid, S. M. (1996). Multiple roles and the self: A theory of role balance. *Journal of Marriage and the Family, 58,* 417–432.

Maruta, T., Colligan, R., Malinchoc, M., & Offord, K. (2000). Optimists versus pessimists: Survival rate among medical patients over 30 year period. *Mayo Clinic Proceedings, 75,* 140–143.

Maslach, C. (2003). Job burnout: New directions in research and intervention. *Current Directions in Psychological Science, 12,* 189–192.

Maslow, A. (1943). A theory of human motivation. *Psychological Review, 50,* 370–396.

McColl, M. A. (2003). *Spirituality and occupational therapy.* Ottawa, ON: CAOT Publications.

McColl, M. A., Bickenbach, J., Johnston, J., Nishihama, S., Shumaker, M., Smith, K., et al. (2000). Changes in spiritual beliefs after traumatic-onset disability. *Archives of Physical Medicine and Rehabilitation, 81,* 817–823.

McColl, M. A., Bickenbach, J., Johnston, J., Schumaker, M., Smith, K., Smith, M., et al. (2000). Spiritual issues associated with traumatic-onset disability. *Disability and Rehabilitation, 22,* 555–564.

Meyer, A. (1922). The philosophy of occupational therapy. *American Journal of Occupational Therapy, 1,* 1–10.

Mezirow, J. (2000). Learning to think like an adult: Core concepts of transformation theory. In J. Mezirow (Ed.), *Learning as transformation: Critical perspectives on a theory in progress* (pp. 1–33). San Francisco: Jossey-Bass.

Monk, T., Essex, M., Smider, N., Klein, N., Lowe, K., & Kupfer, D. (1996). The impact of the birth of a baby on the time structure and social mixture of a couple's life and its consequences for well-being. *Journal of Applied Psychology, 26,* 1237–1258.

Moore, C. (1996). *The mediation process* (2nd ed.). San Francisco: Jossey-Bass.

Palys, T. S., & Little, B. R. (1983). Perceived life satisfaction and the organization of personal project systems. *Journal of Personality and Social Psychology, 44,* 1221–1230.

Pentland, W. (2007). *The meaning of life balance to community-dwelling octogenarians.* Unpublished research.

Pentland, W., Harvey, A. S., Lawton, M. P., & McColl, M. A. (Eds.). (1999). *Time use research in the social sciences.* New York: Kluwer Academic/Plenum.

Pentland, W., Harvey, A. S., Smith, T., & Walker, J. (1999). The time use patterns of men with spinal cord injury. *Journal of Occupational Science, 5,* 14–25.

Perry, R. B. (1968). *Realms of value.* New York: Greenwood Press.

Peterson C., & Seligman, M. E. (2003). Character strengths before and after September 11. *Psychological Science, 14,* 381–384.

Peterson, C., Park, N., & Seligman, M. E. P. (2005). Orientations to happiness and life satisfaction: The full life versus the empty life. *Journal of Happiness Studies, 6,* 25–41.

Primeau, L. A. (1996). Work and leisure: Transcending the dichotomy. *American Journal of Occupational Therapy, 50,* 569–577.

Rohan, M. J. (2000). A rose by any name? The values construct. *Personality and Social Psychology Review, 4,* 255–277.

Riukas, S. (1998, August). *Inherent and instrumental values in ethics. Paper given at the Twentieth World Congress of Philosophy.* Boston. Mass. Retrieved November 27, 2006, from http://www.bu.edu/wcp/MainValu.htm

Ryff, C. (1995). Psychological well–being in adult life. *Current Directions in Psychological Science, 4,* 99–104.

Segerstrom, S, Taylor, S., Kemeny, M., & Fahey, J. (1998). Optimism is associated with mood, coping, and immune change in response to stress. *Journal of Personality and Social Psychology, 74,* 1646–1655.

Scitovsky, T. (1976). *The joyless economy: The psychology of human satisfaction.* Oxford: Oxford University Press.

Siegel, H. (1990). *Educating reason.* New York: Routledge.

Seligman, M. E. P. (2002). *Authentic happiness. Using the new positive psychology to realize your potential for lasting fulfillment.* New York: Free Press.

Seligman M. E. P., & Csikszentmihalyi, M. (2000). Positive psychology: An introduction. *American Psychologist, 55,* 5–14.

Seligman, M. E., Parks, A. C., & Steen, T. (2004). A balanced psychology and a full life. *Philosophical Transactions of the Royal Society of London Biological Sciences, 29,* 1379–1381.

Selye, H. (1974). *Stress without distress.* New York: Lippincott.

Sheldon, K. M., & Niemiec, C. (2006). It's not just the amount that counts: Balanced need-satisfaction also affects well-being. *Journal of Personality and Social Psychology, 91,* 331–341.

Siegel, H. (1990). *Educating reason.* New York: Routledge.

Srivasta, S., & Cooperrider, D. L. (1999). *Appreciative management and leadership: The power of positive and action in organizations.* Euclid, OH: Williams Custom Publishing.

Statistics Canada. (2005). *General Social Survey, 2005 Time Use Survey.* Retrieved August 18, 2006, from http://www40.statcan.ca/l01/cst01/famil36a.htm

Stone, A., Neale, J., Cox, D., & Napoli, A. (1994). Daily events are associated with secretory immune responses to an oral antigen in men. *Health Psychology, 13,* 440–446.

Thurman, R. (2005). *The jewel of Tibet: The enlightenment engine of Tibetan Buddhism.* New York: Free Press.

Townsend, E., & Polatajko, H. (2007). *Enabling occupation II: Advancing an occupational therapy vision for health, well-being & justice through occupation.* Ottawa: CAOT Publications ACE.

VanBoven, L., & Gilovich, T. (2003). To do or to have? That is the question. *Journal of Psychology and Social Psychology, 85,* 1193–1202.

Westhorp, P. (2003). Exploring balance as a concept in occupational science. *Journal of Occupational Science, 10,* 99–106.

Wilcock, A. A., Chelin, M., Hall, M., Hamley, N., Morrison, B., Scrivener, L., et al. (1997). The relationship between occupational balance and health: A pilot study. *Occupational Therapy International, 4,* 17–30.

Zuzanek, J., & Smale, B. J. A. (1997). More work—less leisure? Changes in allocation of time in Canada 1981–1992. *Society and Leisure, 20,* 73–106.

SECTION IV

Life Balance for Specific Populations

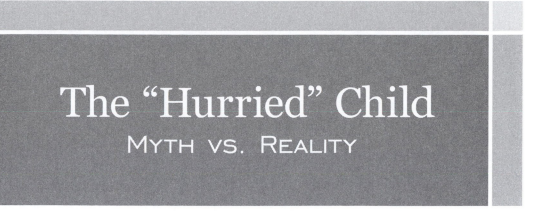

The "Hurried" Child
MYTH VS. REALITY

SANDRA L. HOFFERTH, DAVID A. KINNEY, AND JANET S. DUNN

INTRODUCTION

Recent writings bemoan the loss of childhood. Children are not allowed "to be kids"—to play games at home with friends, siblings, and cousins; to visit family members; to play pick-up ball games in the yard; or to ride bicycles around the neighborhood. Instead, because of the parents' own busy schedules or focus on enrichment, they enroll their children in lessons, team sports, and other scheduled activities outside the neighborhood. The lifestyle in which parents spend their free time driving their children from a swim meet to gymnastics to a soccer match may not only cause adults stress but also result in potential stress and strain for their children, a syndrome some have called "the hurried child" (Elkind, 2001). A recent report by the American Academy of Pediatrics says that a "hurried lifestyle is a source of stress and anxiety and may even contribute to depression" (Ginsburg, 2006, pp. 10–11). Organizations such as Putting Family First have been formed to combat the perceived pressure to overschedule the lives of children and their families (Doherty & Carlson, 2002). In spite of these concerns, little is known about the proportion of children whose involvement in structutred activities may be excessive.

Of course, not all families have such a lifestyle. It has been suggested that scheduling varies by social class, with middle-class families being the most likely to overschedule children (Lareau, 2003). *Social class* can be defined by financial resources or by values and lifestyle. A focus on financial resources implies that families of every class have the same goals but differ in their access to the resources needed to implement these goals. In contrast, if values or knowledge motivate parental actions, that implies differences in objectives resulting from differences in education, occupation, or culture (Lesthaeghe & Surkyn, 1988; Thornton, 2004). Understanding how resources and values drive these differences in family lifestyles helps us evaluate the consequences and develop potential solutions to any problems we identify.

Finally, no systematic studies of children's experience of stress have been reported, which, if prevalent, could imply long-term negative effects of this hurried-child syndrome. We simply do not know whether children are thriving in their activity-rich lifestyle or buckling under the pressure to participate in structured after-school activities. Because structured activity decisions are not random but are based on both parental objectives for children and children's own preferences (Dunn, Kinney, & Hofferth, 2003; Lareau, 2002, 2003), the relationship between structured activities and child stress symptoms may be spurious. Research has examined how families manage the new pressures of structured activities (Arendell, 2001) and adults' experience of time pressure

K. Matuska & C. Christiansen (Eds.)
Life balance: Multidisciplinary theories and research (pp 183–206)
© 2009 SLACK Incorporated and AOTA Press

(Jacobs & Gerson, 2004; Robinson & Godbey, 1997); however, there is little comparable research on children. Research that has been reported was illuminated primarily by conversations with parents as well as observations in the home. Lareau (2003) reported on conversations between children and parents or professionals in 12 families but did not directly interview the children.

This chapter addresses these gaps by focusing on the out-of-school structured activities in which elementary-school-age children are involved, by examining the prevalence of the hurried child and hurried family in the United States today, and by exploring the extent of stress symptoms that children experience. The chapter addresses three questions: (a) What proportion of American children are hurried? (b) Are there differences by social class and family structure in hurriedness, either within or across communities? and (c) Are the most hurried children likely to experience symptoms of stress?

Multiple methods are used to make comparisons by social class in a nationally representative sample and in a qualitative data set collected within and across two communities in the upper Midwest. The quantitative data provide the American national picture, and the qualitative data provide information about how families experience their children's structured activities.

Are Children Participating in Too Many Structured Activities?

That children participate in more before- and after-school care and extracurricular activities and experience increased structure in their lives is well documented (Hofferth & Sandberg, 2001). What is not documented is that a large number of children have high levels of structured activity. Although several theorists (Doherty & Carlson, 2002; Elkind, 2001) argue that too many children have excessive demands placed on them, there is no empirical evidence that this is the case. Lynott and Logue (1993) argued that, from a historical perspective, concern about "lost childhood" is a misreading of history, one that romanticizes an ideal-typical childhood that may have existed in only part of the 20th century in the United States—the 1950s. Before it was made compulsory in the early 20th century, a minority of children attended school, and those who did attended for only a few years. Children participated actively in the business of the family, helping on the farm, providing labor to a family business, or working as indentured servants and apprentices (Mintz, 2004).

Between 1981 and 1997, two major changes in the lives of American children were documented. First, the amount of free time, defined as time not spent in: personal care, eating, sleeping, and school, declined about 7.5 hours per week, from 56.5 hours to 49.0 hours and from about 34% of a child's week to 30% (Hofferth & Sandberg, 2001). Although 7.5 hours in a week may not seem significant, it represents more than an entire school day. Second, children's time became more scheduled and organized, with structured activities such as sports, scouts, ballet, and music lessons taking up an increasing proportion of the after-school hours. For example, between 1981 and 1997, participation in sports rose 35% and participation in the arts (art, music, dance, drama) rose 145% for children between the ages of 9 and 12 (Hofferth & Sandberg, 2001). Thus, there is evidence of a significant increase in children's structured leisure activity over the past several decades. However, the data on hours in specific activities do not provide a sense of how much time individual children spend in extracurricular activities and whether they have too many structured activities or spend too much time in them.

Consequences of Increased Structured Time—Stress

In addition to children being hurried by having too many structured activities, hurriedness may be harmful to children's development (Elkind, 2001). One of the potential consequences of excessive expectations for children's future by parents and perfectionism on the part of children is stress (Luthar & Becker, 2002). From a physiological point of view, a *stress reaction* is the response of an organism to any aversive stimulus (Stefanello, 2004). According to Elkind (2001), "stress is an unusual demand for adaptation that forces us to call upon our energy reserves over and beyond that which we ordinarily expend and replenish in the course of a 24-hour period" (Elkind, 2001, p. 166). In actuality, Elkind defines stress in terms of the number of demands: the greater the number of demands, the greater the stress (p. 165). We add to this the total amount of time, not just the number of activities, because some activities may be quite short. We also argue that control over one's time and activities may be protective against stress (Tansey, Mizelle, Ferrin, Tschopp, & Frain, 2004), whereas pressure to become involved in structured activities in which parents have an interest may increase that stress. A final aspect of hurriedness is whether demands are age appropriate. A narrow range of ages in this study controls somewhat for this; of course, children differ in their ability to manage pressures by individual maturity and temperament. Although checklists to identify a number of stressors in a child's life have been developed, determining stress levels is problematic. However, the literature seems to agree on a set of symptoms, which, if present, are a reasonable indicator of stress-induced psychological problems. These include internalizing problems, such as depression, problems getting along with others, anxiety, crying, stuttering, and sleep problems (Band & Weisz, 1988; Reynolds, O'Koon, Papademetriou, Szczygiel, & Grant, 2001; Stefanello, 2004, p. 294). The most common physical symptoms include stomachache, diarrhea, nervous twitches, headache, hyperactivity, stuttering, muscle tension, and bedwetting (Stefanello, 2004, p. 294). If a child reports or is reported to have some of these symptoms, the child is said to be under stress.

Positive Consequences of Activity Participation

Children do not learn only in formal education settings. At the beginning of the 20th century, social reformers promoted youth organizations, hobbies, and sports to foster development. Over the past century, organizations such as the YMCA, Boy Scouts and Girl Scouts, and Little League have proliferated. They are believed to build character, discourage delinquency, and provide opportunities for growth (Larson, 1994). Two major objectives for participation in these kinds of organized structured activities are that the activities promote integration of youth into the community, peer group, and family and that the activities promote individual personal growth and development, including improving self-concept. Prosocial behavior, social skills, and community involvement are part of the first objective and initiative, and self-regulation and self-esteem part of the second (Larson & Verma, 1999). Research demonstrates that participation in organized activities such as sports teams, lessons, and clubs is associated with lower rates of school failure; higher school achievement, including better grades; and higher rates of attending college (Mahoney, Larson, Eccles, & Lord, 2005). Studies also show that involvement in organized activities reduces problem behavior. Finally, organized activity participation is associated with psychosocial adjustment (Eccles & Gootman, 2002) and it is linked to lower rates of anxiety and depression and higher levels of self-efficacy and self-esteem.

Besides the social benefits of participation in organized activities, theory suggests that organized activities represent a context in which activities are highly valued and exciting, challenge is high, and the opportunity for skill development is equally high. Research shows that the condition of high challenge and high skills (flow) coincides with the most positive moods, self-esteem, high levels of concentration, and motivation and all these experiences are most likely to occur during structured leisure activities (Hektner, Schmidt, & Csikszentmihalyi, 2007). Recent research also shows that one of the physiological indicators of stress, cortisol level, rather than being high, is lower under conditions of enjoyment, mastery, and involvement (Adam, 2005). Cortisol increases under conditions in which challenges are beyond one's skill level (anxiety producing) or when challenge is too low (boring). Adam (2005) states that challenges contribute to health and well-being and are necessary for daily functioning, growth, and development. The proper balance between challenge and skill is key.

Involvement But Not Hurriedness—Balance

Although there is substantial research on the positive aspects of activity participation, there is almost no empirical evidence for the stress and strain part of the hurried-child hypothesis. Work-family studies have focused on adults; no studies have examined children's experiences. In the lone book based on children's reports *(Ask the Children),* children did not express dissatisfaction or unhappiness with their lives (Galinsky, 2002). Although coping skills develop with age, even children as young as 8 and 9 years of age can express the methods they use to cope with everyday stressful events and circumstances (Band & Weisz, 1988; Pincus & Friedman, 2004). The present research makes a unique contribution in that it focuses on the preteen-age years, when excessive structured activity is least developmentally appropriate (Elkind, 2001), and children have the least developed coping skills (Pincus & Friedman, 2004). We asked whether more active children exhibit more symptoms of stress than less-active children. However, we also examined whether activities benefit children's self-esteem, an important measure of psychological health.

Concerted Cultivation and Natural Growth Theories

Although ethnographic research in the 1950s and 1960s was motivated by an interest in the connections between early socialization and adult personality and occupations, recent research has extended this socialization paradigm to contemporary childrearing. Concerned that children develop their potential skills, middle-class parents cultivate their children's verbal skills by spending time with them in extended discussions and negotiations and encourage their extracurricular talents and social skills by enrolling them in sports, lessons, and youth organizations (Dunn et al., 2003; Lareau, 2003). Lareau called this the *concerted cultivation model of parenting* (Lareau, 2003). The result is the transmission of middle-class advantage from parents to their children, because middle-class jobs require such skills. This model is consistent with the earlier socialization paradigm of middle-class parents fostering autonomy and self-direction in their children (Alwin, 2001; Kohn, 1977; Kohn & Schooler, 1983; Schaefer & Edgerton, 1985). The major issue is whether parents are pushing their children too much—pushing them into activities in which they are not interested.

Working-class parents, in contrast, are believed to take a more passive approach to caring for children, allowing them to develop through participation in normal family-based or neighborhood peer-based activities with less structure and adult intrusion. This model of parenting Lareau called the *natural growth model* (Lareau, 2003). In communicating with children, working-class parents are said to be more directive, less skeptical of authority, and less interested in negotiation. As a result, children experience less control over their environments and have a sense of constraint rather than opportunity (Lareau, 2003). This is very much the obedient and conforming-to-authority set of traits discussed by Alwin (2001) and by Kohn and Schooler (1983) that working-class jobs both require and foster.

Additionally, parents are constrained by the settings in which they live and work, in particular by their personal resources and those of their communities. Compared to middle-class parents, working-class parents may be more constrained by their financial resources from making large investments in children's activities. They may depend more on free school-based activities than their middle-class counterparts, although the total number of activities may not vary.

Previous research indicates that children of middle- and working-class parents have become increasingly involved in after-school activities over the past 25 years but that the extent of children's participation still varies by social class.

Objectives of This Chapter

In this chapter, we develop a typology of the structured activity levels of 9- to 12-year-old children and examine its distribution using both a nationally representative sample of American children and two small qualitative samples. We then use statistical techniques to describe the association of social class, maternal employment, and family structure with this activity typology, controlling for gender of the child. We hypothesize that children from middle-class families, defined by education, occupation, income, or community, compared with working-class families, are more likely to fall into the hurried category in terms of activity commitments. Children from two-parent or dual-earner families are also expected to be more likely to be hurried compared to children in single-parent families or single-earner families. We examine evidence as to whether children are reported as experiencing more symptoms of stress as a consequence of being hurried. We also examine levels of self-esteem across activity groups. Finally, returning to the qualitative data, we draw upon children's and parents' in-depth reports to enrich our understanding of the results found in the large-scale data.

DATA AND METHODS

Child Development Supplement to the Panel Study of Income Dynamics

For this study, we drew children 9 to 12 years of age from the nationally representative 2002–2003 Child Development Supplement (CDS) to the Panel Study of Income Dynamics (PSID; see http://psidonline.isr.umich.edu/CDS/ for more information). The CDS is a supplement to a 34-year longitudinal survey of a representative sample of U.S. men, women, children, and the families with which they reside. With funding from the National Institute of Child Health and Human Development, data were collected in 1997 about children younger than age 13 of PSID respondents, with up to two children per household randomly selected for inclusion in the supplement. Data were collected both from the primary caregivers and from the children themselves (for children ages 8 or older). In 1997, interviews were completed with individuals in 2,380 households that contained a total of 3,563 children. The response rate was 88%. Interviews were conducted again over the fall and winter of 2002 to 2003, with a response rate of 91%. Only PSID–CDS non-Hispanic white children ages 9 to 12 years living with their mother and who had time diary information (79%) were included in the present study, a total of 331 children. To match the qualitative component, we also examined a subset of 277 children ages 9 to 12 years living with a mother who had completed 12 years of schooling or more. When poststratification weights based on the 2002 Current Population Survey are used, such as was done here, the PSID has been found to be representative of U.S. individuals and their families (Fitzgerald, Gottschalk, & Moffitt, 1998). Thus, weighted sample characteristics reflect the characteristics of the population of non-Hispanic white children aged 9 to 12 in the United States in late 2002 and early 2003.

Time Spent in Different Activities: Quantitative Data from the CDS

The 2002–2003 CDS collected a complete time diary for one weekday and one weekend day. The time diary, which was interviewer administered either to the parent or to the parent and child, asked questions about the child's flow of activities over a 24-hour period beginning at midnight of a randomly designated day. These questions documented each activity that occurred, when it began and ended, and whether there was another activity at the same time. Children's activities were first assigned to one of 10 general activity categories (e.g., sports, active leisure[1]) and then coded into three-digit subcategories (e.g., playing soccer). Coding was conducted by professional coders employed by the data collection organization; the level of inter-rater reliability

---

[1]Sports included team sports such as football, basketball, baseball, volleyball, hockey, soccer, and field hockey; individual sports such as tennis, squash and racquetball, golf, swimming, skiing, ice or roller skating, sledding, bowling, ping-pong or pinball, judo, weight lifting, jogging or running, bicycling, and gymnastics and other activities such as playing Frisbee or catch, exercises such as yoga, and lessons in any of the above. Youth organizations included participation in Boy/Girl Scouts, Future Farmers of America, YMCA/YWCA, volunteer activities, and helping organizations/clubs in the community or school. Art activities included painting, drawing, sculpture, potting, creative writing, playing a musical instrument, singing, dancing, acting, and related lessons and rehearsals.

exceeded 90%. Time spent traveling for the purpose of engaging in a specific activity was included in that category. The distribution of the total time spent across these 2 days was examined to identify the proportion in the upper tail of the distribution. Across these 2 days, 82% of children spent less than 4 hours in their activities; 4 hours served as the cut-off for low versus high activity levels. Although we do not have data for all 7 days of the week, comparisons across weekdays and weekend days show that weekdays are quite similar to each other in types and times of activities, and weekend days are similar to each other. In other words, these two days provide a reliable representation of a child's typical week.

Child Stress Symptoms

Symptoms of stress or distress are measured in the internalizing items of standard behavior problems measures (Luthar & Becker, 2002). In this study, children's stress symptoms were measured by a subset of items from the 30-item Behavior Problems Index, a standard instrument used in the PSID–CDS and the National Longitudinal Survey of Youth 1979 (NLSY–79) to obtain primary caregiver reports of the incidence and severity of child behavior problems for a wide age range of children (Baker, Keck, Mott, & Quinlan, 1993; Hofferth, Davis-Kean, Davis, & Finkelstein, 1999; Peterson & Zill, 1986). In this scale, the caregiver reports whether a statement was often true, sometimes true, or not true of their child's behavior. Several measures were created. Six items were selected as representing stress symptoms, according to the literature: he or she is high strung and nervous; fearful or anxious; unhappy, sad, or depressed; withdrawn; cries too much; or worries too much. Responses to items (1 = *often true*, 2 = *sometimes true*, and 3 = *not true of child's behavior*) were reverse-coded as (2 = *often true*, 1 = *sometimes true*, and 0 = *not true*) and summed, so that a high value on the scale indicates more and more frequent stress symptoms and 0 means no reported stress symptoms. Means for the full scale averaged 1.9, with a standard deviation of 1.8, $N = 331$. The reliability for the scale, as measured by Cronbach's alpha, was .63. A confirmatory factor analysis was not able to reject the hypothesis that one factor fit the six items. We also used the complete internalizing scale that was constructed by NLSY staff based on 13 items. Besides the items listed above, the complete scale includes items indicating the child has low self-esteem, has difficulty getting along with others, and is highly dependent. The reliability of the complete scale (.80) is higher than the stress subscale. We created two other subscales, an internalizing scale without the stress symptom measures ($\alpha = .74$) and a child-self-esteem subscale ($\alpha = .66$), which consisted of five mother-reported items.

To measure positive aspects of activity participation, we used a six-item scale of child-reported global self-esteem that was included in the PSID–CDS 2002–2003 wave for children ages 8 years and older. It includes items such as: "I can do things as well as most people," I'm as good as most other people," and "when I do something, I do it well." Scored from 1 = *never* to 5 = *always*, a higher score indicates greater self-esteem and has an alpha reliability of .78. Although not the stress construct specified in the literature, a decline in self-esteem is mentioned in the literature as a potential result from overactivity, and the advantage of using this scale is that it is self-reported by the child rather than the mother. The disadvantage is that only 225 of the 331 children answered this self-administered supplement.

QUALITATIVE STUDIES IN RIVERVIEW AND PARKSIDE

The qualitative data presented in this chapter are based on personal interviews conducted with parents and 9- to 12-year-old children from 43 families living in two different Midwestern United States medium-sized communities. Each of these families included at least one school-age child who attended the local public school. Both communities are more than 93% white. Because we had several dimensions of families to examine (family structure, employment, and social class), we decided to include only non-Hispanic white families in this study.[2] In "Riverview" (fictional name), 20 families were interviewed between November 1999 and May 2000; 23 families were interviewed in "Parkside" (fictional name) between May 2000 and February 2001. For seasonal comparability, cross-data comparisons focus on the activities of the 16 Parkside families interviewed in May and June 2000 during the 1999–2000 school year.[3]

We gained access to families through local public elementary and middle schools. Permission to use these schools as sites to recruit parents and children was granted by the superintendent of each public school district. With the assistance of the elementary school and middle school principals, we mailed recruitment letters and brief surveys to 125 families (25 each in grades 3–7) in Riverview and received responses from 42 parents interested in participating in the project, a response rate of about 34%. In Parkside, we mailed letters of information about the research project to parents of 131 children in grades 4–6 and received responses from 25 families, a response rate of 19%.[4] To obtain diversity on our major theoretical concepts (number of earners, education, income, family structure), we interviewed a subsample of 20 Riverview families, whereas we interviewed all but two of the Parkside respondents, for a sample of 23 families. We conducted the interviews ourselves with one parent (usually, but not exclusively, the mother) either at home or in a neutral location such as a coffee shop. Riverview children were interviewed in the school with no parent present. Parkside children were interviewed in the school with no parent present or in the home with parents out of earshot; three of the Parkside children were interviewed with at least one parent present during some of the interview. Interviews of children ranged in length from 30 to 45 minutes. Parent interviews averaged about an 1 ½ hours, but a few lasted more than 2 hours. All interviews except one were taped and transcribed with parental permission and child assent.

The first community, Riverview, is a small city of approximately 40,000 residents (U.S. Census Bureau, 2005). The local economy is largely defined by the presence of several large corporations, a small private university, and a large hospital, all of which provide relatively equal numbers of white-collar and blue-collar jobs. These are linked to the relatively high educational level of its residents; almost 42% of the local population that is 25 years of age or older had a bachelor's degree or higher, compared to only 24.4% for the U.S. adult population of 25 years and older in 2000.

The second community, Parkside, is smaller in population (30,000 residents) and geography than Riverview, and Parkside residents feel a strong sense of community in spite of being surrounded by other suburban communities with similar characteristics. The two communities differ most significantly in terms of their adult members' educational achievement and types of occupation. Adults in the small city of Riverview are four times more likely than parents in the suburban community of Parkside to have completed at least a bachelor's degree. Similarly, Riverview adults are twice as likely to hold white-collar jobs compared to Parkside parents, who are more than twice as likely to hold blue-collar jobs compared to their Riverview counterparts. These significant differences are not reflected in the median family incomes of these two communities, which differ only by about $6,500 ($65,000 in Riverview vs. $58,500 in Parkside in 2000 dollars). We argue that although both of these communities can be considered middle class in terms of income, in terms of occupation and education, Riverview is middle-middle or upper-middle class, and Parkside is more characteristic of the lower-middle or working class. In this chapter we refer to it as *working class*. Similar to Lareau (2003),[5] our definition of social class at the community level is based on the educational and occupational level of parents. At the family level it is based on education and income.

---

[2]Most of the concern to date about hurried children has focused on white middle-class families.

[3]Five of the remaining seven families were interviewed in the summer, when children participated in fewer activities, one was interviewed in early September before activities had begun, and one was interviewed the following year, judged to be too long a time period after the other interviews to include.

[4]The sampling in Parkside was conducted toward the end of the school year, a busy time for families.

[5]In Lareau's conceptualization, middle-class children had a parent who was employed in a managerial position or who used highly complex, educationally certified, college-level skills at work (Lareau, 2003).

Hurriedness and Stress in the Qualitative Data

The interviews were structured around a set of open-ended questions designed to elicit information about each child's daily activities and the family's weekly schedule. For each focal child, we obtained a schedule of activities for the entire week in which the interview took place. We asked parents about aspirations and goals for their children and what worked well in managing their schedules. Interviewing ended when saturation was reached (i.e., when the last parents interviewed added little new information). Parental interviews were transcribed and entered into ATLAS/ti. The interviews were initially coded using an open coding scheme based on the questions used to structure the interview. It was during this coding that we identified the overall activity level of the child and any reports of stress in the present or past.

Axial coding was then conducted to compare the circumstances of families and children who reported experiencing stress symptoms. We attempted to link activity levels to stress symptoms and to identify family strategies for managing them. This led to our typology of hurriedness that included both number of activities and time. Finally, using selective coding we identified specific instances of hurriedness and stress, as well as instances of inactivity, and circumstances surrounding them. We thought that one of the potential sources of stress was extent of control over the activity—whether the child made the decision about participating in the activity or whether it was parent-imposed, so we examined responses to the question "Whose idea was it to be in this activity (or go to this place)?" To gain information on the link between activities and stress from parents, we asked, "What activities that he or she does not now do would you like to see him or her do?" and "How much does he or she like the activity and would he or she like to do something else?" From these questions we were able to determine whether parents and children were thinking of changing or dropping activities and why. To get at the question of how activities are managed, we asked, "Overall, what do you think has really worked well for you in terms of managing your work schedule and your child's school and activity schedule?" The last question was very useful in identifying families who had made changes based on previous difficulties managing their own and their children's schedules.

We were particularly careful about questions asked of children, not wanting to bias their responses with leading questions. Age 8 appears to be a lower limit for children to adequately and comfortably interact with an interviewer about their activities, especially without a parent present. Research has demonstrated that although 9- to 12-year-old children are beginning to learn classification and temporal relations, they have problems with abstract concepts and are very literal in interpretation (Borgers, de Leeuw, & Hox, 1999). They are also very suggestible, want to please the interviewer, and are reluctant to express opinions. We did not ask directly about stress, because it was too abstract a concept. Instead, we asked a number of questions in which respondents could report any symptoms or concerns about their activities without us suggesting or implying they should feel stressed and strained. The following series of questions informed our conclusions about stress symptoms. After getting the complete list of children's weekly activities, we asked the child being interviewed, "Were there other things you wanted to do?" with a probe about how they felt about each activity. We then asked, "Would you have done it [the activity] if you didn't have to?" We also asked, "What are the things you enjoy doing the most outside of school?" "What kinds of things do you like to do with your friends?" "How about when you're by yourself, what do you like to do?" and "How about when you're with your family?" We also asked, "How much time do you have to do the things you want to do: a lot of time, some time, not very much, or hardly any time at all?" We coded instances of not wanting to go to an activity, being tired of the activity, being sore, preferring to do something else or nothing, crying, being overly tired out, and being worried, as symptoms of stress.[6] Child reports were also compared to parent reports in the selective coding phase. The strongest evidence for its existence were reports of stressful periods by both child and parent.

---

[6]Although being sore is not necessarily an indicator of stress, it was significant enough for the child to mention it, and this occurred in the context of multiple overlapping activities in one particularly busy period.

We also numerically coded the social and demographic characteristics of the 36 families in Riverview and Parkside who were interviewed during the 1999–2000 school year to compare their characteristics with those of the national sample of children in the PSID–CDS. Using the data from the two Midwest sites, we regressed (ordered logistic regression) our classification of structured activities in which the children were involved during the week of the interview on maternal education (in years), maternal education squared, maternal employment (employed part-time, employed full-time, or not employed), family income, family structure (two parents vs. one parent), and research site (Parkside vs. Riverview), controlling for the age and gender of the child. A comparable regression was conducted using the national PSID–CDS data without the "site" variable. Child age was never significant and was dropped. Part-time and full-time employment were also never statistically significant and were dropped from the analysis. Using the sample from Parkside and Riverview, additional quantitative analyses were conducted to determine whether the type of structured activity (sports, art activities, and youth groups) engaged in differed by these same variables.

RESULTS

Characteristics of Participants

According to the 2000 U.S. Census, 42% of the population of Riverview had completed a bachelor's degree compared with 9% in Parkside (U.S. Census Bureau, 2005). Our qualitative samples were better educated than the overall population in these two communities. Of the sample we obtained in middle-class Riverview, slightly more than half of the children's mothers and three-quarters of their fathers had completed a college degree. In working-class Parkside, 30% of the mothers and none of the fathers had completed a 4-year degree. Of the national sample of families in which a mother had completed 12 or more years of schooling, 40% of mothers and 50% of fathers had completed a college degree. The paternal education average of 14.5 years of schooling based on the PSID-CDS lies between the Riverview and Parkside averages (16.8 and 13.4 years, respectively), and the maternal average is similar to that of Parkside (Table 13-1).

Community differences are reflected in occupational categories as well. More than two-thirds of mothers in both communities were employed; 40% of the Riverview mothers worked in professional occupations, 25% worked in administrative positions, and 5% were in blue-collar jobs. In Parkside (full sample), 17% worked in professional occupations, 39% worked in administrative positions, and 26% worked in blue-collar jobs. Fathers' occupations differed even more dramatically across the two sites. Three-quarters of the Riverview fathers were employed in professional occupations, 5% were in administrative jobs, and only 15% were in blue-collar jobs. In Parkside, 9% were in professional occupations, 22% were in administrative jobs, and 52% of fathers were in blue-collar jobs. Based on both education and occupation, Parkside is clearly a working-class community and Riverview a middle-class community.

All children lived with their mother; not all lived with their father. In Riverview, 95% of the 20 families were two-parent families. Parkside families were similar to the national average for family structure: 83% of the full sample, 88% of the school-year sample of Parkside families, and 87% of the national sample were two-parent families. Based on Table 13-1, the national sample falls in between the two communities in social characteristics. Table 13-1, last column, shows the full PSID–CDS sample, not restricted by maternal education.

Table 13-1

DESCRIPTIVE CHARACTERISTICS OF DATA SOURCES

	Riverview Proportion/Mean	Parkside Proportion/Mean	Parkside (School Yr) Proportion/Mean	PSID-CDS[a] Proportion/Mean	PSID-CDS[b] Proportion/Mean
Child age (years)	11.35	10.30	10.25	10.89	10.88
Child gender					
Boy	0.45	0.26	0.38	0.54	0.55
Girl	0.55	0.43	0.63	0.46	0.45
Family type					
Two parents	0.95	0.83	0.88	0.86	0.84
Single parent	0.05	0.17	0.13	0.14	0.16
Number of children	2.35	2.50	2.40	2.36	2.40
Maternal education (years)	15.65	14.45	14.34	14.38	13.67
High school (12 years of schooling)	0.10	0.09	0.00	0.26	0.34
Some college (13–15 years)	0.35	0.61	0.69	0.34	0.32
College degree or more	0.55	0.30	0.31	0.40	0.34
Paternal education (years)	16.84	13.40	13.00	14.53	14.23
High school or less	0.00	0.26	0.36	0.26	0.32
Some college	0.20	0.74	0.64	0.25	0.23
College degree or more	0.75	0.00	0.00	0.49	0.45
Maternal Occupation					
1 = Professional	0.40	0.17	0.00	na	na
2 = Administrative	0.25	0.39	0.56	na	na
3 = Blue collar	0.05	0.26	0.25	na	na
Not employed	0.30	0.17	0.19	na	na

continued

Table 13-1 continued

DESCRIPTIVE CHARACTERISTICS OF DATA SOURCES

	Riverview Proportion/Mean	Parkside Proportion/Mean	Parkside (School Yr) Proportion/Mean	PSID-CDS[a] Proportion/Mean	PSID-CDS[b] Proportion/Mean
Maternal work schedule					
Full-time	0.45	0.39	0.38	0.50	0.49
Part-time	0.20	0.43	0.38	0.31	0.31
Not employed	0.35	0.17	0.25	0.19	0.20
Paternal occupation					
1 = Professional	0.75	0.09	0.06	na	na
2 = Administrative	0.05	0.22	0.19	na	na
3 = Blue collar	0.15	0.52	0.63	na	na
4 = No dad/not employed	0.05	0.17	0.13	na	na
Paternal work schedule					
Full-time	0.95	0.83	0.88	0.79	0.79
Part-time	0.00	0.00	0.00	0.05	0.04
No dad/not employed	0.05	0.17	0.13	0.16	0.16
Income (dollars)	100,000	59,350	55,620	91,219	84,314
N	20	23	16	277	331

Note. na = not available

[a]Children whose mother completed 12 or more years of school; [b]Full PSID-CDS sample.

Table 13-2

PERCENTAGE OF CHILDREN PARTICIPATING IN STRUCTURED SPORTS, ART, AND YOUTH ORGANIZATION ACTIVITIES
ONE WEEKDAY AND ONE WEEKEND DAY

Activity Category	Mother Education 12+ years %	Full Sample %
No activities over 2 days	15.4	17.4
Youth organization only, <4 hours	7.5	7.4
Youth organization only, 4+ hours	0	0
Sports only, < 4 hours	20.4	22.4
Sports only, 4+ hours	6.8	6.5
Art only, <4 hours	2.9	3
Art only, 4+ hours	0.4	0.3
Two types of activities, <4 hours	27.3	24.5
Two types of activities, 4+ hours	11.9	12.2
All three types of activities	7.3	6.2
Total	100	100
N	277	331

Note. Data are from 2002/3 PSID-CDS. Data are for non-Hispanic White children ages 9–12 years.

A Typology of Children's Structured Activity Participation

Our activity groups are based on both number of structured activities and time spent in them. Table 13-2 shows the distribution of the PSID–CDS national sample of children by three activity groups (youth organizations, sports, and arts), the number of these activities, and time spent doing them for all white families and just for those in which the mother had completed 12 years of schooling or more. Focusing on the latter for comparison with the community samples, in 2002–2003, 15.4% of non-Hispanic white children ages 9–12 had no structured activities during the 2 days of the school year about which they filled out the diary; these we refer to as "uninvolved." Almost 8% were involved only in youth organizations, 27.2% were involved only in sports, and 3.3% were involved only in structured art activities; 39% were involved in two of the three types of structured activities. The 7.3% who were involved in all three types of activities were defined as *hurried.* Almost one-third of children who participated in a sport and only a small fraction of those in arts activities participated for 4 or more hours over 2 days. Our qualitative research showed that children involved for many hours in an organized sport were those whose families had the most time-management problems. Thus, children who participated in only one or two structured activities but who had high levels of involvement (4 hours or more during the 2 survey days) were added to the hurried category. From this set of structured activities, we classified children into four groups: (1) uninvolved, (2) focused, (3) balanced, and (4) hurried.

Table 13-3

PERCENTAGE OF CHILDREN IN ACTIVITY CATEGORIES,
ONE WEEKDAY AND ONE WEEKEND DAY

Activity Category	PSID–CDS[A]	PSID–CDS[B]	Parkside	Parkside[C]	Riverview
Uninvolved (no structured activities)	15	17	13	13	5
Focused (1 activity & <4 hrs)	31	33	26	25	10
Balanced (2 activities & <4 hrs)	27	25	30	31	40
Hurried (3+ activities or 4+ hrs)	26	25	30	31	45
Total	100	100	99	100	100
N	277	331	23	16	20

[a]Includes only non-Hispanic White children ages 9–12 years, mother has 12+ years of schooling.

[b]Includes only non-Hispanic White children ages 9–12 years, all mothers.

[c]This subsample was interviewed during the 1999–2000 school year.

Table 13-3 shows this typology of structured activities both for the national sample and for the two Midwest sites, Parkside and Riverview. As mentioned previously, 15% of the children in the national sample had no structured activities and were classified as uninvolved. Using the four-category typology described above, 31% of the children in the national sample had only one type of structured activity and spent fewer than 4 hours in this activity during the 2 survey days (focused), 27% of the children had two different types of structured activities and spent fewer than 4 hours in these activities during the 2 survey days (balanced), and 26% of the children either participated in all three types of structured activities or spent more than 4 hours in one or more structured activities during the 2 survey days (hurried).

Of the 16 Parkside children who were interviewed in the 1999–2000 school year, 13% were uninvolved, 25% were focused, 31% were balanced, and 31% were hurried. The distribution of children across the four categories is similar in the full Parkside group. Of the 20 Riverview children, 5% were uninvolved, 10% were focused, 40% were balanced, and 45% were hurried. The proportion of children with balanced and high levels of structured activity was greater in Riverview than in Parkside, and the proportion with no structured activities or a single structured activity was lower in Riverview compared to Parkside.

What Factors Are Associated With Hurriedness?

Table 13-4 presents the ordered logistic regression of our activity typology on education, family structure, site, income, family size, and gender for children ages 9 to 12 years. In contrast to our hypothesis about community class differences, there is no difference in hurriedness between Riverview and Parkside; most of the variation is within rather than between communities. In all three data sets and both models, we see that both measures of family social class—education and income—are significantly associated with a greater chance of being in the high activity category. In the Parkside–Riverview data, we also see that the association between parents' education and activity typology is curvilinear; children's chance of being hurried increases up to 16 years of schooling, after which it declines. In the PSID–CDS, the coefficient for the squared term was never significant (not shown), but this is because mother's education was top-coded at 17, resulting in no variation after 16 years of schooling. Children living with two parents are busier, accord-

Table 13-4

ORDERED LOGISTIC REGRESSION OF ACTIVITY TYPOLOGY ON EDUCATION, FAMILY STRUCTURE, SITE, INCOME, FAMILY SIZE, AND GENDER, CHILDREN AGES 9–12 YEARS

| | Parkside/Riverview[a] | | PSID–CDS, White only | | | |
| | | | Mother High School Grad Plus[b] | | Full Sample[b] | |
Variable	Model 1 Coefficient	Model 2 Coefficient	Model 1 Coefficient	Model 2 Coefficient	Model 1 Coefficient	Model 2 Coefficient
Intercept-Focused	61.248**	8.133	−7.848***	−6.373**	−6.962***	−5.042**
Intercept-Balanced	63.341**	9.939*	−6.585***	−5.105*	−5.8***	−3.876*
Intercept-Hurried	65.844**	12.345*	−4.877***	−3.389*	−4.074*	−2.159
Child gender (male = 1, female = 0)	−1.745*	−1.325*	−0.05	−0.045	−0.004	0.007
Two parents	−3.455	−1.441	0.902*	0.946*	0.629*	0.806*
Mother's education (years)	7.044**	omitted	0.107*	omitted	0.122**	omitted
Mother's education squared	−0.208**	omitted	omitted	omitted	omitted	omitted
Mother completed 12 years	omitted	reference	omitted	reference	omitted	reference
Mother completed 13–15 years	omitted	reference	omitted	0.347	omitted	0.446*
Mother completed 16 years	omitted	2.85**	omitted	0.582*	omitted	0.818**
Mother completed 17+ years	omitted	1.178	omitted	0.601	omitted	0.794*
Log of family income	2.411*	2.961*	0.368*	0.339*	0.325*	0.256
Number of children	0.676	0.345	0.137	0.135	−0.009	−0.038
Site (Parkside = 2, Riverview = 1)	−0.233	0.388	na	na	na	na
N	36	36	277	277	331	331
−2 Log L			733.361	731.94	865.322	866.429

[a]Includes only families interviewed during the 1999–2000 school year.

[b]Mother's education was top-coded at 17 in the PSID–CDS.

*p < .05; **p < .01; ***p < .001, one-tailed test.

ing to the typology, than children who live with only one parent, but this is statistically significant only in the PSID–CDS. The number of children in the family is not linked to the extent of activity in either data set.

Parental Pressure on Children's Activity Participation

One source of stress is lack of control over one's time. How children initially become involved may affect their later willingness to participate and their experience of the activity. Based on the findings of our qualitative study data, there appear to be three general ways children become involved in structured activities: (1) personal interest, (2) parental suggestion and pressure, and (3) the desire to be with friends. Schools send fliers home with the children announcing a variety of events and possible activities. Some flyers are discarded and others prompt action, depending on the child's interest. Parents also may suggest that the child try an activity. Probably the most common source of information and impetus for becoming involved in a particular activity is the desire to be with one's friends. We found all three routes into structured activity reported by the families in our Midwest study.

A number of parents (names have all been changed to protect confidentiality) in our qualitative study were very explicit about their strategies of exposing children to a variety of activities in the hopes that their children could find something they liked and at which they could become skilled. Most seemed very sensitive to the expressed preferences of their children for activity involvement. As one mother explained,

> What I've tried to do is offer the kids a variety of things to try. And then if something is really what they want to do, then we go in that direction. (Billie, mother of Tara [11]—Riverview—2 activities)

This middle-class Riverview parent clearly stated that she explicitly provided or sought out opportunities for her child to participate in structured activities, but then let the child make his or her own decision. In contrast, Ann's mother, Lynn, from working-class Parkside, did not seek out structured activities, but responded to fliers sent from the school if and only if the child showed an interest.

> [With softball] you get the flyers that come home with different activities… She says that she's interested, and if not, we don't worry about it. (Lynn, mother of Ann [12]—Parkside—5 activities)

Of course, this child was already highly active, with five structured activities. Lynn has a more passive approach than Billie, one which fits with the natural growth model, but with sensitivity to the child's preferences and interests, and, in particular, to Ann's tendency to try different activities.

Parents also provide pressure. This is particularly true for children who started a structured activity at an early age. This pressure occurred in both communities. One Parkside child began dance classes in kindergarten and another began soccer at age 5. One Riverview child also began soccer at age 6. It is likely that these were not child-initiated activities. Several children noted that one of their parents used to be involved in a particular activity and wanted the children to try it for themselves.

One of the most common reasons we heard for being involved in a structured activity was to be with friends or because a sibling or other important person in the child's life (such as a father, sister, or cousin) was also involved. This was common in Parkside, the lower-middle-class community, but not as common in Riverview. As this Parkside child explained,

> I used to follow my sister and do whatever she does… So I wanted to try it [soccer] because she played. (Jen [11], daughter of Sally —Parkside—4 activities)

Table 13-5

MEAN VALUES ON DIFFERENT MEASURES OF STRESS SYMPTOMS BY ACTIVITY TYPOLOGY[a]

| Stress Symptoms | Activity Typology | | | | Total | |
	Uninvolved	Focused	Balanced	Hurried	Mean	SD
Parent reported						
Stress symptoms	2.1	1.9	1.9	1.8	1.9	1.8
Internalizing (total)	4.4	3.4	3.0	3.2	3.4	3.3
Internalizing without stress	3.0	2.1	1.8	1.9	2.1	2.3
Low self esteem	1.9	1.3	1.1	1.2	1.3	1.5
N	62	108	77	84	331	
Child reported:						
Self-esteem	24.8	25.0	24.9	24.3	24.7	3.5
N	43	70	51	61	225	

[a]PSID–CDS full sample.

Note. SD = standard deviation.

Hurriedness and Child Stress Symptoms—National Data

Table 13-5 shows means on the various measures of stress symptoms by the typology of hurriedness, using data from the National PSID–CDS. Contrary to our expectations, stress symptoms were found to be highest for the uninvolved children and lowest for those involved in structured activities. In no case did hurried children have the most symptoms.

These results are supported by Table 13-6, which shows the results of regressing the different measures of stress symptoms on categories of the activity typology, controlling for social class, family structure, family size, and child gender. This provides the first quantitative evidence from a large national sample that increased child stress symptoms, as reported by a parent, are not related to hurriedness. Nor is hurriedness linked to low self-esteem as reported by the child (measure E). Contrary to our hypothesis, we found that uninvolved children are the ones who score highest on the internalizing measures. The largest effect was obtained using the total internalizing score. Uninvolved children scored about 1 point higher on the total internalizing scale (measure B), an effect size of one-third of a standard deviation, a substantial effect. The most highly significant association was between inactivity (no structured activities) and low self-esteem (measure D), which included items such as "complains no one loves him/her," "seems to be in a fog," "feels worthless or inferior," "has difficulty getting his/her mind off certain thoughts," and "feels others are out to get him/her."

We also found that children of mothers with more years of education were consistently less likely to show symptoms of stress than children of mothers with fewer years. If more educated mothers were unduly pressuring their children, the latter should show increased symptoms of stress, which was not the case. We explore this further using our qualitative data.

Table 13-6

ORDINARY LEAST SQUARES REGRESSION OF STRESS SYMPTOMS ON SOCIAL CLASS, FAMILY STRUCTURE AND CONTROLS[a]

	Measure A Stress Symptoms		Measure B Internalizing Total		Measure C Internal Without Stress		Measure D Low Self-Esteem (Parent)		Measure E High Self-Esteem (Child)	
	Model 1	Model 2	Model 1	Model 2	Model 1	Model 2	Model 1	Model 2	Model 1	Model 2
Variable	Coeff.	Coeff.	Coeff.	Coeff.	Coeff.	Coeff.	Coeff.	Coeff.	Coeff.	Coeff.
Intercept	4.532**	3.473*	7.506**	4.544	4.557*	2.135	2.607	1.217	21.321***	19.489***
Uninvolved	0.055	0.067	0.928+	0.894+	0.855*	0.823*	0.647**	0.630**	-0.233	-0.150
Hurried	-0.069	-0.090	0.089	0.057	0.052	0.032	0.028	0.020	-0.538	-0.552
Child Gender (M=1, F=0)	0.178	0.172	0.183	0.168	0.028	0.017	0.062	0.057	-0.648	-0.640
Two parents	0.111	-0.046	0.164	-0.144	0.078	-0.128	0.281	0.190	0.234	-0.180
Mother's education (years)	-0.100**		-0.189**		-0.136**		-0.071*		-0.163+	
Mother completed (<13)	reference		reference		reference		reference		reference	
Mother completed (13–15)		-0.414		-0.935*		-0.631*		-0.276		-1.019+
Mother completed (16)		-0.566+		-1.570**		-1.245***		-0.687**		-0.836
Mother completed (17+)		-0.276		-0.493		-0.387		-0.227		-1.427
Log of family income	-0.140	-0.132	-0.156	-0.041	-0.053	0.056	-0.045	0.021	0.442	0.485
Number of children	0.050	0.071	-0.083	-0.030	-0.103	-0.060	-0.077	-0.054	0.433+	0.484+
Site (Parkside = 2, Riverview = 1)										
N	331	331	331	331	331	331	331	331	225	225
R^2	0.037	0.0301	0.050	0.057	0.060	0.072	0.051	0.061	0.048	0.050

Note. Coeff. = coefficient.

$+p < .10$; $*p < .05$; $**p < .01$; $***p < .001$, 2-tailed test

[a]PSID-CDS Full Sample

Hurriedness and Child Stress Symptoms—Qualitative Data

We found evidence in both Riverview and Parkside that children and parents were under occasional stress because of a large number of structured activities or the amount of time spent in them, but this did not appear to be continual or frequent. Out of 43 children, 6 (14%) expressed occasional stress or strain—not wanting to go to an activity, being tired of the activity, preferring to do something else or nothing, crying, being overly tired out, being worried, showing symptoms of depression or anxiety, or having headaches or sore muscles.

For example, a 9-year-old girl in gymnastics 3 hours a day 3 days a week and with two other activities (ballet and ice skating) was pretty tired by Friday:

> Like usually on Fridays I'm like I don't want to be here... [but once I'm there] sometimes I just pep right up. (Serena [9], daughter of Judy—Riverview—hurried)

Another fourth grader with five different structured activities (soccer, scouts, jump rope, recorder, and religious education) said,

> I just like to jump rope once in a while, but now I'm tired of it... Every single time I do it for like 5 minutes and my feet are tired. (Laura [10], daughter of Jeannette—Parkside—hurried)

Given that the children seemed very compliant and only occasionally expressed dissatisfaction with their schedules and activities, we asked parents how they knew when children were doing too much. One Riverview parent offered the following observation:

> I don't believe kids can really articulate that they're stressed. I think it comes about in other ways... My older one was, she seemed like she was tired and distracted and distraught, and so we looked at our activity level and decided we had to cut back (Cathy, mother of Becca [10]—Riverview—balanced)

Billie said that she was very sensitive to her daughter Tara's stress symptoms, such as sleep disturbances, catching a cold, or crying. Tara stopped taking piano lessons because practice led to crying. Eventually they made a conscious decision to cut back to two activities.

There are three possible explanations for the lack of evidence of major problems in terms of child- and parent-reported stress: (1) children and parents under stress were not interviewed, (2) children and parents have gotten used to this lifestyle, and (3) most children are not overly scheduled or stressed.

Nonparticipation by Stressed Families

It is possible that parents who were currently under stress may not have agreed to be interviewed for the qualitative study. Many parents interviewed in Riverview indicated that they had been through a very busy period in the recent past when they felt as though they were overextended in terms of their daily and weekly schedules. This recurrent theme was most often articulated in answers regarding their current weekly schedules, when parents made unsolicited comparisons to how "overwhelmed" or "totally stressed out" they had been a year or 2 earlier when their children were involved in multiple structured activities. For example, Billie noted how she kept track of her daughter's and son's involvement in structured activities along with her husband's after-work commitments, and realized that, because her daughter was moving into the fifth grade with higher academic expectations, she would need "some down time in the evenings." So she discontinued her daughter's piano lessons, took her daughter out of Girl Scouts, and only let her continue basketball and ballet. In her words, Billie "simplified [my family members'] lives" by limiting the number of structured activities her daughter (and son) were involved in.

However, there is little empirical evidence that our interviews captured a particularly low-activity group of families. National data suggest that, to the contrary, our qualitative studies captured more high-activity than low-activity families. Of all the children aged 9 to 12 in the nationally representative PSID–CDS, only 26% fell in the hurried child category, compared with 31% in Parkside (16-case subsample) and 45% in Riverview. According to the PSID–CDS, 15.4% of the national sample had no structured activities, compared with 13% in Parkside and 5% in Riverview.

Families Accustomed to Lifestyle

A second possibility is that parents and children become used to the pace they set and do not evaluate it negatively. One strategy that parents use to justify and to help themselves feel satisfied with their own choices is to continually compare themselves to "other" families. Parents compare their parenting and time-use strategies to those of other families, who are often presented in negative terms. Parents seem to recognize that they could be doing "worse" and use this knowledge to achieve a sense of balance between the conflicting needs of various family members and the desires of parents and their children.

With regard to this second strategy, a number of the parents were asked how they see other families in the community coping with the time crunch. Invariably, the parents interviewed cogently stated that they frequently see other parents in the community "totally stressed out," rushing their children from school to one activity after another, and traveling out of town every weekend for yet another soccer or ice hockey tournament. The following is a typical comment along these lines from a Riverview parent:

> I know some people…the parents really push the kids to get involved in not just school activities, but two or three other extracurricular activities at a real young age. And the kids end up being very burned out, and then don't want to do anything. And [the parents say] "I've invested all this time and energy and money into dance lessons over the last four years and you will continue on." And then who is actually doing it? Is it the parents living through the child? Or is it because the kids want to learn a skill? (Erin, mother of Judy [11]—Riverview—balanced)

It appears that parents draw on these vivid accounts of their harried neighbors to gain a sense of calm and contentment from their belief that, although they are busy, they are not "overdoing" it like some of the other parents in the community. Regardless of how hectic their lives were, every family could identify another family that was busier.

Children Not Overscheduled

Finally, a third possibility is that children are not all that busy. This interpretation is consistent with the results from the quantitative study. Children averaged two to three structured activities per week in both Riverview and Parkside. Most children were involved in a sport (or art activity) and one school or nonschool club. The third activity could be a second sport or an art activity. Riverview children were more likely than Parkside children to be in art activities, and Parkside children were significantly more likely than Riverview children to be involved in scouts and somewhat more likely to be enrolled in religious education. Although the average number of organized activities was the same across the two communities, the distribution of activity levels differed (see Table 13-3). Riverview children were more likely to be hurried and less likely to be uninvolved than Parkside children and the national sample. This is because they spent more time in their structured activities. Riverview children were more likely than Parkside children to be involved in multiple sports during a week; the children involved in multiple sports activities were the ones most likely to complain of being tired.

Parental Pressure and Activity Level

Based on our qualitative data, we found little evidence that parental pressure was the major force leading to child participation in structured activities. There appear to be three general ways children become involved in structured activities: desire to be with friends was the major factor leading to participation, followed by personal interest, and finally, by parental encouragement. Even when the latter was operative, it took child motivation to stick with the activity.

In fact, children with no structured activities caused considerable parent concern; 15% of the national sample, 13% of Parkside children interviewed during the school year, and 5% of Riverview children had no structured activities. For the most part, these children spent their after-school time riding their bicycles, playing with friends, reading, watching TV, playing basketball or pick-up hockey games, Rollerblading, and roller skating. Parents worried when children did not have any structured activities.

One child (David from Parkside) was in sixth grade, and his only structured activity earlier during the school year was a church group. He played handheld video games (e.g., Playstation) a lot. David's father (Robert) was concerned that his son did not want to do any organized activities. Robert commented that he was disappointed that his son had stopped taking guitar lessons and thought his son would benefit from the social aspect of being involved in a team sport. Yet, he also was concerned about pushing his son:

> I'm trying, you know, my wife and I fight back and forth a little bit about that nudge...
> And I don't want to push him, then I think as soon as you push, they push back.
> (Robert, father of David [12]—Parkside—uninvolved)

Characteristic of several other children with low levels of structured activity was shyness or introversion. For example, Susan explained why her daughter, now involved in one after-school activity, stopped participating in gymnastics:

> Holly is really shy. And it's hard to get her involved in things, even with school, let alone outside of school. (Susan, mother of Holly [10]—Parkside—focused)

In both communities, parents whose children had many structured activities worked hard to keep them within limits, and parents whose children were participating in few or no extracurricular activities worried that their children might be missing something important.

DISCUSSION AND CONCLUSIONS

The structure of children's lives has changed over the past several decades. The number of after-school activities and weekend meets and games and the time spent in them have expanded greatly (Crosnoe, 2001; Hofferth & Sandberg, 2001). As a result, many families wonder whether they are making the right decisions for their children and themselves. This research addressed, first, how active American children are; second, whether there is evidence that children from upper-middle-class families are more active than those from working-class families and third, whether children are overscheduled to the extent that they exhibit stress symptoms.

The strength of this study is that we were able to use data from a large national sample of families and quantitative and qualitative data for the same age-group of children from two different communities in the Midwest, one an upper-middle-class community and the other a working-class community. We had a particularly large sample size for qualitative interviews, 43 families. The different samples are similar in characteristics. This means that we could use the qualitative data from the community samples to provide more depth to data from quantitative analyses. The limited age range was useful in keeping variability by maturity relatively low and its effects insignificant; we were unable to directly adjust for differential maturity. The major limitation of the community samples is that they were restricted to white working-class and middle-class families. However, we argue that the hurried child is a white middle-class issue, and proposed solutions are focused on white middle-class families, not minority or low-income families. In addition, low-income families are more likely to be female-headed, which makes the resource constraints substantially unequal and confounds class with family structure, a problem for earlier research. This research avoids that pitfall.

The first question is whether a large proportion of children are overscheduled or hurried. The current study found about 26% of American children ages 9 to 12 years had three or more structured activities or were involved in one or two structured activities for 4 or more hours on 2 days in the week. This group exemplifies what Elkind (2001) called hurried children. The majority of children (58%) are either focused or balanced in their structured activities, and 15% are uninvolved.

Are structured activities a function of social class of the community or the family? Because of differences in parental education between our upper-middle-class and working-class communities, we expected that there would be variations in the childrearing beliefs and values of parents across communities and that these different beliefs would lead to differential involvement of their children in structured activities. However, our initial assumptions were wrong. Although children were definitely more hurried in the middle-class community, children were active in both communities. Rather than activity differences being primarily *between* communities, we found that the major activity differences were *within* each community. Maternal education was more closely linked to the child's structured activities than any other factor, but it was not linear, rising and then falling as maternal education rose. There are two possible reasons for this nonlinearity. First, in highly educated families, such as the medical doctor married to a medical doctor, parents may be too busy to involve the children in multiple structured activities. Second, highly educated mothers may be more knowledgeable regarding professional concerns about the effects of excessive activities and limit their children's activities accordingly. This relationship between education and activities was similar in Riverview and Parkside. In interviews with parents in both communities, parents saw education as key to the future. However, higher family income and having two parents were also linked to more structured activity. Besides education, financial and parental resources at home are critical to participation in activities. Both the national and community studies supported these conclusions.

The third question is whether children who are more hurried experience stress because of their schedules. We expected to find children with many structured activities to experience greater stress symptoms. However, we found little evidence for this hurried-child hypothesis. In the national data set we did not find hurried children to be more likely to exhibit symptoms of stress or have low self-esteem. Instead, those *least involved in organized activities exhibited more symptoms* of withdrawal, inability to get along with others, and lower self-esteem.

The results of the qualitative analyses support our conclusion that children are, for the most part, engaged voluntarily in healthy levels of structured activities and that their parents are wary and watchful for stress symptoms. The parents in our studies cut back their children's schedules when these occurred. The most interesting reports were that parents of children who did not participate in structured activities were quite concerned about it. Qualitative reports from parents and children suggest that children who have problems getting along with others, low self-esteem, or who are socially immature are those who rarely participate in organized extracurricular activities.

We argue that there are three reasons why we failed to find much evidence for excessive activities. First, those families whose children are overly hurried may not have participated in our studies. However, this explanation is not likely because both Riverview and Parkside children were *more,* not *less,* active than the average child ages 9 to 12 years in the national sample. Second, families may be used to a busy schedule or may have been through a busy time and had subsequently cut back on their activities by the time of the interviews. As evidence, we found that some families reported that they had recently scaled back their activities; perhaps we were seeing families who had already gone through the overly stressed phase and not those who were experiencing very busy times. In addition, families saw themselves as normal, whereas they could point out other families who had too many structured activities and seemed to be overly stressed.

However, the third possibility is that it is normal for healthy children to have lots of structured activities. The direction of causality is reversed; those who have adjustment problems are the ones who are uninvolved. Children today may be busier than they were in the recent past; however, that does not necessarily mean that this has caused them or their families excessive stress and strain.

Attaining Balance

The majority of children and their families in our study had attained a measure of balance, meaning that they were involved in activities and organizations beyond the family, but within reasonable limits. Children's stresses were lowest in the focused and balanced categories. According to our definitions, such children had one or two structured activities, and the total weekly time in such activities was less than 4 hours over the 2 diary days. Such involvement appears to be both normal and valuable to child development; it was associated with lower stress and higher self-esteem on a variety of measures. Other research shows long-term benefits of organized activities as well (Mahoney et al., 2005).

What is important is that these activities not strain family members beyond their capacities. Besides each individual child's activities, parents need to balance the activities of other children and their own activities. Of the various strategies used, the most important we found was to reduce the mother's employment schedule from full-time to part-time, or, in some cases, to work at home. Mothers were most likely to alter their schedules, but fathers also made decisions to forgo promotions that would have increased their work time. Flexibility at work was helpful to both parents. The second major strategy was organization, including setting priorities and using technology, such as cell phones. Communication among family members was critical. A third strategy was to enlist others as backup, including carpooling and getting help from relatives and neighbors. Siblings often attended each other's practices and lessons. The fourth strategy, involving the children in family routines and chores, facilitated the smooth running of the family. Finally, parents involved themselves in their children's structured activities—as coach, den leader, parent–teacher organization leader, and volunteer. Parents were aware of the dangers of too much activity and appeared relatively successful in managing their family's schedule. As one Parkside mother put it:

> I think we've got enough going on and all the right things going on... so I think we've got a pretty good balance on everything right now. (Joanne, mother of Michael [9]—Parkside—hurried)

REFERENCES

Adam, E. K. (2005). Momentary emotion and cortisol levels in the everyday lives of working parents. In B. Schneider & L. J. Waite (Eds.), *Being together, working apart: Dual-career families and the work–life balance* (pp. 105–133). Cambridge, UK: Cambridge University Press.

Alwin, D. F. (2001). Parental values, beliefs, and behavior: A review and promulga for research into the new century. In T. Owens & S. Hofferth (Eds.), *Children at the millennium: Where did we come from, where are we going?* (pp. 97–139). New York: Elsevier Science.

Arendell, T. (2001). The new care work of middle-class mothers: Managing childrearing, employment, and time. In K. Daly (Ed.), *Minding the time in family experience* (pp. 163–204). London: Elsevier Science.

Baker, P. C., Keck, C. K., Mott, F. L., & Quinlan, S. V. (1993). *NLSY child handbook* (rev. ed.). Columbus: Center for Human Resource Research, Ohio State University.

Band, E. B., & Weisz, J. R. (1988). How to feel better when it feels bad: Children's perspectives on coping with everyday stress. *Developmental Psychology, 24,* 247–253.

Borgers, N., de Leeuw, E., & Hox, J. (1999). Surveying children: Cognitive development and response quality in questionnaire research. In A. Christianson et al. (Eds.), *Official statistics in a changing world* (pp. 133–140). Stockholm: Statistics Sweden.

Crosnoe, R. (2001). The social world of male and female athletes in high school. In D. A. Kinney (Ed.), *Sociological studies of children and youth* (pp. 89–110). Oxford, UK: Elsevier.

Doherty, W. J., & Carlson, B. (2002). *Putting family first: Successful strategies for reclaiming family life in a hurry-up world.* Minneapolis, MN: University of Minnesota.

Dunn, J. S., Kinney, D. A., & Hofferth, S. L. (2003). Parental ideologies and children's after-school activities. *American Behavioral Scientist, 46,* 1359–1386.

Eccles, J., & Gootman, J. A. (2002). *Community programs to promote youth development.* Washington, DC: National Academy Press.

Elkind, D. (2001). *The hurried child.* Cambridge, MA: Perseus.

Fitzgerald, J., Gottschalk, P., & Moffitt, R. (1998). An analysis of sample attrition in panel data: The Michigan Panel Study of Income Dynamics. *Journal of Human Resources 33,* 251–299.

Galinsky, E. (2002). *Ask the children.* New York: Families and Work Institute.

Ginsburg, K. R. (2006). *The importance of play in promoting healthy child development and maintaining strong parent-child bonds* [Clinical report]. Chicago: American Academy of Pediatrics.

Hektner, J., Schmidt, J., & Csikszentmihalyi, M. (2007). *Experience sampling method.* Thousand Oaks, CA: Sage.

Hofferth, S., Davis-Kean, P., Davis, J., & Finkelstein, J. (1999). *1997 user guide: The child development supplement to the panel study of income dynamics.* Ann Arbor, MI: Institute for Social Research, University of Michigan.

Hofferth, S. L., & Sandberg, J. F. (2001). Changes in American children's time, 1981–1997. In S. Hofferth & T. Owens (Eds.), *Children at the millennium: Where did we come from, where are we going?* (pp. 193–229). New York: Elsevier Science.

Jacobs, J. A., & Gerson, K. (2004). *The time divide: Work, family, and gender inequality.* Cambridge, MA: Harvard University Press.

Kohn, M. L. (1977). *Class and conformity.* Chicago: University of Chicago Press.

Kohn, M., & Schooler, C. (1983). *Work and personality: An inquiry into the impact of social stratification.* Norwood, NJ: Ablex.

Lareau, A. (2002). Invisible inequality: Social class and childrearing in black families and white families. *American Sociological Review, 67,* 747–776.

Lareau, A. (2003). *Unequal childhoods: Class, race, and family life.* Berkeley: University of California Press.

Larson, R. (1994). Youth organizations, hobbies, and sports as developmental contexts. In R. Silbereisen & E. Todt (Eds.), *Adolescence in context: The interplay of family, school, peers, and work in adjustment* (pp. 46–65). New York: Springer-Verlag.

Larson, R., & Verma, S. (1999). How children and adolescents spend time across the world: Work, play, and developmental opportunities. *Psychological Bulletin, 125,* 701–736.

Lesthaeghe, R., & Surkyn, J. (1988). Cultural dynamics and economic theories of fertility change. *Population and Development Review, 14,* 1–45.

Luthar, S. S., & Becker, B. E. (2002). Privileged but pressured? A study of affluent youth. *Child Development, 73,* 1593–1610.

Lynott, P. P., & Logue, B. J. (1993). The "hurried child": The myth of lost childhood in contemporary American society. *Sociological Forum, 8,* 471–491.

Mahoney, J. L., Larson, R. W., Eccles, J. S., & Lord, H. (2005). Organized activities as developmental contexts for children and adolescents. In J. L. Mahoney, R. W. Larson, & J. S. Eccles (Eds.), *Organized activities as contexts of development* (pp. 3–22). Mahwah, NJ: Lawrence Erlbaum.

Mintz, S. (2004). *Huck's raft: A history of American childhood.* Cambridge, MA: Harvard University Press.

Peterson, J. L., & Zill, N. (1986). Marital disruption, parent–child relationships, and behavioral problems in children. *Journal of Marriage and the Family, 48,* 295–307.

Pincus, D. B., & Friedman, A. G. (2004). Improving children's coping with everyday stress: Transporting treatment interventions to the school setting. *Clinical Child and Family Psychology Review, 7,* 223–240.

Reynolds, L. K., O'Koon, J. H., Papademetriou, E., Szczygiel, S., & Grant, K. E. (2001). Stress and somatic complaints in low-income urban adolescents. *Journal of Youth and Adolescence, 30,* 499–514.

Robinson, J. P., & Godbey, G. (1997). *Time for life: The surprising ways Americans use their time.* University Park: Pennsylvania State University Press.

Schaefer, E., & Edgerton, M. (1985). Parental and child correlates of parental modernity. In I. Sigel (Ed.), *Parental belief systems: The psychological consequences for children* (pp. 287–318). Hillsdale, NJ: Lawrence Erlbaum.

Stefanello, R. (2004). Short communication: A preliminary study of stress symptoms and nutritional state in children. *Stress and Health, 20,* 293–299.

Tansey, T., Mizelle, N., Ferrin, J., Tschopp, M., & Frain, M. (2004). Work-related stress and the demand-control-support framework: Implications for the P x E fit model. *Journal of Rehabilitation, 70,* 34–41.

Thornton, A. (2004). *Reading history sideways: The fallacy and enduring impact of the developmental paradigm on family life.* Chicago: University of Chicago.

U.S. Census Bureau. (2005). Retrieved February 25, 2005, from http://factfinder.census.gov/home/saff/main.html?_lang=en

Time Use Imbalance
DEVELOPMENTAL AND EMOTIONAL COSTS

JIRI ZUZANEK

INTRODUCTION

I would like to start my comments about life balance with quotations from two books written more than a century apart. The first book is *Robinson Crusoe* by Daniel Defoe. It was published in 1719 and probably needs no comment. The second is Wilkie Collins' *The Moonstone*, published in 1868 and called by T. S. Eliot, "the first, the longest, and the best of modern English detective novels." It is *The Moonstone* that drew my attention to *Robinson Crusoe*. One of *Moonstone's* main characters, House-Stewart Gabriel Betteredge, insists that he can find answers to all his questions in *Robinson Crusoe*: "I have tried that book for years, and I have found it in need in all the necessities of the mortal life. When my spirits are bad—*Robinson Crusoe*. When I want advice—*Robinson Crusoe*."

So, when I was asked to contribute a chapter to this book on life balance, I decided to put Betteredge's words to the test and pulled off my library shelf an old copy of *Robinson Crusoe* that had followed me on my journeys from China, where I was born; to Czechoslovakia, where I lived for a time; and then to Canada, where I now live. The book did not fail me. Here is what I found on page 12, where Robinson's father tries to dissuade his son from the "rambling thoughts" of going to sea, and in doing so touches upon the very problem of interest to us—life balance.

> My father asked me what reasons, more than a mere wandering inclination, I had for leaving his house, and my native country, where I might be well introduced, and had a prospect of raising my fortune, by application and industry, with a life of ease and pleasure. He told me that it was men of desperate fortunes, on the one hand, or of the superior fortunes, on the other, who went abroad upon adventures, aspiring to rise by enterprise and make themselves famous in undertakings of nature out of the common road; that these things were either too far above me, or too far below me; that mine was the middle state, or what might be called the upper station of low life, which he had found, by long experience, was the best state of the world, the most suited to human happiness; not exposed to the miseries and hardships, the labor and sufferings of the mechanic part of mankind, and not embarrassed with the pride, luxury, ambition and envy of the upper part of mankind.[1]

---

[1]Quotation from *Robinson Crusoe* is taken from Daniel Defoe, *Life and Adventures of Robinson Crusoe* (London: Ward, Lock & Co, undated), p. 12. Quotations from *The Moonstone* and T. S. Eliot are taken from Wilkie Collins, *The Moonstone* (Ware, Hertfordshire, UK: Wordsworth Classics, 1993), p. 16 and the cover, respectively.

K. Matuska & C. Christiansen (Eds.)
Life balance: Multidisciplinary theories and research (pp 207–222)
© 2009 SLACK Incorporated and AOTA Press

RESEARCH PROBLEM:
AGAINST THE CONFINES OF LINEAR THINKING

The problem of life balance has long intrigued men of letters, as well as men of affairs and men of ordinary ways of life. The notion of balance can be found in the famous lines from Ecclesiastes, that there is a time to every purpose under heaven—"a time to weep and a time to laugh, a time to mourn, and a time to dance." It is present in Ovid's verse that the "middle course is the safest for you to take," the Aristotelian notion of the "golden mean," and a French-language line in one of Alexander Pushkin's letters, "Il n'est de bonheur que dans les voies communes" (There is no happiness outside of the common road).[2] The notions of balance, common road, and golden mean have, however, one common problem—disagreement on what constitutes the extremes. A comparison of time-use patterns of today with those of a century ago makes this clearer. In 1918, a 6-day, 48-hour workweek was a desirable norm and an acceptable mean. Today, its imposition on the North American worker would be certainly resisted and condemned as excessive. In short, *balance* and *mean* are time and situation specific and therefore hard to define. In the words of Robert Burns:

> Then at the balance let's be mute...
> What done we partly may compute,
> But know not what's resisted.[3]

Methodologically, the social sciences—unlike the arts—are poorly equipped for dealing with the problem of life balance. Much of modern-era social discourse is dominated by linear thinking. The notion of life balance, however, defies linear explanations.

Examples of this linear thinking include the overly optimistic forecasts of the imminent growth of leisure and its beneficial effects that were popular in the 1960s. In 1962, Joffre Dumazedier published his trend-setting book, *Vers une civilisation du loisir? (Toward a Society of Leisure?)*. It was translated into English and published with a highly supportive introduction by David Riesman. Jean Fourastie predicted in 1965 that by the mid-1980s people would work only one-third of their lives, the length of the workweek would not exceed 30 hours, and 12 weeks of vacation would be guaranteed. Articles published at that time abound with statements about the multiplication of "leisure opportunities," "development of new values," "valorization of self-expression," and even an "aesthetic-ethical revolution" (taken from the review *Society and Leisure*, 1975, No. 1).

The situation has changed, however, since the 1970s. The buzzwords in the 1980s and particularly the 1990s were not "the promise of leisure" but "time pressure," "time scarcity," and "life stress." Linder (1971), Wilensky (1981), and Schor (1991) argued that people in rich societies are confronted with a shortage rather than an abundance of leisure, and Robinson (1977) observed that shorter working hours and more free time, contrary to popular expectations, do not always make people happier. These findings gradually tempered hopes about the impending leisure bliss, and people were urged to look at leisure and work as complementary parts of modern life rather than opposites. A balance of work and leisure rather than a "society of leisure" was put on the research and policy agenda.

There are other examples of linear thinking. According to Phillips and Sandstrom (1990); Clausen (1991); and Mortimer, Harley, and Aronson (1999), paid work helps adolescents learn useful skills, better manage their time, and be prepared for a successful transition to adulthood. This position is countered by critics who claim that teens' part-time work consists mostly of menial jobs, carries few experiential benefits, and takes time away from schoolwork, physically active

---

[2]Quotations from Ecclesiastes, Ovid, Aristotle, and Pushkin are from Ecclesiastes, 3:1; Ovid's *Metamorphose*, Book 2; Aristotle's *Nicomachean Ethics*, Translated by Harris Rackham (Cambridge, MA: Harvard University Press, 1926); and Pushkin's letter to N. I. Krivtsov written on February 10, 1831 (Complete works, volume X, Russian Edition, 1951), p. 338.

[3]The Robert Burns quotation is from "Address to the Unco Guid," in *The Complete Poetical Works* (Edinburgh: William P. Nimmo, 1866), p. 91.

leisure, and sleep (Greenberger & Steinberg, 1986; Steinberg & Cauffman, 1995). Regretfully, this debate paid little attention to the effects of different amounts of teens' paid work, missing the point that, apart from the quality of the jobs, the effects of part-time work depend on its varying amounts—that is, on the balancing of time.

An artificial juxtaposition of arguments can also be found in regard to teens' homework. Publications such as Kralovec and Buell's *The End of Homework* (2000) and Bennett and Kalish's *The Case Against Homework* (2006) single out homework as the underlying reason for adolescent stress, disruption of family relationships, and questionable academic results rather than acknowledge its contribution to students' successful functioning in knowledge-driven economies. Whether homework interferes with teens' well-being is again, among other things, a question of its amount.

The role of unstructured leisure activities (e.g., mass media, hanging around with friends) in the lives of teens, as opposed to structured leisure (e.g., physically active leisure, extracurricular activities) is likewise often presented as an either–or dilemma, and it too can benefit from a more calibrated approach.

Increasing amounts of television viewing had originally been greeted as venues for greater family togetherness, providing an opportunity for family members, parents, and children to spend time together (Riley, Cantwell, & Ruttiger, 1949; Katz & Gurevitch, 1976; Robinson, 1972). Today, this position is not widely shared. Attention has shifted to the sedentary nature of television viewing and its *displacement effects* or taking time away from developmentally more challenging activities (Jordan & Robinson, 2008; Neuman, 1988). For most researchers, television viewing is essentially a passive experience that offers little challenge, requires little attention, and provides limited venues for personal growth or emotional togetherness (Kubey & Csikszentmihalyi, 1990). Yet it remains one of teenagers' favorite activities. Should it be hailed or damned? The answer to this question depends, again, on how much television viewing is involved—on time balance. The time balance approach pertains to the contacts with friends as well.

The famous question from Shakespeare's *As You Like It,* "Can one desire too much of a good thing?" applies to all human activities.[4] Time use is the very core of life balance. It is therefore surprising that time-diary data, collected over the past several decades by statistical agencies and researchers in different countries, have been rarely used to address the life–balance issue.

METHOD

Analyses reported in this chapter are based on time-diary data collected as part of the 1998 Canadian General Social Survey (GSS) and the Ontario Survey of Adolescent Time Use (OATUS) conducted in 2002–2003 by the Research Group on Leisure and Cultural Development of the University of Waterloo.

According to Robinson and Converse (1972), time-diary data offer "a unique view of the intersection between the imperatives of the human condition and the range of individual behavioral choice" (p. 19). A 24-hour day can be visualized, according to those authors, as an available input of lifestyle resources, with the output represented by the time allocated to and the choice of different activities. By reporting time use for a specific day (usually yesterday) in short time intervals (5 or 10 minutes) and by focusing on the entire range of daily behavior rather than a single group of activities (e.g., leisure, sports), time diaries reduce recall errors and make the reporting of activities less susceptible to a social desirability bias.

The 1998 GSS used a national probability sample to collect time-diary information for population ages 15 years or older ($n = 10,749$). The survey included a subsample of 414 high school students ages 15 to 19 years. In addition to time diaries, the survey collected rich information about adults' and adolescents' sense of well-being, life satisfaction, and health.

---

[4]William Shakespeare, *As You Like It*, act IV, scene 1, line 1623.

The OATUS was administered in 13 Ontario schools selected from different neighborhoods in small and medium-size Ontario cities as well as in metropolitan Toronto ($n = 2,213$). A time diary for the day preceding the survey was filled out in class. It was accompanied by questions about adolescents' academic performance, lifestyle preferences, relationship with parents, expectations of the future, emotional well-being, and health. The 219 teens who participated in the time diary part of the study formed the sample of a subsequent experience sampling survey (ESM). Using a method originally developed at the University of Chicago (Csikszentmihalyi & Larson, 1987), respondents were signaled several times a day by a preprogrammed digital wristwatch during the course of a week. In a short self-report form that was filled out at the time of the beep, they identified their main activity at the time of the beep as well as a number of accompanying emotional and experiential states.

The combination of time diary, well-being, experiential, and health data in the surveys used for the analyses reported in this chapter provides a unique opportunity to identify time arrangements that best correspond with desirable well-being and health outcomes for adults and adolescents. Life balance in this chapter is thus operationalized, in essence, as an optimal time-use configuration that best suits human developmental, emotional, and health needs.

How Much Free Time Is Too Much?

As indicated, greater amounts of leisure have in the past been associated with higher levels of well-being. Campbell et al. (1976) saw access to time as an important resource for well-being. This assumption was questioned by Robinson (1977), who noticed that "contrary to the positive value placed on free time in our society, greater life satisfaction generally was associated with less rather than more available free time" (p. 168). This observation is corroborated by Argyle (1987), for whom satisfaction with different forms of leisure is "not closely related to the amount of time spent" (p. 67).

The implications of greater access to free time among teenagers have been of particular interest to educators, parents, and researchers. Concerns with adolescents' emotional well-being and health require paying attention to the overall patterns of teens' daily life, including their access to free time. Findings reported in Table 14-1 summarize academic and well-being effects of access to free time on school days and Sundays among Ontario high school students ages 12 to 18 years. Having more than 4 hours of free time on school days or more than 6 hours on Sundays spells poorer grades. This is not unexpected. What is more surprising is that excessive amounts of free time on school days and Sundays carry a negative emotional toll.

Students with more than 7 hours of free time on school days (21% of the sample) scored higher on the emotional problem scale (composite of feeling lonely, bored, and unhappy; $\alpha = .76$) than students with 4 to 7 hours of free time (54% of the sample). This pattern held true for Sundays as well. Students with more than 11 hours of free time on Sundays (18% of the sample) and students with fewer than 6 hours of free time (22% of the sample) scored higher on the emotional problem scale (6.3 and 6.7, respectively) than students in the 6 to 11 hours in-between group, who scored the lowest (mean 6.0). In short, emotionally the middle ground wins.

Data in Table 14-2 are taken from the 1998 Canadian National Time Use Survey (GSS, Cycle 12) and refer to the adult population ages 25 to 64 years. Findings reported in this table support the contention that greater amounts of free time do not correlate with higher levels of life satisfaction or happiness. A breakdown of respondents' access to free time shows that access to more than 4 hours of free time on weekdays is associated, at the very best, with average levels of life satisfaction and perceived happiness. On Sundays, moderate amounts of free time (3–7 hours) are associated with higher levels of life satisfaction and perceived happiness than excessive or limited amounts of free time. Again, emotionally the in-between group is better off.

Findings reported in Tables 14-1 and 14-2 suggest that the relationships between access to free time and well being are not linear. Optimal well-being outcomes are associated with a balanced

Table 14-1

HOW DOES AMOUNT OF FREE TIME AFFECT TEENS' ACADEMIC PERFORMANCE AND EMOTIONAL WELL-BEING?
(OATUS; CORRELATIONS AND MEAN SCORES)

DAILY ACTIVITIES (HOURS PER DAY)	GRADE AVERAGE (OUT OF 100) PEARSON r*	EMOTIONAL PROBLEMS (2–15) PEARSON r*
Free time on school days	−.22	ns
Free time on Sundays	−.23	−.09
Free time on school days	Means	Means
Less than 4 hours	74.0	6.37
4–7 hours	73.4	5.97
More than 7 hours	70.2	6.41
Total	72.9	6.16
Free time on Sundays		
Less than 6 hours	72.4	6.73
6–11 hours	72.1	6.00
11 hours or more	69.2	6.32
Total	71.5	6.20

Note. Emotional problems computed as a sum of feeling lonely, depressed and unhappy (α = .76). Significant at .005 level. NS = not significant.

use of free time that is commensurate with specific time and situational expectations (for a more detailed analysis of this issue, see the discussion).

Students' Part-Time Work: Costs and Benefits

Analyses of adolescent time-use trends indicate that part-time work is in many countries competing with school-related activities, sleep, and leisure. There is anecdotal evidence that teens in Canada occasionally skip classes to work in fast-food outlets. Parents and educators, obviously, are concerned with the implications of this trend. Analyses of Canadian and Ontario data, collected as part of the 1998 GSS and OATUS, show that most jobs performed by teens are not attractive developmentally. According to OATUS, 35% of Ontario high school students ages 15 years or older, worked in sales and 28% in fast-food outlets and restaurants. Among girls ages 12–14 years older, the most popular job was babysitting (32%) and among boys of the same age, paper routes (26%). Not surprisingly, friends, family, access to time, and leisure rank much higher than work on the list of teens' life priorities. The main attraction of part-time work for the teens seems to be easier access to discretionary money.[5]

The key to the paid-work issue, as in many other areas of time use, is an ability to maintain balance. Both abstention from part-time work and excessive amounts of it carry negative emotional implications. According to the 1998 GSS, teens who did not work at all or worked more than 7

Table 14-2

RELATIONSHIP BETWEEN AMOUNT OF FREE TIME, LENGTH OF VACATION, LIFE SATISFACTION, FEELING OF HAPPINESS, AND STRESS
(GSS, 1998; CORRELATIONS AND MEAN SCORES)

	LIFE SATISFACTION (1-5) PEARSON r	HAPPINESS (1-5) PEARSON r
Amount of free time: all days	−.01	−.02
Length of paid vacation	.05	.04
	Mean Scores	Mean Scores
Amount of free time: weekdays		
Fewer than 2 hours	3.24	3.34
2–4 hours	3.29	3.35
4 hours or more	3.22	3.32
Total	3.24	3.33
Amount of free time: Sundays		
Fewer than 3 hours	3.10	3.21
3–7 hours	3.31	3.39
7 hours or more	3.17	3.28
Total	3.23	3.32

Note. Correlations calculated for employed population only.
Means calculated for population ages 25–64 years.

---

hours per week felt less happy, less satisfied with their life, and more stressed than students who reported moderate levels of paid work (Table 14-3).

Analyses of OATUS data produce similar findings. Students who worked fewer than 12 hours per week (the mean for this group was 8 hours) obtained higher grades, felt happier, healthier, less depressed, and foresaw a brighter future than adolescents who did not work at all or who worked more than 12 hours per week (Table 14-4).

Research evidence from Canadian population health surveys (Statistics Canada, 1996; not reported in the tables) suggests that teens' longer hours of part-time work correlate with higher levels of alcohol consumption and smoking. In view of the fact that most part-time jobs available to the youth are not particularly challenging, parents, educators, and policy makers should direct their attention toward the length of teens' working hours. The fact that Ontario students ages 17–19 years report, on average, over 15 hours of paid work per week, certainly, reflects an off-balance situation (OATUS).

---

[5]Correlation between estimated weekly hours of adolescents' paid work and satisfaction with finances was, according to GSS 1998, positive ($r = .12$). No such association was found with life satisfaction or satisfaction with the use of time.

Table 14-3

HOW DOES TEENS' PART-TIME WORK AFFECT THEIR EMOTIONAL WELL-BEING? (GSS 1998; MEAN SCORES)

PART-TIME WORK (HOURS PER WEEK)	SATISFIED WITH LIFE	FEELING HAPPY	FEELING STRESSED
1 hour or less	3.3	3.3	3.5
2 to 6 hours	3.8	3.6	3.3
7 hours or more	3.4	3.4	3.6
Total	3.3	3.4	3.5

Table 14-4

RELATIONSHIP BETWEEN TEENS' WEEKLY HOURS OF PAID WORK, ACADEMIC PERFORMANCE, EMOTIONAL WELL-BEING, AND HEALTH (OATUS; MEAN SCORES)

PAID WORK (HOURS PER WEEK)	GRADE AVERAGE	EXPECTATION OF BRIGHT FUTURE	EMOTIONAL PROBLEMS (COMPOSITE OF LONELY, DEPRESSED, UNHAPPY)	SELF-ASSESSED HEALTH
No work reported	71	4.0	5.9	3.7
1 to 12 hours	75	4.2	6.0	3.9
12 hours or more	73	4.0	6.7	3.6
Total	73	4.1	6.2	3.8

Is There a Homework Threshold?

Although concerns with students' homework have been voiced primarily in North America, the workloads of U.S. and Canadian high school students do not appear excessively heavy. In 2003, U.S. students reported 56 minutes of homework on school days, and the Canadian figure in 2005 (GSS Cycle 19) was 70 minutes, which is about the same or less than in most other countries. Although these data suggest that U.S. and Canadian students are not overburdened with homework, the "homework problem" continues to worry parents and educators. Teens' high levels of reported time pressure, obesity, and growing frequency of emotional and behavioral problems draw public attention, but is homework to blame?

GSS and OATUS data show that longer hours of homework take time away from virtually all daily activities, but most time is taken away from watching television, computer and video games, socializing with friends, and sports. The losses are thus mainly among less structured and arguably developmentally less-beneficial activities (with the exception of physically active leisure).

According to OATUS data (not reported in the tables), heavier homework loads are associated with less boredom, brighter perceptions of teens' future, less smoking, and fewer bodily aches, yet

Table 14-5

DOES THE AMOUNT OF TIME SPENT DOING HOMEWORK AFFECT TEENS' ACADEMIC PERFORMANCE AND THEIR EMOTIONAL WELL-BEING?
(OATUS; MEAN SCORES)

ACTIVITIES (MINUTES PER DAY)	GRADE AVERAGE (OUT OF 100)	EMOTIONAL PROBLEMS (RANGE 2–15)
Homework on school days		
Less than 30 minutes	71.0	6.41
30–60 minutes	74.9	6.06
61–120 minutes	75.3	6.23
121 minutes or more	77.2	6.41
Homework on Sundays		
None reported	70.8	6.37
1–60 minutes	73.8	5.65
61–180 minutes	77.6	6.28
181 minutes or more	80.5	6.88

Note. Emotional problems computed as a sum of feeling lonely, depressed, and unhappy ($\alpha = .76$)

---

they also correlate with considerably higher levels of anxiety (composite of feeling worried, upset, and tense), and lower levels of affect (feeling good, happy, and cheerful).[6] It thus appears that positive correlates of homework (good academic performance) are not matched by teens' subjective feelings. In short, homework may be developmentally useful but is perceived by adolescents as stressful and emotionally unattractive.

The picture gets more nuanced, however, when we examine the effects of different amounts of homework. Table 14-5 shows that an extra 30 minutes of homework on school days or an extra hour on Sundays can beef up students' grade average by 3% to 4%. The effects of additional homework time on emotional well-being are more complex. Allocating more time to homework—up to a point—contributes to fewer emotional problems (feeling lonely, depressed, unhappy), but over 2 hours of homework on weekdays or over 3 hours on Sundays turns the clock around, and teens begin to feel more troubled, which brings us back to the issue of balance.

Time With Friends and Parents: Two Poles Apart?

Developmental psychologists agree that play, talk, and interaction with family members and friends "may be among the most important contexts of learning" (Larson & Verma, 1999, p. 702). As teens grow older, peers begin to play a more prominent role in their lives, while the influence of the family diminishes (Zani, 1993). According to the 1998 GSS data, 30% of adolescents ages

---

[6]Alphas for the composite scales of both anxiety and affect were .83.

Table 14-6

EFFECTS OF SOCIALIZING WITH PEERS ON ADOLESCENTS' ACADEMIC PERFORMANCE, EMOTIONAL WELL-BEING, AND HEALTH (OATUS; MEAN SCORES)

	GRADE AVERAGE PEARSON r*	EXPECTATION OF BRIGHT FUTURE PEARSON r*	FEELING HAPPY PEARSON r*	SELF-ASSESSED HEALTH PEARSON r*
School day socializing with friends	−.21	−.07	0.06	ns
Sunday socializing with friends	−.06	−.07	ns	ns
	Mean Score	Mean Score	Mean Score	Mean Score
School day socializing with friends				
None reported	76.1	4.12	3.90	3.60
1 hour or less	76.2	4.21	4.11	3.83
More than 1 hour	72.8	3.99	4.10	3.60
Sunday socializing with friends				
None reported	73.4	4.14	3.87	3.63
1–2 hours	77.2	4.23	4.09	3.81
2–6 hours	75.9	4.20	4.11	3.72
6 hours or more	72.5	3.86	3.84	3.60

15 to 19 years did not report any contact with parents on school days, and 40% did not do so on weekends.[7] Personal contact with parents, reported by the teens in the OATUS as the main activity (talking, reading, playing with parents), occupied very little after-school time on school days (around 20 minutes) and, surprisingly, even less on Sundays (15 minutes). Socializing with friends, on the other hand, amounted to 70 minutes on school days and close to 80 minutes on Sundays.

According to OATUS, parents' opinions count more than peers' when teens make important decisions, but interacting with parents is almost entirely missing from the list of teens' favorite daily activities (4% of first and second choices). Interacting with friends, on the other hand, is at the top of the list, with 54% of adolescents listing it as their favorite way of spending time (OATUS).

Analyses of OATUS data show that, similar to free time, long hours of socializing or hanging around with friends on school days and Sundays are associated with poorer academic performance and negative rather than positive emotional and health outcomes (Table 14-6). Interestingly, however, the same is true of teens that do not socialize with friends and peers at all. They also report poorer grades, have lower expectations of the future, and feel less happy and healthy than students with a moderate amount of peer contacts.

---

[7]Time diaries usually underestimate the amount of contact with parents because short encounters or brief verbal exchanges are often overlooked when reconstructing the sequence of daily activities.

Table 14-7

EFFECTS OF TEENS' SOCIALIZING WITH PEERS AND PARENTS ON THEIR EMOTIONAL WELL-BEING (GSS 1998; MEAN SCORES)

	Satisfied With Life	*Feeling Happy*
Socializing with friends: weekdays		
No socializing reported	3.3	3.3
10–60 minutes	3.7	3.6
61–180 minutes	3.3	3.4
181 minutes or more	3.0	3.3
Socializing with friends: weekends		
No socializing reported	3.4	3.4
10–180 minutes	3.3	3.3
181 minutes or more	3.5	3.4
Contact with parents: weekends		
No contact reported	3.3	3.3
10–150 minutes	3.6	3.5
151 minutes or more	3.3	3.4

If one were to draw a recommendation from the data reported in Table 14-6, one would have to say that around 1 hour of socializing with friends on school days and 1 to 6 hours on Sundays is about right, while doing things alone or being with friends for too long does not pay off.

Analyzing the GSS data about the well-being effects of teens' school-day socializing with friends produces results similar to OATUS (Table 14-7). Teens spending, on school days, 1 hour or less with friends are emotionally better off than students reporting no contact at all or more than an hour of contact. Interestingly, the negative effects of longer hours of socializing with friends disappear on Sundays.

In *Being Adolescent,* Csikszentmihalyi and Larson (1984) make a poignant observation:

> In all societies since the beginning of time, adolescents have learned to become adults by observing, imitating, and interacting with grown-ups around them. It is therefore startling how little time these teenagers [in the U.S.] spend in the company of adults. (p. 73)

The reasons for the decline of contacts between adolescents and parents are manifold. Parents' busy lifestyles are often quoted as an explanation, but the deepening of the communication gap between adolescents and parents has sociocultural reasons as well, with teens trying to achieve greater independence earlier, often with the encouragement of mass media and business interests, who consider youth an important and burgeoning market. GSS data indicate that teens are comfortable with only so much contact time with parents. On weekends, 1 or 1 1/2 hours of contact time made them happy, but beyond that, their levels of life satisfaction and happiness dropped (see Table 14-7).

Table 14-8

HOW DOES SLEEP CORRELATE WITH ADOLESCENTS' EMOTIONAL WELL-BEING? (GSS 1998; MEAN SCORES)

DURATION OF SLEEP ON SCHOOL DAYS	SATISFIED WITH LIFE (1–4)	SATISFIED WITH TIME USE (1–4)	SELF-ASSESSED HEALTH (1–5)	FEELING OF TIME PRESSURE (1–27)	PERCEIVED STRESS (1–5)
7.5 hours or less	3.36	3.20	3.66	13.7	3.82
7.5–8 hours	3.40	3.54	3.82	13.1	3.41
More than 8 hours	3.34	3.20	3.80	11.9	3.27
Total	3.36	3.25	3.76	12.7	3.47

As in other areas of life, teens' relationships with parents and peers should be kept in balance. One has to agree with Larson (1983) that,

> the functional constraints of family interactions and the generative excitement of friends, both have their roles to play in development. The most fortunate adolescents are those who find ways to benefit from the constraints and potentials of both. (p. 748)

How Long Will Thou Sleep?

Concerns about the potential ill-effects of adolescents' short sleep during the school week have been voiced for quite some time (Carscadon, 1990; National Sleep Foundation, 2000; Tynjala, 1999). Educators, physicians, and researchers are alarmed by teens' short hours of sleep. According to Mercer, Meritt, and Cowell (1998),

> While the biological need for sleep is increasing, psychosocial pressures of homework, sports, jobs, and social activities, and decreases in parental control over bedtime combine to reduce the amount of time adolescents spend sleeping. (p. 259)

Health specialists believe that adolescents need around 9 hours of sleep to remain healthy and function effectively (Carscadon, 1990), yet in most countries teens sleep much less, particularly on school days. According to the 1998 GSS, 45% of Canadian students slept fewer than 8 hours on school days. The OATUS findings are even more worrisome. In 2003, by 11:30 p.m., over 26% of Ontario adolescents were still not in bed, and 14% went to bed after midnight. Two-thirds of the 15- to 19-year-olds slept less than 8 hours on school days, and, of these, almost half slept fewer than 7 hours. The most important factors contributing to shorter sleep are, according to OATUS, surfing the Internet, having a computer in the bedroom, and playing computer and video games.[8]

Sleep deprivation may be, according to researchers, at the root of poorer school performance, negative moods, increased risk of accidents due to fatigue, and increased likelihood of stimulant use (Wolfson & Carscadon, 1998). GSS data show that in 1998, almost 30% of Canadian adolescents reported having sleeping problems. Students who slept on school days fewer than 7.5 hours (over one-third of the GSS sample) experienced above average levels of time pressure and stress and reported below average levels of health (Table 14-8). This is not unexpected. More surprising is that longer hours of sleep (8 hours of more) did not raise teens' levels of life satisfaction or their satisfaction with time use.

---

[8]The respective bivariate correlations are .18, .14, and .09.

Table 14-9

ADOLESCENTS' SLEEP: EMOTIONAL AND HEALTH CORRELATES (OATUS; MEAN SCORES)

	GRADE AVERAGE	EXPECTATION OF BRIGHT FUTURE	FEELING TIRED ON WAY TO SCHOOL	FEELING HAPPY	FEELING DEPRESSED
7.5 hours or less	75.1	4.12	4.24	3.95	2.39
7.5–8.5 hours	75.4	4.13	3.90	4.08	2.06
8.5–9 hours	74.2	4.01	3.84	4.10	2.01
9 hours or more	72.7	4.03	3.65	4.07	2.00
Total	74.8	4.09	3.97	4.04	2.15

It is, of course, possible that students are (subconsciously?) aware of some of the negative implications of the proverbial wisdom "How long will thou sleep, O sluggard?"[9]

OATUS findings reported in Table 14-9 suggest that more than 8.5 hours of sleep on school days result in poorer grades and lowers expectations of a bright future. Yet having a long sleep makes teens less fatigued on the way to school, less depressed, and perhaps even happier. In short, good sleep delivers good moods but not necessarily good grades. This is not big news, but there is no simple answer to this conundrum either.

Balancing recommended sleep requirements with good academic performance and teens' leisure interests (e.g., mass media, socializing, Internet) is a tricky task. Adolescents are trying to compensate for the shortage of sleep on school days by longer hours of sleep on weekends. On Sundays, 35% of Ontario teens stay in bed until after 10:00 a.m. and 6% past midday (OATUS). However, this "compensation," according to experts, does not provide them with much-needed developmental and health balance (Dahl & Carscadon, 1995, pp. 354–359).[10] Sleep is an important as well as a fragile part of life balance. Balancing health and well-being concerns with the requirements of a successful academic or professional career is one of the great challenges of modern times. The sleep equilibrium of adults and teens is threatened by the sped-up rhythms of modern life and competitive demands of globalized economies that may require new personal time-management strategies as well as social interventions.

DISCUSSION AND CONCLUSION

Time balance, as already said, is in essence a time-use configuration that optimizes positive developmental and emotional outcomes. Several points can be made based about it on the analyses reported in this chapter: (1) greater access to free time is not synonymous with optimal time-use configuration, (2) time balance is not a universal, one-size-fits-all state but is variable and situation specific, (3) comprehension of time balance is not well served by linear or exponential thinking, (4) achievement of time balance is a personal as well as a social matter.

---

[9]Proverbs 24:33.

[10]According to Dahl and Carscadon (1995) irregular sleep schedules, including significant discrepancies between weekdays and weekends, contribute to trouble falling asleep and poor quality of sleep.

Balance Against Excess

Analyses of GSS and OATSUS data show that access to greater amounts of free or enjoyable time does not always go hand in hand with higher levels of emotional well-being and health. Although free time activities, socializing with friends, and watching television are invariably listed by respondents among their most enjoyed daily activities,[11] a cumulative exposure to greater amounts of free time or mass media seems to carry negative rather than positive emotional outcomes. Based on findings that over one-third of all free time in modern societies is spent watching television and most people enjoy it, some authors concluded that "people who spend a lot of time watching TV derive much happiness from it" (Eysenck, 1990). A closer look at time use data shows, however, that this conclusion is wrong.

A sum of enjoyable episodes does not make a person happy or satisfied with life. People who report a lot of free time or TV viewing are not necessarily a happy lot. In Canada, correlations between the amounts of reported free time, time spent watching TV, and feelings of happiness were negative in GSS 1986, 1998, and 2005.[12]

Analyses of OATUS data also show that students who hang around with friends a lot may be emotionally more troubled than teens reporting moderate amounts of contact with peers. Excessive amounts of overstructured and unstructured activities contribute to stress and emotional discomfort alike. In other words, too much of a good thing does not necessarily result in a positive outcome. Human happiness and life satisfaction hinge on equilibriums of work and nonwork, committed and discretionary time, and structured and unstructured activities rather than on excessive amounts of any one of them.

Balance as a Match

An important condition for achieving time balance is tailoring time use to specific circumstances and the needs or expectations of a particular population. In discussing the notion of the golden mean, Aristotle defined *equilibrium* as the right feeling at the right time, about the right things, about right people, for the right end, and in the right way.[13] Much of what Aristotle said applies to lifestyle and time balance. *Time balance*, defined as a configuration of time use that maximizes positive emotional and developmental outcomes, differs for an employed father, a student, a retired person, on a weekday, and on a Sunday. The answer to the question of how much work or free time constitutes a balance differs depending on an array of normative, situational, demographic, and psychological factors. It takes much more free time to turn teens apprehensive on Sunday than on school days. Additional analyses (not reported in this chapter) show that optimal configurations of time use vary for men and women, different life-cycle and occupational groups, as well as different historical periods or cultures.

Data reported in Table 14-2 show that the form of time use rather than the amounts of time may determine well-being outcomes. According to Canadian GSS and U.S. time-use surveys, greater access to free time during the workweek does not make people more satisfied with life, but longer paid vacations do. People clearly prefer "bunched" forms of leisure to "intermittent" ones.[14] In sum, desirable emotional and developmental outcomes are predicated on commensurate rather than inflexible time-use arrangements.

In Favor of a Nonlinear Approach

A sense of balance and feelings of happiness are contextual. The equations on which they stand are formed in part by objective conditions of life and in part by personal and social expectations.

---

[11]In GSS 1998, 62% of respondents listed free time as their most enjoyed activity. Social leisure and physically active leisure were both listed by 12% of respondents and watching television and videos by 11%.

Social expectations of what is fair or acceptable, as far as work or leisure are concerned, change in time. This being said, in a given period of time and for a given population, one can usually define the dividing line between extremes and find a sound configuration of time use. We will probably never find the ultimate key to human happiness, but we may provide a useful operational hint on how much of what is too much and what direction to take to reach a more balanced lifestyle.

Achievement of lifestyle balance or time balance is often hindered by linear or more-of-the-same thinking. Unfortunately, we seem to be cursed with such thinking. Investing more money in leisure infrastructures improves the quality of human life—does it not? Opening the doors to cultural events free of charge (as attempted in the Netherlands in the 1980s) brings more people to art events—does it not? Reducing hours of paid work and house chores will direct human curiosity and energy to challenging activities—and so it goes on. When one magical solution turns stale, we begin to look for another. Like the alchemists of the middle ages, we search for a magic and invigorating elixir of life rather than for the right mixture or balance of things that are handy and within our reach.

We seem to ignore the fact that there is a middle ground between the Protestant work ethic and hedonism, between instrumental and expressive activities, between being a TV addict or a bookworm, a hermit or a social butterfly, or extrinsically or intrinsically motivated. The question is: why do we extol the virtues of the extremes? After all, is not the middle ground, as suggested by Crusoe's father, the most rewarding and most helpful way to a "life of ease and pleasure"?

Lifestyle Balance in Social Context

One serious concern facing modern societies is the accelerated rhythms of daily life that are putting considerable pressure on human well-being and health. Most commentators agree that we live in an era marked by rising levels of time pressure and psychological stress (Robinson & Godbey, 1997; Schor, 1991). Numerous polls conducted in the United States and other industrialized nations indicate that people experienced higher levels of time pressure in the 1980s and 1990s than they did in previous decades.

According to Robinson (1993), more people in the United States reported that they were "always rushed" in 1985 than in 1975 or 1965. Bondl, Galinsky, and Swanberg (1997) wrote that the proportion of Americans who felt that they "never had enough time" to get everything done on the job rose from 40% in 1977 to 60% in 1997. Canadian GSS data show that, in 1992, 47% of Canadians felt more rushed than they did "5 years ago," while in 1998 this figure rose to 50% (Zuzanek, 2000). These trends affect the adult as well as adolescent populations. In 1992, 62% of Canadian adolescents ages 15 to 19 years, attending school and living with parents, reported feeling rushed every day or a few times a week. By 1998, this figure had climbed to 68%, that is, a higher proportion than for the adult population (Zuzanek, 2005).

Analyses of OATUS data (not reported in the tables) show that people feel better when the time is flying fast than when it is creeping slowly. According to OATUS, the correlation between the perception of how fast time is passing and affect (composite of how happy, good, and cheerful the respondent felt; $\alpha = .83$) was positive, $r = .17$. Higher levels of time pressure are, on the other hand, associated with negative emotional outcomes. The correlation between feeling pressed for time and affect was negative, $r = -.29$. The critical difference between positive emotional correlates of time passage and negative correlates of time pressure rests with the respondents' control of the situation. Fast passage of time is associated with being in control of the situation, while feelings

---

[12]In 1986, the correlation between TV viewing and feeling happy was −.06; in 1998 it was −.02, and in 2005 −.06. Correlations between the amount of free time and feeling happy ranged from −.06 to −.01.

[13]Aristotle's observation is paraphrased from *Nicomachean Ethics*, edited by H. Rackham; Book 2, 1106b.

[14]According to the 1975 U.S. time-use survey, correlation between diary hours of free time and life satisfaction was negative ($r = -.22$), but between life satisfaction and the length of paid vacation it was positive ($r = .21$).

of time pressure occur when such control is missing.[15] In a way, people do not like to stand still, but they do not like to be pushed to run either. Balancing time requires first and foremost being in control of the situation. This task is however often hampered by the prevailing and socially sanctioned patterns of time use that confront us.

Contract arrangements limiting annual number of working hours, yet allowing employers to lay workers off when market demand slows take control over time out of employees' and their families' hands. The same is true of the late and night-shift work that proliferated with the move toward a 24-hour society. A fluid labor market, frequently changing job requirements, interrupted career trajectories, technological innovations, compression of simultaneous activities into single time slots, the use of electronic media and mobile phones, frequent interruptions of television programs by commercials—all require constant change of attention and a fast reaction. Under these conditions, aiming at lifestyle balance or opting for a slower rhythm of life cannot succeed without structural societal changes.

We hope that greater acceptance of flexible working hours, longer paid and unpaid leaves, later start times at some schools, social movements such as Slow Cities in Italy (for more detail see Honoré, 2004), or the fact that the percentage of Canadian teens who planned to slow down increased between 1992 and 1998 from 11% to 22% (Zuzanek, 2000) foreshadow policy shifts and value changes that will help redress negative emotional, social, and health effects of time pressure and will create conditions more favorable for lifestyle balance.

REFERENCES

Argyle, M. (1987). *The psychology of happiness*. New York: Routledge.

Bennett, S., & Kalish, N. (2006). *The case against homework: How homework is hurting our children*. New York: Crown.

Bondl, J. T., Galinsky, E., & Swanberg, J. E. (1997). *The 1997 national study of the changing workforce*. New York: Families and Work Institute.

Campbell, A., Converse, P. E., & Rodgers, W. L. (1976). *The quality of American life: Perceptions, evaluations, and satisfactions*. New York: Russell Sage Foundation.

Carscadon, M. A. (1990). Patterns of sleep and sleepiness in adolescents. *Pediatrician 17*, 5–12.

Clausen, J. (1991). Adolescent competence and the shaping of the life course. *American Journal of Sociology, 96*, 805–842.

Csikszentmihalyi, M., & Larson, R. (1984). *Being adolescent: Conflict and growth in the teenage years*. New York: Basic Books.

Csikszentmihalyi, M., & Larson, R. (1987). Validity and reliability of the experience sampling method. *Journal of Nervous and Mental Disease, 175*, 526–537.

Dahl, R. E., & Carscadon, M. A. (1995). Sleep and its disorders in adolescence. In R. Ferber & M. Kryger (Eds.), *Principles and practices of sleep medicine in the child* (pp. 354–359). Philadelphia: W. B. Saunders.

Dumazedier, J. (1962). *Vers une civilisation du loisir?* Paris: Editions du Soleil.

Eysenck, M. W. (1990). *Happiness: Facts and myths*. East Sussex: Lawrence Erlbaum.

Fourastie, J. (1965). *Les 40,000 Heures*. Paris: Editions Gonthier.

Greenberger, E., & Steinberg, L. D. (1986). *When teenagers work: The psychological and social costs of teenage employment*. New York: Basic Books.

Honoré, C. (2004). *In praise of slow*. Toronto: Alfred A. Knopf.

Jordan, A. B., & Robinson, T. (2008). Children, television viewing, and weight status: Summary and recommendations from an expert panel meeting. *Annals of the American Academy of Political and Social Science, 616*, 119–132.

Katz, E., & Gurevitch, M. (1976). *The secularisation of leisure: Culture and communication in Israel*. Cambridge, MA: Harvard University Press.

Kralovec, E., & Buell, J. (2000). *The end of homework: How homework disrupts families, overburdens children, and limits learning*. Boston: Beacon Press.

Kubey, R. W. & Csikszentmihalyi, M. (1990). *Television and the quality of life: How viewing shapes everyday experience*. Mahwah, NJ: Lawrence Erlbaum.

---

[15]Analyses of OATUS and National Population Health Survey (Statistics Canada, 1996) data (not reported in the tables) show that respondents who worked long hours and felt in control of the situation experienced less time pressure and stress than respondents who worked shorter hours but lacked control (Zuzanek, 2004).

Larson, R. W. (1983, November). Adolescents' daily experience with family and friends: Contrasting opportunity systems. *Journal of Marriage and Family, 45,* 739–750.

Larson, R. W., & Verma, S. (1999). How children and adolescents spend time across the world: Work, play, and developmental opportunities. *Psychological Bulletin, 125,* 701–736.

Linder, S. B. (1971). *The harried leisure class.* New York: Columbia University Press.

Mercer, P. A., Meritt, S. L., & Cowell, J. M. (1998). Differences in reported sleep need among adolescents. *Journal of Adolescent Health, 23,* 259–263.

Mortimer, J. T., Harley, C., & Aronson, P. (1999). How do prior experiences in the workplace set the stage for the transition to adulthood? In A. Booth, A. C. Crouter, & M. S. Shanahan (Eds.), *Transitions to adulthood in a changing economy* (pp. 131–159). Westport, CT: Praeger.

National Sleep Foundation. (2000). *Adolescent sleep needs and patterns: Research report and resource guide.* Washington, DC: Author.

Neuman, S. B. (1988). The displacement effect: Assessing the relation between television viewing and reading performance. *Reading Research Quarterly, 23,* 414–440.

Phillips, S., & Sandstrom, K. L. (1990). Parental attitudes toward youth work. *Youth and Society, 22,* 160–183.

Riley, J., Cantwell, R., & Ruttiger, K. (1949). Some observations on the social effects of television. *Public Opinion Quarterly, 13,* 223–224.

Robinson, J. P. (1972). Towards defining the functions of television. In E. Rubinstein, G. Comstock, & J. Murray (Eds.), *Television and social behavior: Vol. 4. Television in day-to-day life: Patterns of use.* Washington, DC: U.S. Government Printing Office.

Robinson, J. P. (1977). *How Americans use time. A social–psychological analysis of everyday behavior.* New York: Praeger.

Robinson, J. P. (1993). The time squeeze. *American Demographics, 12,* 12–13.

Robinson, J., & Converse, P. (1972). Social change reflected in the use of time. In A. Campbell & P. Converse (Eds.), *The human meaning of social change.* New York: Russell Sage Foundation.

Robinson, J. P., & Godbey, G. (1997). *Time for life: The surprising ways Americans use their time.* University Park, PA: Pennsylvania State University Press.

Schor, J. B. (1991). *The overworked American: The unexpected decline of leisure.* New York: Basic Books.

Statistics Canada. (1996). National Population Health Survey. Retrieved on February 11, 2003, from http://www.statcan.ca/english/survey/household/health/health.htm

Steinberg, L., & Cauffman, E. (1995). The impact of employment on adolescent development. *Annals of Child Development, 11,* 131–166.

Tynjala, J. (1999). *Sleep habits, perceived sleep quality and tiredness among adolescents.* Jyväskylä, Finland: University of Jyväskylä.

Wilensky, H. L. (1981). *Family life-cycle, work, and the quality of life: Reflections on the roots of happiness, despair, and indifference in modern society.* Berkley: Institute of Industrial Relations.

Wolfson, K. L., & Carscadon, M. A. (1998). Sleep schedules and daytime functioning in adolescents. *Child Development, 69,* 875–887.

Zani, B. (1993). Dating and interpersonal relationships in adolescence. In S. Jackson & H. Rodrigues-Tome (Eds.), *Adolescence and its social worlds* (pp. 95–119). Hillsdale, NJ: Lawrence Erlbaum.

Zuzanek, J. (2000). *The effects of time use and time pressure on child–parent relationship.* Waterloo, Onatario: Otium Publications.

Zuzanek, J. (2004).Work, leisure, time pressure, and stress. In J. T. Haworth & A. J. Veal (Eds.), *Work and leisure* (pp. 123–144). New York: Routledge.

Zuzanek, J. (2005). Adolescent time use and well-being from a comparative perspective. *Loisir et Societe [Society and Leisure] 29,* 379–423.

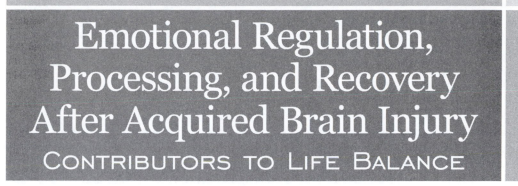

Emotional Regulation, Processing, and Recovery After Acquired Brain Injury
CONTRIBUTORS TO LIFE BALANCE

BEATRIZ C. ABREU, DENNIS ZGALJARDIC, JOAN C. BOROD,
GARY SEALE, RICHARD O. TEMPLE, GLENN V. OSTIR,
AND KENNETH J. OTTENBACHER

INTRODUCTION

Life balance is an elusive term used to describe the personal satisfaction that an individual experiences when his or her obligations, rules, and duties are in harmony. The social sciences literature suggests that life balance is important for healthy living (Christiansen & Matuska, 2006; Drago, 2007). In today's frenetically paced world, life balance is a challenge and a very unique construct when we consider that it represents one's satisfying arrangement of personally meaningful roles and occupational choices. Life-balance conflict is largely seen as connected to the difficulty posed when fulfilling commitments to family, friends, and community in a world in which one feels pressured to work and produce more and more (Bloom & Van Reenen, 2006; Premeaux, Adkins, & Mossholder, 2007). The identification of variables affecting life balance can help us explore lifestyle patterns in health promotion, disease prevention, and social policy (Allan, Loudoun, & Peetz, 2007; Bryson, Warner-Smith, Brown, & Fray, 2007; Christiansen & Matuska, 2006). Life balance describes a subjective human condition shaped by ethical, political, economic, and psychological perspectives.

In this chapter, we will portray life balance as an emotional cultural judgment in individuals with and without acquired brain injury (ABI). Quality-of-life assessments are important to enhance understanding of the benefits of health promotion and rehabilitation. We will suggest that the emotional regulation and emotional processing deficits frequent in persons with ABI might affect subjective and objective well-being and life-balance appraisals.

ACQUIRED BRAIN INJURY (ABI)

ABI includes the diagnoses of traumatic brain injury and stroke. In the brain injury literature, quality of life is associated with positive emotion (Ergh, Hanks, Rapport, & Coleman, 2003; Gordon et al., 2006), but frequently ABI is characterized by an inability to regulate positive and negative emotions (Bay, Hagerty, Williams, & Kirsch, 2005; Wilz, 2007). This lack of emotional regulation influences individual coping and adaptation strategies after trauma as well as their

K. Matuska & C. Christiansen (Eds.)
Life balance: Multidisciplinary theories and research (pp 223–240)
© 2009 SLACK Incorporated and AOTA Press

well-being and quality-of-life appraisals (Finset & Andersson, 2000; Schultz, 2007). In general, rehabilitation researchers have studied negative consequences after brain injury, such as anxiety and depression (Cicerone et al., 2005; Gordon et al., 2006). Published narratives of individuals with ABI provide a window into clients' struggles to meet goals that contribute to well-being and life balance. The narratives of clients, families, and caretakers generally reveal a conspicuous negative portrait of life balance (Jongbloed, 1994; Krefting, 1989). Frequently, individuals are unable to attain a sense of belonging and a high quality of life due to multiple factors, including loss of relationships, friendships, and spouses (Djikers, 2004). Indeed, there is overwhelming evidence that ABI can produce numerous losses.

Significantly less attention has been paid to the perceived positive consequences after brain injury, such as making sense of one's losses and the growth of positive emotions from coping with that loss. Some investigations have reported that clients awaken at a deep level that sustains them in a positive manner even when they appear to struggle with personal roles and occupational choices (Faircloth, Boylstein, Rittman, Young, & Gubrium, 2004; Gillen, 2005; McColl et al., 2000).

Life-balance conflicts between home and work in people with and without ABI can exhibit different adaptation issues.

LIFE BALANCE

Several studies that assess life balance have placed a focus on the association between home and work (Loretto et al., 2005; Steptoe, Cropley, & Joekes, 1999). In particular, some studies report that personal dissatisfaction can be created as a function of the time spent engaged in activities at work versus in the home or by the intensity of work versus the intensity of conflicts in the home (Sverko, Arambasiic, & Galesic, 2002). Voydanoff (2005) suggests that work–life harmony involves a cognitive (subjective) appraisal of the balance between demands and resources. He posited that when demands exceed resources, one could experience strain, stress, or even physical illness. On the other hand, when resources meet or exceed demands, a positive state of mental and physical health may follow. Some believe that life balance will be experienced when work and family resources, such as skills, aptitudes, coping strategies, time, and energy, are sufficient to meet demands and when participation is effective in both domains (Sverko et al., 2002). In addition, it is important to note that demographics and sociocultural factors such as age, gender, ethnicity, marital status, and disability influence work–life balance (MacDonald, Phipps, & Lethbridge, 2005).

The meaning of work changes after brain injury. Some individuals with ABI no longer experience work as the primary event in life, and the social dimension becomes much more important (Johansson & Tham, 2006). Many individuals can achieve life balance without reentering the workforce. Therefore, instead of examining the relationship between work and family life following brain injury or the opportunities for work after community reintegration, our team has chosen to examine the social and neuropsychological underpinnings of emotion and how they may contribute to the understanding of life balance after brain injury.

Life balance has been viewed from a time-use perspective by determining the percentages of a 24-hour day spent in various categories of occupations and the level of intensity of each activity (Christiansen, 1996). Although occupational scientists suggest that structured and balanced daily activities may result in improved well-being, researchers have been unable to support this assumption (Leufstadius, Erlandsson, & Eklund, 2006). Life balance can also be appraised from the emotional regulation perspective by analyzing the manner in which a person processes and experiences positive and negative emotions. The exploration of emotional regulation deficits following ABI is critical for a better understanding of objective and subjective well-being and life balance appraisals.

In the following section, we will review emotional processing deficits following brain insult.

EMOTIONAL PROCESSING DEFICITS AND ABI

Emotional disturbance is common following ABI. Individuals with ABI typically report symptoms related to depression and anxiety, although increases in levels of aggression, agitation, and apathy are also common (for a review, see Prigatano, 1992). With time, pathological levels of emotionality can diminish; however, residual symptoms could persist (Lippert-Grüner, Kuchta, Hellmich, & Klug, 2006). These disturbances in emotion can either occur secondary to one's reaction to a brain injury (i.e., exogenous) or be intrinsic factors that are involuntary (i.e., endogenous). The following section will discuss the latter as it pertains to deficits in emotional processing in individuals with ABI. More specifically, inter- and intrahemispheric theories of emotional processing will be reviewed, as well as recent findings on the recovery of emotional processing deficits secondary to ABI. Here, we will consider emotions as being distinct from affective traits or moods (Alpert & Rosen, 1990; Borod, 1993; Rosenberg, 1998; Ross, 1985).

From a neuropsychological perspective, the term *emotion* is defined as an individual's reactions to appropriately evocative stimuli that include appraisal, expression, experience, arousal, and goal-directed activity (Plutchik, 1984). By *emotional processing,* we refer to the ability to perceive, express, or experience emotions (e.g., happiness, sadness) across multiple channels of communication involving the face, *prosody* (i.e., vocal intonation), gesture, and speech content (Borod, 1992). Traditionally, the literature has placed emotional processing within subcortical regions of the brain, such as the limbic system (e.g., MacLean, 1958; Papez, 1937); however, more contemporary work suggests that the grey matter of the brain (i.e., neocortex) also maintains a significant role in emotional processing (Adolphs, 2002; Borod, 1992). This is a crucial point to consider, because diffuse cortical and subcortical structures can be damaged following ABI, which may in turn lead to emotional processing deficits and subsequently disrupted life balance.

In conjunction with theories on hemispheric dominance for language, a considerable focus in the emotional processing literature has been placed on hemispheric lateralization for emotion (for reviews, see Borod, 2000; Borod, Bloom, Brickman, Nakhutina, & Curko, 2002; Borod, Zgaljardic, Tabert, & Koff, 2001; Heilman, Blonder, Bowers, & Valanstein, 2003; Rogers, Borod, & Ramig, 2008). Hemispheric lateralization is important to address in this context because ABI does not discriminate. In other words, individuals can sustain left- or right-sided brain injuries. Lesion location (right or left side) is a strong indicator of the type of cognitive, functional, and emotional deficits observed in those who have sustained ABI.

Specific lesion areas may be likewise related to particular dysfunctional strategies that can limit or disrupt an individual's emotional interpretation and reaction to a given environment or situation. Folkman, Lazarus, Gruen, and Delongis (1986) defined *coping* as "the person's cognitive and behavioral efforts to manage (reduce, minimize, master, or tolerate) the internal and external demands of the person–environment transaction that is appraised in taxing or exceeding the resources of the person" (p. 572).

Hence, psychological, cognitive, and behavioral sequelae secondary to ABI can very well lead to difficulty in gauging, monitoring, and self-regulating one's ability to cope with life stressors, which can, in turn, lead to emotional dysregulation.

Finset and Andersson (2000) assessed coping strategy styles in 70 individuals who had sustained ABI (e.g., due to stroke, anoxia, and/or trauma) and in a group of 71 healthy volunteers. In their study, Finset and Andersson (2000) used the COPE (Carver, Scheier, & Weintraub, 1989) to establish participants' coping styles. In addition to the COPE, measures that assess symptoms related to depression and apathy were also administered. Their findings indicated that brain-damaged individuals displayed coping strategies similar to the sample of healthy volunteers; however, patients with brain damage tended to use approach strategies relatively less frequently. With regard to lesion laterality, there was no significant evidence to support an association between coping strategy style and the hemisphere of a brain lesion. Furthermore, brain-damaged individuals with significant levels of apathy were less likely to use an active coping approach style, whereas a more passive/avoidant approach was associated with brain-damaged individuals with significant levels of depressive symptomatology. Significant levels of apathy in participants were associated with right-hemisphere lesions, whereas significant levels of depressed mood were related to left-hemisphere or bilateral lesions. Although these findings do not support a relationship between lesion lateralization and coping strategy per se, they do provide evidence that certain affective states (e.g., apathy, depression) may influence one's approach to the formation of coping strategies and should be considered when studying emotional processing deficits in individuals with ABI. This is crucial because, as mentioned above, changes in affective states are common following brain damage and may potentially influence the profile of deficits related to emotional processing.

Emotion Processing Theories

Investigations using patients with ABI have resulted in the development of several neuropsychological theories regarding hemispheric mechanisms underlying emotional processing (for reviews, see Borod, 1992, 1996; Heilman, Blonder, Bowers, & Crucian, 2000; Mandal et al., 1999). In the following section, we will briefly address two hypotheses pertaining to cerebral lateralization of emotion: (1) the right hemisphere hypothesis and (2) the valence hypothesis.

The right-hemisphere hypothesis maintains that the right cerebral hemisphere is dominant for emotional processing regardless of the *valence* (i.e., the pleasantness level) of the emotion (Borod, 1992; Borod et al., 2002). Support for this hypothesis, on a psychological level, is based on the assumption that processing emotion, in general, entails strategies (e.g., integrative, holistic) and functions (e.g., nonverbal, visuospatial) for which the right hemisphere of the brain is considered to be superior (Borod, 1992). From a neuroanatomical perspective, the cytoarchitecture of the right hemisphere is seen as supporting the strategies and functions associated with emotional processing (Borod, 1992; Borod, Bloom, & Haywood, 1998).

The valence hypothesis, on the other hand, posits two versions and incorporates both hemispheres. In one version, it is proposed that the right cerebral hemisphere is specialized for negative emotions (e.g., sadness) and the left for positive emotions (e.g., happiness), regardless of processing mode (e.g., perception, expression; see for example, Sackeim, Greenberg, Weiman, Hungerbuhler, & Geschwind, 1982; Sato & Aoki, 2006; Silberman & Weingarten, 1986). In a second version of the valence hypothesis (Borod, 1992; Davidson, 1984), it is proposed that differential hemispheric specialization (i.e., left or right) occurs for the expression and experience of emotion as a function of valence but that the right hemisphere is dominant for the perception of emotions of both valences. Moreover, in this version, differential specialization for the expression and experience of emotions occurs within anterior (i.e., motor) regions of the brain, whereas right-hemisphere dominance is specific to posterior (i.e., sensory) regions of the brain (Davidson, 1984).

Although we can only speculate about how differential effects of valence may have evolved, there has been discussion of how particular emotions might have come to be linked with particular behaviors (see Borod, 1992). Because negative emotions are associated with survival (e.g., with removing the organism from danger), a system that is sensitive to multimodal inputs and is able to quickly scan and evaluate the environment would be to the organism's advantage. This ability to quickly evaluate the environment would also be beneficial in tailoring an individual's approach in a given emotionally charged situation or environment. According to Borod (1992), such behaviors seem more compatible with gestalt, synthetic processing (a right-hemisphere approach) than with discrete, focused analysis (a left-hemisphere approach). Positive emotions, by contrast, may be more linguistic and communicative than reactive and potentially more strongly associated with the left hemisphere (Borod, Caron, & Koff, 1981). As regions for language processing are typically located in the dominant (left) hemisphere, the expression and perception of positive emotions may be diminished in those individuals experiencing an aphasia syndrome secondary to ABI.

In compartmentalizing emotional processing theory even further, we must also consider processing modes (mentioned earlier) and communication channels of emotion. Emotional processing modes are likely governed by separate neuroanatomical regions, suggesting intrahemispheric (not interhemispheric) specialization (Borod, 1993). Lesions toward the front of the brain have been shown to have a greater effect on emotional expression, whereas lesions toward the back have a greater impact on emotional perception (e.g., Ross & Monnot, 2007). This notion of emotional processing mode complements the motor (i.e., anterior) and sensory (i.e., posterior) intrahemispheric neuroanatomical layout of the neocortex.

Nonetheless, whether people are in the process of expressing or perceiving emotion, they do so via a single or a combination of communication channels (e.g., facial, prosodic, lexical). For the *facial channel*, the most frequently used behavioral measures in research investigations are visual-field differences in response to tachistoscopic or computerized presentation of facial emotional expressions and hemispace advantages in free-field viewing paradigms. For the *prosodic channel*, the most commonly used measures are ear differences in response to dichotic presentation of emotionally intoned verbal (e.g., speech) or nonverbal (e.g., environmental sounds) stimuli. Similar to the facial channel, measures of the *lexical channel* are visual-field differences to tachistoscopic or computerized presentation of emotionally meaningful verbal materials, most typically words imbued with emotional meaning.

Borod and colleagues (2001) conducted a review of the literature from a 12-year period (1987–1998) assessing emotion laterality in healthy individuals. The studies that were reviewed employed various techniques assessing processing mode (expression and perception) and communication channel (facial, prosodic, and lexical). Right-hemisphere dominance for the perception of emotion, regardless of valence, was found for the facial and prosodic channels but not for the lexical channel. For the lexical channel, greater left-hemisphere involvement than right was discovered. This finding perhaps reflects the language aspect of this channel and, hence, mediation by the left hemisphere. As for emotional expression studies, only the facial channel was examined, as it is the only channel amenable to behavioral lateralization research protocols. For facial expression, the findings revealed left hemiface dominance (i.e., a right hemisphere advantage) for the expression of emotion. Findings from this review of the normal literature were generally similar to those observed by Borod and colleagues (2002) in their review of the literature assessing emotion laterality in individuals with unilateral brain damage. The findings from the Borod and colleagues' review indicated that patients with right-hemisphere brain damage demonstrate specific deficits in the expression and perception of emotion via the facial and prosodic channels compared to patients with left-hemisphere brain damage and healthy volunteers. Further, the perception of emotional materials via the lexical channel was also implicated as being subserved by the right hemisphere. This is in contrast to findings from the review of emotional processing in the healthy adults by Borod and colleagues (2001) suggesting a left-hemisphere advantage for emotional perception via the lexical channel.

Emotional Recovery

The recovery from emotional processing deficits secondary to ABI is a topic that has received very little attention in the literature. On the other hand, an extensive amount of the research investigating functional recovery subsequent to ABI has been conducted on speech and language functions. Research using patients with aphasia (Fazzini, Bachman, & Alpert, 1986; Kertesz, 1993) has shown that most spontaneous recovery occurs within the first 6 months after left-hemisphere stroke onset (Kertesz, 1993). As to the possible neuronal mechanisms, there are both behavioral and brain injury explanations (Fazzini et al., 1986), with some theories proposing a reorganization or substitution of right-hemisphere (Kinsbourne, 1971) or subcortical (Geschwind, 1974) substrates for damaged left-hemisphere ones. Hence, we can hypothesize that a reorganization or substitution of left-hemisphere structures may occur for individuals with unilateral right-hemisphere brain damage who experience emotional processing deficits.

In another interpretation of inter-hemispheric differences with regard to lesion location (Zgaljardic, Borod, & Sliwinski, 2002), impairments subsequent to right-hemisphere damage, such as visuospatial deficits and unilateral neglect, have often been associated with poor functional outcome (Sterzi et al., 1993). Liotti and Tucker (1992) reported that individuals experiencing depression often have left visual-field impairments that are indicative of some type of right-hemisphere dysfunction, perhaps by interfering with right-hemisphere arousal mechanisms. Similarly, previous research has attributed deficits in arousal and attention to functional recovery outcome. Robertson, Ridgeway, Greenfield, and Parr (1997) reported that patients with right-hemisphere damage demonstrated less recovery of motor functions over a 2-year period than did patients with left-hemisphere damage. These differences were attributed to a greater incidence of attentional impairments in the patients with right-brain damage. Nelson, Cicchetto, Satz, Sowa, and Mitrushina (1994) reported that patients with left-brain damage demonstrated mood stabilization 6 months after stroke onset, whereas patients with right brain damage tended to become progressively worse over time, suggesting that additional factors might impede emotional recovery in individuals with right-brain damage.

More recent work has assessed recovery of emotional perception and expression in individuals who experienced unilateral strokes (Nakhutina, Borod, & Zgaljardic, 2006; Zgaljardic et al., 2002). Zgaljardic and colleagues (2002) administered the New York Emotion Battery (NYEB; Borod, Welkowitz, & Obler, 1992) to 23 participants, including 9 with right-brain damage, 7 with left-brain damage, and 7 healthy volunteers. Emotional perception tasks, including non-emotional control, (assessing facial, prosodic, and lexical communication channels) were administered at two separate time points, with a median interval of approximately 2 years. The three subject groups were well matched on demographic, screening, and non-emotional control variables. Individuals with right- or left-brain injury performed significantly worse on the emotional tasks compared to healthy volunteers. For the three communication channels, there was no evidence of recovery of emotional perception in patients with either right- or left-brain damage. However, when sex differences were taken into account, men with right-hemisphere brain damage demonstrated improved performance over time on emotional tasks within the lexical channel (i.e., for both sentence and word identification tasks). Using the same sample of participants, Nakhutina and colleagues (2006) assessed recovery of posed prosodic emotional expression. Posers (study participants who produced the prosodic emotional expressions) were required to produce neutral-content sentences using four different emotional tones (happiness, sadness, anger, and fear). Raters (undergraduate students) were trained to judge poser output for accuracy and intensity and to evaluate the confidence with which they (i.e., the raters) made their accuracy judgments. The findings from this study revealed limited recovery in individuals with left-brain damage and significant declines in performance for individuals with right-brain damage. Inspection of group means suggested that frontal lobe lesions had a particularly negative impact on performance for individuals with right-brain damage. This is not surprising given that emotional expression is thought to be governed by anterior brain regions, especially within the right-hemisphere (Pick, Borod, Ehrlichman, & Bloom, 2003; Wasserman, Borod, & Winnick, 1998).

The next section will highlight positive as well as negative emotion regulation.

POSITIVE AND NEGATIVE EMOTION REGULATION

Positive and negative emotions are distinct from each other, and it is difficult to describe their role under one theoretical framework (Aspinwall, 1998; Isen, 2001). Nearly 60 years ago, the World Health Organization (WHO; 1948) defined *health* as "a state of complete physical, mental, and social well-being and not merely the absence of disease or infirmity." This definition constitutes a positive perspective on human function, but most of the literature in emotional regulation after ABI primarily focuses on negative outcomes. Some researchers suggest that negative emotions have a strong survival value, are more urgent than positive emotions, and can be powerful enough to override positive emotions in case of immediate problems or objective dangers (Seligman, 2005; Seligman & Csikszentmihalyi, 2000). Nevertheless, positive affect expressed by clients and caretakers plays a role in health outcomes. Adams (1996) showed that the use of positive emotions during reframing, adaptation, and growth after ABI does not take away the suffering but makes the tragedy more bearable. Two examples of positive emotional responses are optimism and post-traumatic growth.

Optimism is the tendency to look on and expect the most positive results regarding events and conditions. Optimism can affect the adaptation capacity to adjust and modify behavior readily after trauma and disability (Grote, Bledsoe, Larkin, Lemay, & Brown, 2007). According to Isen and Reeve (2005), optimism depends on a combination of factors, including an individual's goals, judgments, and expectations about situations (Isen, 2000a, 2000b). Interestingly, optimistic individuals use different coping methods than pessimistic individuals (Scheier & Carver, 1992). Optimists used more planning, problem-focused coping, reframing, and acceptance and were at much less risk of developing clinical depression compared with those who were pessimists (Isaacowitz & Seligman, 2001; Scheier, Weintraub, & Carver, 1986). In contrast, pessimists are more likely to use denial and avoidance (Scheier & Carver, 1992). Interestingly, Peterson (2000) suggests that unrealistic optimism can lead to increased personal risk for illness and injury.

The second positive emotional response is *post-traumatic growth*. This growth is viewed as the perception of benefits after trauma, such as improved interpersonal relationships, positive change in the perception of self, and a positive philosophy of life (Tedeschi & Calhoun, 1996, 2004). McGrath and Linley (2006) examined the degree and time course of positive psychological change among persons with ABI. They studied individuals both in the early (i.e., acute) and chronic stages of recovery. The chronic group reported higher levels of anxiety and depression but also higher levels of positive change than the acute group, indicating that it may take time for post-traumatic growth to take place. Post-traumatic growth is not precluded by severe brain injury. Optimism and post-traumatic growth are important constructs that require further investigation (Westphal & Bonanno, 2007).

The relationship between positive emotions and psychological well-being is complex and creates interesting challenges for researchers and clinicians. Researchers continue to explore the differentiation between the cognitive and action components of post-traumatic growth (Pat-Horenczyk & Brom, 2007; Westphal & Bonanno, 2007). Hobfoll and colleagues (2007) found that, within the context of terrorism, post-traumatic growth was related to negative outcomes such as psychological distress and support for radical political attitudes and retaliatory violence.

We believe that to optimize rehabilitation and healthcare outcomes, practitioners need to understand and promote adaptive processes after trauma that facilitate resilient and positive outcomes. This perspective in research and clinical practice is derived from the new discipline, *positive psychology* (Csikszentmihalyi & Csikszentmihalyi, 2006; Eid & Larsen, 2008), which is largely dedicated to expanding theory, practice, and social policy to amplify the individual's strengths rather than repair the weaknesses (Diener & Seligman, 2002; Seligman, 2005; Seligman & Csikszentmihalyi, 2000). We advocate the identification and analysis of both positive and negative emotion regulation in rehabilitation and health care.

Investigations on the physiological connections among life experience, emotion, and health outcomes have also focused on the negative or stress-related factors (Ryff & Singer, 1998). In the next section, we provide an overview of physiological indicators of stress.

Physiological Indicators of Stress

Stress has been defined as an actual or perceived threat to the body's ability to maintain stability or homeostasis (Szanton, Gill, & Allen, 2005). The responses and adaptation to stress supplied by the sympathetic nervous system, the neuroendocrine system, and the immune system have been described as allostatic systems (McEwen & Stellar, 1993; Selye, 1976; Sterling & Eyer, 1981).

The cognitive activation theory of stress postulates that the stress response produces a general activation of increased arousal (Ursin & Ericksen, 2004). This response is essential and presents no threat to health, and it is indeed the process used to adapt to events in daily life. Individuals can have a positive response to stress (e.g., coping), a negative response (e.g., hopelessness), or no response (Ursin & Ericksen, 2004).

Allostatic load refers to the quantification of prolonged or chronic stress and was originally introduced by Sterling and Eyer in 1988. In 1993, McEwen and Stellar proposed the construct as a cumulative measure of physiologic dysregulation. Examining the allostatic load of individuals with ABI may help researchers understand stress and coping during the rehabilitation and community-integration process (McEwen, 2003; Szanton et al., 2005).

The brain interprets experiences as stressful or nonstressful and determines the behavioral and physiological responses to each situation (McEwen, 2007). There are cortical and subcortical structures related to stress. Arousal activity depends on the brainstem reticular activating system but also includes limbic structures and the frontal lobes. The limbic system is a functional arrangement of brain structures associated with memory, learning, motivation, visceral functions, and a wide range of emotional processes. The limbic system regulates personal drive, automatic responses, and hormonal activity; it also has connections to the frontal lobe and other regions of the brain. This widespread network integrates information and mediates physiological, behavioral, and psychological responses (Flannelly, Koenig, Galek, & Ellison, 2007; White et al., 2008). The limbic system includes the amygdala, hippocampus, and hypothalamus, which are structures believed to be involved with helplessness, hopelessness, fear, and pain (LeDoux, 1993; White et al., 2008). These structures interpret and regulate stress. The amygdala has been found to be hyperactive in post-traumatic disorders and depressive illness (McEwen, 2003). The *hypothalamus*, which is a small cluster of nuclei, influences body physiology and sits below the thalamus along the wall of the third ventricle. These structures communicate with neurons all over the body and brain, helping the individual maintain a state of homeostasis by controlling blood pressure, metabolic rate, and body temperature. The *pituitary gland* exists underneath the hypothalamus. Damage in the pituitary gland after brain injury can lead to a hormonal deficiency called *hypopituitarism* (Masel, 2004). This hormonal deficiency may be confused with the sequelae of brain injury; therefore, all patients with ABI should be evaluated for hypopituitarism, which can lead to further complications, such as sleep disorders and post-traumatic hypersomnia, that can affect stress (Masel, 2004). A characteristic of the stress response is the activation of the autonomic nervous system and hypothalamo–pituitary–adrenal axis (HPA). Depression and chronic stress have been associated with HPA and the hypothalamus–pituitary–thyroid axis (HPT; Olff, Güzelcan, de Vries, Assies, & Gersons, 2006; Simeon et al., 2007).

All individuals, including those with ABI, display a variety of neurobiological alterations due to emotional dysregulation that can cause stress and illness. This point further emphasizes the importance of continued study of changes in biomarkers after stress.

Variations of Biomarkers in Stress

Some researchers have attempted to measure allostatic load based on a summary indicator comprising a group of biomarkers that reflect alterations in levels of activity that have been linked to increased disease and stress. Allostatic load measures include, but are not limited to, multiple variables such as saliva, urine, blood cortisol, epinephrine, norepinephrine, dopamine, insulin-like growth factors, metabolic markers, and cardiovascular markers such as systolic and diastolic blood pressure. It is not clear which is the best way to combine the allostatic load markers that predict health risks (Karlamangla, Singer, McEwen, Rowe, & Seeman, 2002). A number of studies have examined the association between cortisol, one of the biomarkers, and three factors: age, gender, and work stressors. Some researchers have supported the opinion that biomarkers of stress can vary with age. Crimmins, Johnston, Hayward, and Seeman (2003) used a sample of over

18,000 U.S. noninstitutionalized people ages 20 years or older to examine age differences in 13 allostatic load markers including cortisol. Their findings showed that all the static loads increased up to about age 60 and then the loads decreased and remained stable through the 70s, 80s, and 90s. They found that the allostatic load noted in all age groups participating in the study indicated either lower stress or increased frailty linked to mortality in this population.

The second association that has been investigated by rehabilitation scientists is gender and cortisol levels. Although there has been some support of the notion that men and women differ in their levels of how they experience and interpret anxiety (Jones & Cale, 1989), researchers have not found clear evidence of gender differences and cortisol levels (Thatcher, Thatcher, & Dorling, 2004). Masi, Rickett, Hawkley, and Cacioppo (2004) examined gender and ethnic differences in overnight urinary cortisol and other biomarkers of stress in a sample of 229 adults in an urban community. They found no gender or ethnic differences in cortisol production. They attributed their findings to the different urine and hormone calculations in their studies. In another study of 12 adult field-hockey players (6 women, 6 men), Thatcher and colleagues (2004) investigated gender differences in hormonal responses to competitive sport stressors. Their findings also did not support the gender differences suggested by previous research. Further investigations are needed to clarify the gender association with cortisol.

The third factor related to cortisol levels is work-related stress. There is some suggestion that there is a link between work-related stress and cortisol. Morning cortisol is believed to be a sensitive indicator of work overload in women. Lundberg and Hellström (2002) investigated the association between workload and morning cortisol in women. They analyzed saliva cortisol collected 15, 30, and 45 minutes after awakening on the morning of a nonworking day in 2,000 full-time workers. They found that women working more than 10 hours overtime per week had significantly higher cortisol levels than women working regular hours. In another study, Wellens and Smith (2006) investigated 84 white-collar workers divided into four groups: those (1) with no stressors, (2) with temporal stressors only, (3) with physical stressors only, and (4) with both temporal and physical stressors. They found that the participants exposed to a combination of stressors had significantly elevated levels of both blood pressure and salivary cortisol levels. Additional research is needed to understand the association of cortisol with age, gender, and work.

Cortisol Levels and Brain Injury

Investigations of biomarkers of stress and depression, as measured by cortisol levels after brain injury, are limited and show conflicting results (Tchiteya, Lecours, Elie, & Lupien, 2003). In 1989, Jackson and Mysiw demonstrated that cortisol levels were lower in people with ABI who did not respond to antidepressants when compared to people who responded well to antidepressants. Bay and colleagues (2002) found that stress created a high level of cortisol but in 2005, they did not support their previous findings. They attributed the lack of support to their measurement protocol. Researchers have found that brain lesions impact cortisol secretion and have attempted to relate cortisol levels to specific brain areas. Wittling and Pfluger (1990) have suggested that regulation of cortical secretion is under primary control of the right-hemisphere. In 2005, Wolf, Fujiwara, Luwinski, Kirschbaum, and Markowitsch found that patients with severe global amnesia had no morning cortisol response when compared with a without brain injury control group. They speculated that the possible underlying mechanism for this lack of cortisol response could be related to hippocampus and prefrontal cortex damage as frequently seen in amnesic patients. Tchiteya and colleagues (2003) showed that frontal lesions produced higher levels of cortisol than posterior ones.

There is growing support for the view that biomarkers such as cortisol are of key importance for explaining behavioral factors and quality-of-life judgments. The understanding of the effect of cortisol levels in brain injury may contribute to the understanding of life balance. Cortisol levels have been related to negative emotions such as stress. However, further studies are needed to understand the possible role of positive emotions with respect to biomarkers and health outcomes.

EMOTION AND HEALTH OUTCOMES

In this section, we will review selected evidence on emotion and health outcomes. Some researchers posit that the overall balance of positive and negative emotions in daily life predict the individual's level of subjective well-being (Csikszentmihalyi & Csikszentmihalyi 2006; Eid & Larsen, 2008; Gross, 2007). Subjective well-being includes a broad collection of constructs that relate to the individual's evaluative judgments of the quality of his or her life (Diener, 2000; Diener, Lucas, & Scollon, 2006; Eid & Larsen, 2008; Fredrickson, 2004, 2006).

Researchers have studied positive affect (PA) and negative affect (NA) and their effect on health outcomes. PA and NA are dispositional personality dimensions. *NA* is indicative of subjective distress and unpleasurable engagement, and PA reflects the extent to which an individual experiences pleasurable engagement with the environment (Crawford & Henry, 2004). NA and PA have been demonstrated to be orthogonal constructs; in other words, being high on one of the constructs does not necessarily indicate that the individual is low on the other. For example, an individual can experience a high level of pleasurable and unpleasurable engagement within the same environment.

One of the most widely used instruments for measuring positive and negative emotion is the Positive and Negative Affect Schedule (PANAS; Crawford & Henry, 2004; Kennedy-Moore, Greenberg, Newman, & Stone, 1992; Murray et al., 2007; Watson, Clark, & Tellegen, 1988). The PANAS has shown excellent reliability in medical rehabilitation (Ostir, Smith, Smith, & Ottenbacher, 2005). The relationships among PA, NA, and health outcomes have been well documented using the PANAS, and in particular, the benefits of high PA have been demonstrated across a number of studies.

Bood, Archer, and Norlander (2004) examined the relationship between PA and quality-of-life appraisals after brain injury. They reported that individuals with a combination of high PA and low NA showed a more psychologically healthy and self-actualizing profile than did individuals with a combination of low PA and high NA, who showed a self-destructive profile. In another study, Man and colleagues (2004), using a Chinese version of the PANAS, demonstrated that PA scores correlated significantly with overall quality of life in material well-being, health, productivity, safety, intimacy, and emotional well-being. In addition, they found that clients tended to have a higher intimacy score during the first 5 years post-injury rather than later in recovery. There is limited information regarding the association of PA and NA and functional outcomes following ABI.

Ostir and colleagues conducted a series of four studies that supported the relationship between PA and functional outcomes as measured by the Center for Epidemiological Studies Depression Scale (CES–D; Fisher, Al Snih, Ostir, & Goodwin, 2004; Ostir, Berges, Markides, & Ottenbacher, 2006; Ostir, Markides, Blank, & Goodwin, 2000; Ostir, Markides, Peek, & Goodwin, 2001). Ostir and colleagues (2006) used a 4-item positive affect scale created from the 20-item CES–D items to load onto a single positive emotion factor that showed high internal consistency. (Radloff, 1977; Sheehan, Fiffield, Reisine, & Tennen, 1995). The Ostir and colleagues study in 2000 was a prospective cohort study of 2,282 Mexican Americans, ages 65 to 99 years, with no reported activities of daily living limitations at baseline interview. They investigated the relationship between PA and subsequent functional ability and survival in this older population. When they reinterviewed 2 years later, they found that higher PA scores at baseline interview predicted a lower incidence of functional disability, faster walking speed, and a lower likelihood of having died compared to people with low PA.

In 2001, the same group conducted a second prospective cohort study of 2,478 older people who reported no history of strokes at the baseline interview. They assessed whether PA, NA, or both predicted the risk of stroke. Their findings indicated that higher PA scores were significantly associated with a reduced risk of stroke over a 6-year follow-up period. These researchers suggested that PA seemed to protect against stroke in older adults.

In the Fisher and colleagues study in 2004, the team examined the relationship between PA and subsequent functional ability in 1,084 older Mexican Americans with arthritis. They found that higher PA scores at baseline interview were associated with a lower incidence of functional disability two years later.

In the Ostir and colleagues study in 2006, the team investigated the role of PA and hypertension in older adults. They conducted a cross-sectional study of 2,564 Mexican Americans ages 65 years and older. They found that higher PA scores were significantly associated with lower continuous systolic and diastolic blood pressure for those not on hypertensive medications. They also found that higher PA was also significantly associated with lower continuous diastolic blood pressure for those on hypertensive medication. An emerging literature suggests that PA may play a protective role in health and lead to less vulnerability to inflammatory diseases (Prather, Marsland, Muldoon, & Manuck, 2007).

Benyamini, Idler, Leventhal, and Leventhal (2000), in a longitudinal study of 851 elderly residents (ages 70–80 years) of a retirement community, found that PA influenced residents' perceptions of health. These studies provide support for a relationship between PA and health outcomes.

In summary, the notion that positive emotions are markers of optimal well-being is evident in the social sciences literature (Diener, 2000, 2008; Fredrickson 2001, 2006, 2008). The foregoing studies support the notion that positive emotions improve health outcomes. We would also suggest that positive and negative emotion regulation might moderate life-balance appraisals. In the following section, we will review qualitative evidence supporting positive emotion regulation after ABI.

QUALITATIVE EVIDENCE

Disability and illness have an impact on subjective well-being and quality-of-life appraisals, including life balance. Societal perceptions of disability may present barriers to participation in meaningful life activities, creating a sense of imbalance that can lead to negative self-appraisals. Some qualitative studies support the fact that many individuals who have experienced ABI struggle to attain a high quality of life and a sense of belonging that can contribute to their subjective well-being, while others show that some individuals can accept limitations and restrictions in a positive manner, even when they appear to struggle with limited personal roles and occupational choices. This form of positive emotional regulation is likely to improve their well-being and be a contributor to enhanced quality-of-life appraisals (Phillips, Henry, Hosie, & Milne, 2006).

There are several personal accounts in the qualitative brain injury literature that demonstrate some positive life changes after brain injury. Stone (2005) studied a group of women 3 years post-stroke. Many of the women found a new appreciation of life and worked to minimize the stress that was part of their pre-injury lifestyle. Some became less controlling and practiced letting go of worries and burdens. Gillen (2005) asked stroke survivors if they could identify any positive consequences of their injury. Of those interviewed, 63% were able to identify some positive consequences, including improving relationships with family, increasing awareness of the need to engage in a healthy lifestyle, feeling more religious, developing unselfish concern for others, and reprioritizing what was important in life.

McColl and colleagues (2000) found that individuals 2 years post-traumatic brain injury or spinal cord injury reported changes in spirituality. Williams, Rittman, Boylstein, Faircloth, and Haijing (2005) reported that veterans who were not diagnosed with depression following stroke tended to face adversity with strength, tried to find meaning in their stroke (e.g., the stroke slowed them down and caused them to appreciate family more), tried to focus on the present rather than think about the past or worry about the future, and were more hopeful about the future and expected further functional recovery. The effects of stroke were not as devastating for those who viewed it as a normal part of life or for those who had prior experience (e.g., they had watched family or friends struggle and eventually cope following a stroke). Positive psychological change can occur following onset of disability, and this type of change has been studied in individuals with ABI. Clinicians often neglect to identify positive emotions during the rehabilitation process. Limited understanding of positive affect hinders a holistic treatment approach; therefore, more research is needed to explore how positive affect influences functional recovery (McGrath & Linley, 2006).

Two processes that may reshape personal loss are finding meaning and finding benefits after trauma (Davis, Nolen-Hoeksema, & Larson, 1998; Davis, Wortman, Lehman, & Silver, 2000). An example of finding meaning has been described in the qualitative brain injury literature as when an individual views having a stroke as a natural part of the whole life cycle (Faircloth, Boylstein, Rittman, & Gubrium, 2005; Williams et al., 2005). Other narratives have described how individuals after brain injury shift their roles and self-perception, which can lead to a growth in character (McGrath & Linley, 2006). Religious belief appeared to help many participants find meaning and understanding about their loss (McColl et al., 2000). These are examples of how individuals can reconstruct the world after disability (Lopez & Snyder, 2003; Snyder & Lopez, 2005).

There is also support for the value of negative emotions in health outcomes. Tyerman and Humphrey (1984) confirmed that there were profound changes in self-concept in 25 individuals with severe head injury. Their findings suggested that people with severe head injury frequently show insight and self-awareness. Other people with brain injury may show continued reliance on unrealistic expectations that possibly can initially protect and motivate but can also constrain the rehabilitation and adjustment process (Tyerman & Humphrey, 1984). McGrath (2000) reported that NA was associated with emotionalism and tearfulness in a sample of individuals undergoing rehabilitation following severe brain injury.

CONCLUSIONS

Our review and attempt to describe emotional regulation, processing, and recovery after ABI as contributors to life balance appraisals suggests three major conclusions. First, the existing definitions and measurement of life balance are vague, conceptually complex, and not explicitly differentiated. Developing consistent definitions and measurements is never easy but may facilitate a clearer understanding of quality-of-life appraisals. Second, the methodological differences reflected in the cited investigations impede the interpretation of findings. The potential sources of variance among the studies of emotional regulation, processing, and recovery after ABI are enormous. Some studies were based on small sample sizes, and participants sustained diverse brain lesions and cognitive impairments. In addition, quasi-experimental designs were used; studies showed limitations in randomization, used different outcome measures, and collected biomarkers samples using different time frames and protocols. These variables clearly limit the generalization of the studies reviewed. Third, the social science literature and rehabilitation data-mining observational studies strongly suggest that emotional regulation, in particular PA, has a protective and buffering effect on health. Additional quantitative and qualitative studies investigating the positive and negative effects of acute and chronic stress, biomarkers, and rehabilitation outcomes are needed.

Life balance is a multilevel, multifactor term requiring an interdisciplinary, global perspective to understand its implications, validity, measurement, and use with healthy, as well as ABI, populations. Life balance needs to be studied as a personal and public health issue.

ACKNOWLEDGEMENTS

This work was supported in part by NIH R01 Grant DC01150 subcontract and professional staff congress—City University of New York Research Award, 69683-0038 for Queens College; by the National Institute on Aging, Grant K02-AG019736; by the National Institute of Child Health and Human Development, Grant K01-HD046682; and by the Moody Foundation, Grant 2005-24. We also gratefully acknowledge Renee Pearcy for her research assistance.

REFERENCES

Abreu, B. C., Reistetter, T. A., Ottenbacher, K. J., & Sangole, A. P. (2006, April). *Meta-analysis: Qualitative and quantitative evidence-based practice for direct care practitioners.* Paper presented at the 86th Annual AOTA Conference & Expo, Charolotte, NC.

Adams, N. (1996). Positive outcomes in families following traumatic brain injury. *Australian and New Zealand Journal of Family Therapy, 18,* 75–84.

Adolphs, R. (2002). Recognizing emotion from facial expressions: Psychological and neurological mechanisms. *Behavioral and Cognitive Neuroscience Reviews, 1,* 21–62.

Allan, C., Loudoun, R., & Peetz, D. (2007). Influences on work/non-work conflict. *Journal of Sociology, 43,* 219–239.

Alpert, M., & Rosen, A. (1990). A semantic analysis of the various ways that the terms affect, emotion, and mood are used. *Journal of Communication Disorders, 23,* 237–246.

Aspinwall, L. G. (1998). Rethinking the role of positive affect in self-regulation. *Motivation and Emotion, 22,* 1–32.

Bay, E., Hagerty, B. M., Williams, R. A., Kirsch, N., & Gillespie, B. (2002). Chronic stress, sense of belonging, and depression among survivors of traumatic brain injury. *Journal of Nursing Scholarship, 34,* 221–226.

Bay, E., Hagerty, B., Williams, R. A., & Kirsch, N. (2005). Chronic stress, salivary cortisol response, interpersonal relatedness, and depression among community-dwelling survivors of traumatic brain injury. *Journal of Neuroscience Nursing, 37,* 4–14.

Benyamini, Y., Idler, E. L., Leventhal, H., & Leventhal, E. A. (2000). Positive affect and function as influences on self-assessments of health: Expanding our view beyond illness and disability. *Journal of Gerontology: Psychological Sciences, 55B,* P107–P116.

Bloom, N., & Van Reenen, J. (2006). Management practices, work–life balance, and productivity: A review of some recent evidence. *Oxford Review of Economic Policy, 22,* 457–482.

Bood, S., Archer, T., & Norlander, T. (2004). Affective personality in relation to general personality, self-reported stress, coping, and optimism. *Individual Differences Research, 2,* 26–37.

Borod, J. (1992). Interhemispheric and intrahemispheric control of emotion: A focus on unilateral brain damage. *Journal of Consulting and Clinical Psychology, 60,* 339–348.

Borod, J. (1993). Cerebral mechanisms underlying facial, prosodic, and lexical emotional expression: A review of neuropsychological studies and methodological issues. *Neuropsychology, 7,* 445–463.

Borod, J. (1996). Emotional disorders/emotion. In J. G. Beaumont, P. Kenealy, & M. Rogers (Eds.), *The Blackwell dictionary of neuropsychology* (pp. 312–320). Oxford: Blackwell.

Borod, J. (Ed.). (2000). *The neuropsychology of emotion.* New York: Oxford University Press.

Borod, J., Bloom, R. L., Brickman, A. M., Nakhutina, L., & Curko, E. A. (2002). Emotional processing deficits in individuals with unilateral brain damage. *Applied Neuropsychology, 9,* 23–36.

Borod, J., Bloom, R. L., & Haywood, C. S. (1998). Verbal aspects of emotional communication. In C. Chiarello (Ed.), *Right-hemisphere language comprehension: Perspectives from cognitive neuroscience* (pp. 285–308). Mahwah, NJ: Lawrence Erlbaum.

Borod, J., Caron, H., & Koff, E. (1981). Facial asymmetry for positive and negative expressions: Sex differences. *Neuropsychology, 19,* 819–824.

Borod, J., Welkowitz, J., & Obler, L. (1992). *The New York Emotion Battery.* Unpublished manuscript, Mount Sinai Medical Center, Department of Neurology, New York.

Borod, J., Zgaljardic, D. J., Tabert, M. H., & Koff, E. (2001). Asymmetries of emotional perception and expression in normal adults. In G. Gainotti (Ed.), *Handbook of neuropsychology: Emotional behavior and its disorders.* Amsterdam: Elseiver Science.

Bryson, L., Warner-Smith, P., Brown, P., & Fray, L. (2007). Managing the work–life roller-coaster: Private stress or public health issue? *Social Science and Medicine, 65,* 1142–1153.

Carver, C. S., Scheier, M. F., & Weintraub, J. K. (1989). Assessing coping strategies: A theoretically based approach. *Journal of Personality and Social Psychology, 56,* 267–283.

Christiansen, C. (1996). Three perspectives on balance in occupation. In R. Zemke & F. Clark (Eds.), *Occupational science: The evolving discipline* (pp. 431–451). Philadelphia: F. A. Davis.

Christiansen, C. H., & Matuska, K. M. (2006). Lifestyle balance: A review of concepts and research. *Journal of Occupational Science, 13,* 49–61.

Cicerone, K. D., Dahlberg, C., Malec, J. F., Langenbahn, D. M., Felicetti, T., Kneipp, S., et al. (2005). Evidence-based cognitive rehabilitation: Updated review of the literature from 1998 through 2002. *Archives of Physical Medicine and Rehabilitation, 86,* 1681–1692.

Crawford, J. R., & Henry, J. D. (2004). The Positive and Negative Affect Schedule (PANAS): Construct validity, measurement properties, and normative data in a large non-clinical sample. *British Journal of Clinical Psychology, 43,* 245–265.

Crimmins, E. M., Johnston, M., Hayward, M., & Seeman, T. (2003). Age differences in allostatic load: An index of physiological dysregulation. *Experimental Gerontology, 38,* 731–734.

Csikszentmihalyi, M., & Csikszentmihalyi, I. S. (Eds.). (2006). *A life worth living: Contributions to positive psychology.* New York: Oxford University Press.

Davidson, R. J. (1984). Affect, cognition, and hemispheric specialization. In C. E. Izard, J. Kagan, & R. Zajonc (Eds.), *Emotion, cognition, and behavior* (pp. 320–365). New York: Cambridge University Press.

Davis, C. G., Nolen-Hoeksema, S., & Larson, J. (1998). Making sense of loss and benefiting from the experience: Two construals of meaning. *Journal of Personality and Social Psychology, 75,* 561–574.

Davis, C. G., Wortman, C. B., Lehman, D. R., & Silver, R. C. (2000). Searching for meaning in loss: Are clinical assumptions correct? *Death Studies, 24,* 497–540.

Diener, E. (2000). Subjective well-being: The science of happiness and a proposal for a national index. *American Psychologist, 55,* 34–43.

Diener, E. (2008). Myths in the science of happiness, and directions for future research. In M. Eid & R. J. Larsen (Eds.), *The science of subjective well-being* (pp. 493–514). New York: Guilford Press.

Diener, E., Lucas, R. E., & Scollon, C. N. (2006). Beyond the hedonic treadmill: Revising the adaptation theory of well-being. *American Psychologist, 61,* 305–314.

Diener, E., & Seligman, M. E. P. (2002). Very happy people. *Psychological Science, 13,* 81–84.

Djikers, M. P. (2004). Quality of life after traumatic brain injury: A review of research approaches and findings. *Archives of Physical Medicine and Rehabilitation, 85,* S21–S35.

Drago, R. W. (2007). *Striking a balance: Work, family, life.* Boston: Dollars & Sense.

Eid, M., & Larsen, R. J. (Eds.). (2008). *The science of subjective well-being.* New York: Guilford Press.

Ergh, T. C., Hanks, R. A., Rapport, L. J., & Coleman, R. D. (2003). Social support moderates caregiver life satisfaction following traumatic brain injury. *Journal of Clinical and Experimental Neuropsychology, 25,* 1090–1101.

Faircloth, C. A., Boylstein, C., Rittman, M., & Gubrium, J. F. (2005). Constructing the stroke: Sudden-onset narratives of stroke survivors. *Qualitative Health Research, 15,* 928–941.

Faircloth, C. A., Boylstein, C., Rittman, M., Young, M. E., & Gubrium, J. F. (2004). Sudden illness and biographical flow in narratives of stroke recovery. *Sociology of Health and Illness, 26,* 242–261.

Fazzini, E., Bachman, D., & Alpert, M. (1986). Recovery of function in aphasia. *Journal of Neurolinguistics, 2,* 15–46.

Finset, A., & Andersson, S. (2000). Coping strategies in patients with acquired brain injury: Relationships between coping, apathy, depression, and lesion location. *Brain Injury, 14,* 887–905.

Fisher, M., Al Snih, S., Ostir, G. V., & Goodwin, J. S. (2004). Positive affect and disability among older Mexican Americans with arthritis. *Arthritis and Rheumatism, 51,* 34–39.

Flannelly, K., Koenig, H. G. M., Galek, K., & Ellison, C. G. (2007). Beliefs, mental health, and evolutionary threat assessment systems in the brain. *Journal of Nervous and Mental Disease December, 195,* 996–1003.

Folkman, S., Lazarus, R. S., Gruen, R. J., & Delongis, A. (1986). Appraisal, coping, health-status, and psychological symptoms. *Journal of Personality and Social Psychology, 50,* 571–579.

Fredrickson, B. L. (2001). The role of positive emotions in positive psychology: The broaden-and-build theory of positive emotions. *American Psychologist, 56,* 218–226.

Fredrickson, B. L. (2004). The broaden-and-build theory of positive emotions. *Philosophical Transactions of the Royal Society of London Series B: Biological Sciences, 359,* 1367–1378.

Fredrickson, B. L. (2006). The broaden-and-build theory of positive emotion. In M. Csikszentmihalyi & I. S. Csikszentmihalyi (Eds.), *A life worth living: Contributions to positive psychology* (pp. 85–103). New York: Oxford University Press.

Fredrickson, B. L. (2008). Promoting positive affect. In M. Eid & R. J. Larsen (Eds.), *The science of subjective well-being* (pp. 449–468). New York: Guilford Press.

Geschwind, N. (1974). Late changes in the nervous system: An overview. In N. Butters (Ed.), *Plasticity and recovery of function in the central nervous system* (pp. 467–471). New York: Academic.

Gillen, G. (2005). Positive consequences of surviving a stroke. *American Journal of Occupational Therapy, 59,* 346–350.

Gordon, W. A., Zafonte, R., Cicerone, K. D., Cantor, J., Brown, M., Lombard, L., et al. (2006). Traumatic brain injury rehabilitation: State of the science. *American Journal of Physical Medicine and Rehabilitation, 85,* 343–382.

Gross, J. J. (Ed.). (2007). *Handbook of emotion regulation.* New York: Guilford Press.

Grote, N. K., Bledsoe, S. E., Larkin, J., Lemay, E. P., & Brown, C. (2007). Stress exposure and depression in disadvantaged women: The protective effects of optimism and perceived control. *Social Work Research, 31,* 19–33.

Heilman, K. M., Blonder, L. X., Bowers, D., & Crucian, G. P. (2000). Neurological disorders and emotional dysfunction. In J. Borod (Ed.), *The neuropsychology of emotion* (pp. 367–413). New York: Oxford University Press.

Heilman, K. M., Blonder, L. X., Bowers, D., & Valenstein, E. (2003). Emotional disorders associated with neurological diseases. In K. M. Heilman & E. Valenstein (Eds.), *Clinical neuropsychology* (4th ed.). New York: Oxford University Press.

Hobfoll, S. E., Hall, B. J., Canetti-Nisim, D., Galea, S., Johnson, R. J., & Palmieri, P. A. (2007). Refining our understanding of traumatic growth in the face of terrorism: Moving from meaning cognitions to doing what is meaningful. *Applied Psychology—An International Review, 56,* 345–366.

Isaacowitz, D. M., & Seligman, M. E. P. (2001). Is pessimism a risk factor for depressive mood among community-dwelling older adults? *Behavior Research and Therapy, 39,* 255–272.

Isen, A. M. (2000a). Positive affect and decision making. In M. Lewis & J. M. Haviland-Jones (Eds.), *Handbook of Emotions* (2nd ed., pp. 417–435). New York: Guilford Press.

Isen, A. M. (2000b). Some perspectives on positive affect and self-regulation. *Psychological Inquiry, 11,* 184–187.

Isen, A. M. (2001). An influence of positive affect on decision making in complex situations: Theoretical issues with practical implications. *Journal of Consumer Psychology, 11,* 75–85.

Isen, A. M., & Reeve, J. (2005). The influence of positive affect on intrinsic and extrinsic motivation: Facilitating enjoyment of play, responsible work behavior, and self-control. *Motivation and Emotion, 29,* 297–325.

Jackson, R. D., & Mysiw, W. J. (1989). Abnormal cortisol dynamics after traumatic brain injury: Lack of utility in predicting agitation or therapeutic response to tricyclic antidepressants. *American Journal of Physical Medicine and Rehabilitation, 68,* 18–23.

Johansson, U., & Tham, K. (2006). The meaning of work after acquired brain injury. *American Journal of Occupational Therapy, 60,* 60–69.

Jones, G., & Cale, A. (1989). Precompetition temporal patterning of anxiety and self-confidence in males and females. *Journal of Sports Behavior, 12,* 183–195.

Jongbloed, L. (1994). Adaptation to a stroke: The experience of one couple. *American Journal of Occupational Therapy, 48,* 1006–1013.

Karlamangla, A. S., Singer, B. H., McEwen, B. S., Rowe, J. W., & Seeman, T. E. (2002). Allostatic load as a predictor of functional decline—MacArthur studies of successful aging. *Journal of Clinical Epidemiology, 55,* 696–710.

Kennedy-Moore, E. I., Greenberg, M. A., Newman, M. G., & Stone, A. A. (1992). The relationship between daily events and mood: The mood measure may matter. *Motivation and Emotion, 16,* 135–155.

Kertesz, A. (1993). Recovery and treatment. In E. Valenstein (Ed.), *Clinical neuropsychology* (pp. 647–661). New York: Oxford University Press.

Kinsbourne, M. (1971). The minor cerebral hemisphere as a source of aphasic speech. *Archives of Neurology, 25,* 302–306.

Krefting, L. (1989). Reintegration into the community after head injury: The results of an ethnographic study. *Occupational Therapy Journal of Research, 9,* 67–83.

LeDoux, J. E. (1993). Emotional memory: In search of systems and synapses. *Annals New York Academy of Sciences, 17,* 149–157.

Leufstadius, C., Erlandsson, L.-K., & Eklund, M. (2006). Time use and daily activities in people with persistent mental illness. *Occupational Therapy International, 13,* 123–141.

Liotti, M., & Tucker, D. M. (1992). Right-hemisphere sensitivity to arousal and depression. *Brain and Cognition, 18,* 138–151.

Lippert-Grüner, M., Kuchta, J., Hellmich, M., & Klug, N. (2006). Neurobehavioural deficits after severe traumatic brain injury (TBI). *Brain Injury, 20,* 569–574.

Lopez, S. J., & Snyder, C. R. (Eds.). (2003). *Positive psychological assessment: A handbook of models and measures.* Washington, DC: American Psychological Association.

Loretto, W., Popham, F., Platt, S., Pavis, S., Hardy, G., MacLeod, L., et al. (2005). Assessing psychological well-being: A holistic investigation of NHS employees. *International Review of Psychiatry, 17,* 329–336.

Lundberg, U., & Hellström, B. (2002). Workload and morning salivary cortisol in women. *Work and Stress, 16,* 356–363.

MacDonald, M., Phipps, S., & Lethbridge, L. (2005). Taking its toll: The influence of paid and unpaid work on women's well-being. *Feminist Economics, 11,* 63–94.

MacLean, P. (1958). The limbic system with respect to self-preservation and the preservation of the species. *Journal of Nervous and Mental Disease, 127,* 1–11.

Man, D. W., Lee, E. W., Tong, E. C., Yip, S. C., Lui, W. F., & Lam, C. S. (2004). Health services needs and quality of life assessment of individuals with brain injuries: A pilot cross-sectional study. *Brain Injury, 18,* 577–591.

Mandal, M. K., Borod, J., Asthana, H. S., Mohanty, A., Mohanty, S., & Koff, E. (1999). Effects of lesion variables and emotion type on the perception of facial expression. *Journal of Nervous and Mental Disease, 187,* 603–609.

Masel, B. E. (2004). Rehabilitation and hypopituitarism after traumatic brain injury. *Growth Hormone and IGF Research, 14,* S108–S113.

Masi, C. M., Rickett, E. M., Hawkley, L. C., & Cacioppo, J. T. (2004). Gender and ethnic differences in urinary stress hormones: The population-based Chicago health, aging, and social relations study. *Journal of Applied Physiology, 97,* 941–947.

McColl, M. A., Bickenbach, J., Johnston, J., Nishihama, S., Schumaker, M., Smith, K., et al. (2000). Changes in spiritual beliefs after traumatic brain injury. *Archives of Physical Medicine and Rehabilitation, 81,* 817–823.

McEwen, B. S. (2003). Mood disorders and allostatic load. *Biological Psychiatry, 54,* 200–207.

McEwen, B. S. (2007). Physiology and neurobiology of stress and adaptation: Central role of the brain. *Physiological Reviews, 87,* 873–904.

McEwen, B. S., & Stellar, E. (1993). Stress and the individual: Mechanisms leading to disease. *Archives of Internal Medicine, 153,* 2093–2101.

McGrath, J. C., & Linley, P. A. (2006). Post-traumatic growth in acquired brain injury: A preliminary small scale study. *Brain Injury, 20,* 767–773.

McGrath, J. J. (2000). A study of emotionalism in patients undergoing rehabilitation following severe acquired brain injury. *Behavioural Neurology, 12,* 201–207.

Murray, G., Judd, F., Jackson, H., Fraser, C., Komiti, A., Pattison, P., et al. (2007). Ceremonies of the whole: Does social participation moderate the mood consequences of neuroticism? *Social Psychiatry and Psychiatric Epidemiology, 42,* 173–180.

Nakhutina, L., Borod, J. C., & Zgaljardic, D. J. (2006). Posed prosodic emotional expression in unilateral stroke patients: Recovery, lesion location, and emotional perception. *Archives of Clinical Neuropsychology, 21,* 1–13.

Nelson, L. D., Cicchetti, D., Satz, P., Sowa, M., & Mitrushina, M. (1994). Emotional sequelae of stroke: A longitudinal perspective. *Journal of Clinical and Experimental Neuropsychology, 16,* 796–806.

Olff, M., Güzelcan, Y., de Vries, G.-J., Assies, J., & Gersons, B. P. R. (2006). HPA- and HPT-axis alterations in chronic posttraumatic stress disorder. *Psychoneuroendocrinology, 31,* 1220–1230.

Ostir, G. V., Berges, I. M., Markides, K. S., & Ottenbacher, K. J. (2006). Hypertension in older adults and the role of positive emotions. *Psychosomatic Medicine, 68,* 727–733.

Ostir, G. V., Markides, K. S., Blank, S. A., & Goodwin, J. S. (2000). Emotional well-being predicts subsequent functional independence and survival. *Journal of American Geriatrics Society, 48,* 473–478.

Ostir, G. V., Markides, K. S., Peek, M. K., & Goodwin, J. S. (2001). The association between emotional well-being and the incidence of stroke in older adults. *Psychosomatic Medicine, 63,* 210–215.

Ostir, G. V., Smith, P. M., Smith, D., & Ottenbacher, K. J. (2005). Reliability of the Positive and Negative Affect Schedule (PANAS) in medical rehabilitation. *Clinical Rehabilitation, 19,* 767–769.

Papez, J. W. (1937). A proposed mechanism of emotion. *Archives of Neurology and Psychiatry, 38,* 725–743.

Pat-Horenczyk, R., & Brom, D. (2007). The multiple faces of post-traumatic growth. *Applied Psychology: An International Review, 56,* 379–385.

Peterson, C. (2000). The future of optimism. *American Journal of Psychology, 55,* 44–55.

Phillips, L. H., Henry, J. D., Hosie, J. A., & Milne, A. B. (2006). Age, anger regulation, and well-being. *Aging and Mental Health, 10,* 250–256.

Pick, L. H., Borod, J. C., Ehrlichman, H., & Bloom, R. (2003). Lexical expression of emotion in stroke: Intra- and inter-hemispheric effects [Abstract]. *Journal of the International Neuropsychological Society, 9,* 185–186.

Plutchik, R. (1984). Emotions: A general psychoevolutionary theory. In K. R. Scherer & P. Ekman (Eds.), *Approaches to emotion* (pp. 197–219). Hillsdale, NJ: Erlbaum.

Prather, A. A., Marsland, A. L., Muldoon, M. F., & Manuck, S. B. (2007). Positive affective style covaries with stimulated IL-6 and IL-10 production in a middle-aged community sample. *Brain, Behavior, and Immunity, 21,* 1033–1037.

Premeaux, S. F., Adkins, C. L., & Mossholder, K. W. (2007). Balancing work and family: A field study of multi-dimensional, multi-role work–family conflict. *Journal of Organizational Behavior, 28,* 705–727.

Prigatano, G. P. (1992). Personality disturbances associated with traumatic brain injury. *Journal of Consulting and Clinical Psychology, 60,* 360–368.

Radloff, L. S. (1977). The CES–D Scale: A self-report depression scale for research in the general population. *Applied Psychological Measurement, 1,* 385–401.

Robertson, I. H., Ridgeway, V., Greenfield, E., & Parr, A. (1997). Motor recovery after stroke depends on intact sustained attention: A 2-year follow-up study. *Neuropsychology, 11,* 290–295.

Rogers, K., Borod, J., & Ramig, L. (2008). Side bias: Cerebral hemisphere asymmetry in emotion and social cognition. In R. Adams, N. Amady, K. Nakayama, & S. Shimojo (Eds.), *People watching : The psychology of social vision.* New York: Oxford University Press.

Rosenberg, E. L. (1998). Levels of analysis and the organization of affect. *Review of General Psychology, 2,* 247–270.

Ross, E. (1985). Modulation of affect and nonverbal communication by the right hemisphere. In M.-M. Mesulam (Ed.), *Principles of behavioral neurology* (pp. 239– 257). Philadelphia: F. A. Davis.

Ross, E. D., & Monnot, M. (2007). Neurology of affective prosody and its functional–anatomic organization in right hemisphere. *Brain and Language.*

Ryff, C. D., & Singer, B. H. (1998). The contours of positive human health. *Psychological Inquiry, 9,* 1–28.

Sackeim, H. A., Greenberg, M. S., Weiman, A. L., Hungerbuhler, J. P., & Geschwind, N. (1982). Hemispheric asymmetry in the expression of positive and negative emotions: Neurologic evidence. *Archives of Neurology, 39,* 210–218.

Sato, W., & Aoki, S. (2006). Right hemispheric dominance in processing of unconscious negative emotion. *Brain and Cognition, 62,* 261–266.

Scheier, M. F., & Carver, C. S. (1992). Effects of optimism on psychological and physical well-being: Theoretical overview and empirical update. *Cognitive Therapy and Research, 16,* 201–228.

Scheier, M. F., Weintraub, J. K., & Carver, C. S. (1986). Coping with stress: Divergent strategies of optimists and pessimists. *Journal of Personality and Social Psychology, 51,* 1257–1264.

Schultz, L. E. (2007). Models of exceptional adaptation in recovery after traumatic brain injury: A case series. *Journal of Head Trauma Rehabilitation, 22,* 48–55.

Seligman, M. E. P. (2005). Positive psychology, positive prevention, and positive therapy. In C. R. R. Snyder & S. J. Lopez (Eds.), *Handbook of positive psychology* (pp. 3–9). New York: Oxford University Press.

Seligman, M. E. P., & Csikszentmihalyi, M. (2000). Positive psychology: An introduction. *American Psychologist, 55,* 5–14.

Selye, H. (1976). 40 years of stress research: Principal remaining problems and misconceptions. *Canadian Medical Association Journal, 115,* 53–56.

Sheehan, T. J., Fifield, J., Reisine, S., & Tennen, H. (1995). The measurement structure of the Center for Epidemiologic Studies Depression Scale. *Journal of Personality Assessment, 64,* 507–521.

Silberman, E. K., & Weingartner, H. (1986). Hemispheric lateralization of functions related to emotion. *Brain and Cognition, 5,* 322–353.

Simeon, D., Knutelska, M., Yehuda, R., Putnam, F., Schmeidler, J., & Smith, L. M. (2007). Hypothalamic–pituitary–adrenal axis function in dissociative disorders, post-traumatic stress disorder, and healthy volunteers. *Biological Psychiatry, 61,* 966–973.

Snyder, C. R. R., & Lopez, S. J. (Eds.). (2005). *Handbook of positive psychology.* New York: Oxford University Press.

Steptoe, A., Cropley, M., & Joekes, K. (1999). Job strain, blood pressure, and response to uncontrollable stress. *Journal of Hypertension, 17,* 193–200.

Sterling, P., & Eyer, J. (1981). Biological basis of stress-related mortality. *Social Science and Medicine, 15E,* 3–42.

Sterling, P., & Eyer, J. (1988). Allostasis: A new paradigm to explain arousal pathology. In S. Fisher & J. Reason (Eds.), *Handbook of life stress, cognition, and health* (pp. 629–649). New York: John Wiley & Sons.

Sterzi, R., Bottini, G., Celani, M. G., Righetti, E., Lamassa, M., Ricci, S., et al. (1993). Hemianopia, hemianaesthesia, and hemiplegia after right- and left-hemisphere damage. A hemispheric difference. *Journal of Neurology, Neurosurgery and Psychiatry, 56,* 308–310.

Stone, S. D. (2005). Being as doing: Occupational perspectives of women survivors of hemorrhagic stroke. *Journal of Occupational Science, 12,* 17–25.

Sverko, B., Arambasiic, L., & Galesic, M. (2002). Work–life balance among Croatian employees: Role time commitment, work–home interference, and well-being. *Social Science Information/Information sur les Sciences Sociales, 41,* 281–301.

Szanton, S. L., Gill, J. M., & Allen, J. K. (2005). Allostatic load: A mechanism of socioeconomic health disparities? *Biological Research for Nursing, 7,* 7–15.

Tchiteya, B. M., Lecours, A. R., Elie, R., & Lupien, S. J. (2003). Impact of a unilateral brain lesion on cortisol secretion and emotional state: Anterior/posterior dissociation in humans. *Psychoneuroendocrinology, 28,* 674–686.

Tedeschi, R. G., & Calhoun, L. G. (1996). The Post-Traumatic Growth Inventory: Measuring the positive legacy of trauma. *Journal of Traumatic Stress, 9,* 455–471.

Tedeschi, R. G., & Calhoun, L. G. (2004). Posttraumatic growth: Conceptual foundations and empirical evidence. *Psychological Inquiry, 15,* 1–18.

Thatcher, J., Thatcher, R., & Dorling, D. (2004). Gender differences in the pre-competition temporal patterning of anxiety and hormonal responses. *Journal of Sports Medicine and Physical Fitness, 44,* 300–308.

Tyerman, A., & Humphrey, M. (1984). Changes in self-concept following severe head injury. *International Journal of Rehabilitation Research, 7,* 11–23.

Ursin, H., & Eriksen, H. R. (2004). Review: The cognitive activation theory of stress. *Psychoneuroendocrinology, 29,* 567–592.

Voydanoff, P. (2005). Toward a conceptualization of perceived work–family fit and balance: A demands and resources approach. *Journal of Marriage and Family, 67,* 822–836.

Wasserman, S., Borod, J., & Winnick, W. (1998). *Memory of emotional and neutral words in patients with unilateral brain damage.* Paper presented at the International Neuropsychological Society, Honolulu, HI.

Watson, D., Clark, L. A., & Tellegen, A. (1988). Development and validation of brief measures of positive and negative affect: The PANAS Scales. *Journal of Personality and Social Psychology, 54,* 1063–1070.

Wellens, B. T., & Smith, A. P. (2006). Combined workplace stressors and their relationship with mood, physiology, and performance. *Work and Stress, 20,* 245–258.

Westphal, M., & Bonanno, G. A. (2007). Posttraumatic growth and resilience to trauma: Different sides of the same coin or different coins? *Applied Psychology: An International Review, 56,* 417–427.

White, T., Cullen, K., Rohrer, L. M., Karatekin, C., Luciana, M., Schmidt, M., et al. (2008). Limbic structures and networks in children and adolescents with schizophrenia. *Schizophrenia Bulletin, 34,* 18–29.

Williams, C. L., Rittman, M., Boylstein, C., Faircloth, C. A., & Haijing, Q. (2005). Qualitative and quantitative measurement of depression in veterans recovering from stroke. *Journal of Rehabilitation Research and Development, 42,* 277–290.

Wilz, G. (2007). Predictors of subjective impairment after stroke: Influence of depression, gender, and severity of stroke. *Brain Injury, 21,* 39–45.

Wittling, W., & Pfluger, M. (1990). Neuroendocrine hemisphere asymmetries: Salivary cortisol secretion during lateralized viewing of emotion-related and neutral films. *Brain and Cognition, 14,* 243–265.

Wolf, O. T., Fujiwara, E., Luwinski, G., Kirschbaum, C., & Markowitsch, H. J. (2005). No morning cortisol response in patients with severe global amnesia. *Psychoneuroendocrinology, 30,* 101–105.

World Health Organization. (1948). Preamble to the Constitution of the World Health Organization. *Official Records of the World Health Organization, 2,* 100.

Zgaljardic, D. J., Borod, J. C., Foldi, N. S., & Mattis, P. J. (2003). A review of the cognitive and behavioral sequelae of Parkinson's disease: Relationship to frontostriatal circuitry. *Cognitive and Behavioral Neurology, 16,* 193–210.

Zgaljardic, D. J., Borod, J. C., & Sliwinski, M. (2002). Emotional perception in unilateral stroke patients: Recovery, test stability, and interchannel relationships. *Applied Neuropsychology, 9,* 159–172.

Professional Coaching for Life Balance

AMY HEINZ AND WENDY PENTLAND

INTRODUCTION

Although defining *life balance* is difficult, as many of the chapters in this book show, achieving life balance is even more challenging. Many lament that with the fast pace of Western society— busy schedules, multiple demands, and seemingly limited time—the idea of achieving life balance is nothing more than a concept too far out on the horizon to realize. We hear other people, or even ourselves, speak of life balance and perhaps fantasize about it, making statements such as "Someday I will have more balance in my life" or "When I finish this, I will have life balance." In the meantime, someday is now, and as we promise ourselves life balance, our lives are ticking by.

On the face of it, restoring and sustaining life balance would seem to be relatively simple and straightforward. Unfortunately, research and collective experience show that people, while they have little difficulty recognizing when their lives feel imbalanced, have far more difficulty achieving and maintaining what they consider a balanced state. Professional coaching can be a powerful resource for the journey to life balance. This chapter is organized into two general sections. First, we begin with an explanation of the coaching approach and process, its theoretical underpinnings, and its relevance to issues of life balance. Second, we provide a description of the current nature of the coaching profession, including coach training, preparation, and competencies.

PROFESSIONAL COACHING FOR LIFE BALANCE: APPROACH AND PROCESS

Professional coaching is a process engaged in by persons who want to make changes in their lives. The process occurs over time and is facilitated by a coach. The coach works with the client in a conversation- and question-based process to foster client self-awareness and assessment of current behaviors, definition of personal values, and recognition of strengths that in turn foster self-directed client learning. Coaching takes an appreciative approach in that it focuses on the individual's strengths and builds on what is working in his or her life (Cooperrider & Whitney, 1999). In this way, coaching assists clients to make lasting lifestyle changes that enhance well-being and health. In the professional coaching relationship, clients are considered partners, or

K. Matuska & C. Christiansen (Eds.)
Life balance: Multidisciplinary theories and research (pp 241–254)
© 2009 SLACK Incorporated and AOTA Press

equals, with the coach. Clients are supported in clarifying what is important to them, recognizing their beliefs and assumptions about who they are in the world, expanding their options, and choosing and making desired life changes—all with the overall aim of moving in the direction of a more balanced, effective, and personally meaningful life.

Although no universal definitions of *life balance* or *life imbalance* exist, there seems to be consensus that it refers to what people do in their lives, how they have constructed their lifestyle, and how they feel about it. Hence, at least part of the process of improving or restoring life balance will involve making changes in that lifestyle. When people report feeling that their lives are out of balance, they will make comments like "I don't know what I want anymore" or "But I have no choice right now." In other words, while people easily identify when their lives feel imbalanced, they reveal significant difficulty or inertia with actually making changes to improve their lives. We have all heard the expression, "If nothing changes, then nothing changes." Coaching is a talk-based intervention, different than therapy, and specifically about assisting people to identify and make the requisite changes to move from their current state to a more desired future state. Consequently, it is a powerful resource for people wanting to improve their life balance.

What Is Professional Coaching?

Although for the purposes of this chapter we will use the term *professional coach* or *coach*, it is important to note that the concept of coaching goes by many titles. Common terms used in the literature and popular press include *life coach, wellness coach, executive coach, personal coach, peer coach,* and *mentor.* Definitions of coaching vary, but "the contemporary use of the term coaching has moved well beyond the traditional references to sports or educational coaching" (Cavanagh, Grant, & Kemp, 2005, p. 2). The International Coach Federation (ICF) describes coaching as

> partnering with clients in a thought-provoking and creative process that inspires them to maximize their personal and professional potential. Professional coaches provide an ongoing partnership designed to help clients produce fulfilling results in their personal and professional lives. Coaches help people improve their performances and enhance the quality of their lives. (ICF, 2007a)

Approaches taken by individual coaches range from an instructional approach to a more facilitative approach. Despite differences in definitions, there are common core features across most coaching approaches, including a focus on the egalitarian and collaborative relationship of the coach and the client, a focus on goal attainment, and an emphasis on the process of coaching being systematic and involving personal growth and self-direction on the part of the client (Stober & Grant, 2006). Professional coaching focuses on questions such as "Who am I at my best?" "What is most energizing and meaningful to me?" "What do I want to do with my life?" and "How can I go about creating the life I want?" The coach uses questions, tools, and techniques to help clients gain the necessary clarity about their lives that will allow them to find their own unique answers. The coach assists clients in designing plans and strategies to enhance their lives in accordance with these insights and supports them through the process of putting the plans and strategies into action. Unlike much of the information provided in self-help books, videos, and workshops, professional coaches assist clients to take these strategies and techniques beyond knowledge and actually integrate them into daily life. Ultimately, coaching is about assisting clients to take action (Yousey, 2001). Professional coaches assist individuals to increase their self-awareness, identify their choices, and develop strategies to deal with what gets in their way of moving forward. It is a method that draws on the holistic view of the individual by using the individual's life experiences and strengths. As is the case with therapy, in which highly personal or sensitive information is explored, the quality of the relationship between the coach and the client is a key factor in the process.

Another way to describe coaching is to be clear about what coaching is not. First, coaching is not counseling, therapy, consulting, or educating. Coaching clients are not considered patients or students. The coach is not in a position of power and does not instruct or give advice. Rather, coaching is a partnership where the clients are the experts on their own lives and the coach helps clients come up with their own answers. In coaching, the client (not the coach) is viewed as the agent of change. In other words, the client is responsible for identifying where change is needed and how to go about making that change. Second, coaching is not about analyzing or healing the past or judging past behaviors; instead, coaching is future oriented and goal directed. Coaches challenge clients to focus on the present and to invent their future rather than trying to justify or make up for the past. Finally, coaching is not about the coach being an expert, giving advice, or having a particular agenda. In the coaching relationship, it is the clients who set the agenda and drives the process toward reaching their goals. This is also described as the coach "dancing in the moment" (Whitworth, Kimsy-House, Kimsey-House, & Sandahl, 2007). The coach asks nonjudgmental questions and listens at a deep, intuitive level, guiding the session and process on the basis of the information the client provides. In this way, it is as if the client and the coach are engaged in an intimate dance, with the client leading. The coach's role is to support, stretch, and challenge the client toward achieving his or her goals—whatever they may be.

Theoretical Underpinnings

Those working in professional coaching are currently in the process of consolidating its theoretical foundations and expanding its empirical evidence base. Like most of the human services professions, it borrows its theoretical foundations from a wide range of fields, including human development, psychology, philosophy, and education.

At the core of coaching is recognizing the importance of the dynamic between the human desire for differentiation and unique self-expression on the one hand and the need for integration, connection, and meeting the expectations and demands of the environment on the other. The coaching approach adopts the perspective that we need to help people discover how to bring their choices and actions more in line with their unique "best self" and to connect more creatively with the deep human desire to make a contribution to the betterment of humanity. The success that we have in resolving this paradoxical tension between self and others determines, to a significant extent, our success and satisfaction in life (Sinclair & Russell, 2002). Perspectives on adult development and life stages suggest that the nature and extent of the resolution of this paradox will differ at different life stages (Kegan, 1982, 1994; Vaillant, 2002). For example, developing a career and adapting to and meeting social expectations are more typically regarded as tasks of young adulthood. These tasks assist in attaining work and income and establishing relationships necessary to create and support stable social structures to raise children and thus sustain society. Individuation and authentic self-expression have been regarded by some human-development theorists, such as Carl Jung, as tasks associated more with the midlife stage and beyond (Hollis, 2001). In this context, the challenge for the coach is to work with clients to help them discover what their optimal resolution to this dynamic between differentiation and integration is at their particular stage of life.

A number of important notions underpin the coaching approach. One is based in learning theory, particularly *transformative learning theory*, which focuses on those aspects of adult learning and knowledge construction that entail making meaning, particularly through becoming aware of the assumptions, values, expectations, and purposes assimilated from others (Mezirow, 2000). Through powerful open questioning, coaches assist clients to become aware of their own values, assumptions, and expectations and how they currently frame their issues and choices. This enhanced self-awareness is often sufficient to precipitate new awarenesses, options, choices, and possibilities that were previously not seen by the client.

A second and related notion that informs the coaching process is that there is no single true reality; rather, we as humans create our own reality with our thinking. Consequently we can re-create or change our reality by choosing either to change our thinking or how we respond to it. This notion is not new and pervades various fields, including psychology (e.g., logotherapy; see Frankl, 1984; Glasser, 2000; May, 1953, 1975, 1983), Eastern religions such as Buddhism (Thurman, 2005), and qualitative research methods such as the phenomenological and narrative approaches (DePoy & Gitlin, 2005).

Victor Frankl (1984) gives a powerful illustration of this ability of humans to create their own reality on the basis of his experience as a prisoner in a German concentration camp in World War II. Regarding suffering, Frankl states, "If it is avoidable, the meaningful thing to do is to remove its cause, for unnecessary suffering is masochistic rather than heroic. If, on the other hand, one cannot change a situation that causes his suffering, he can still choose his attitude" (p. 172). He refers to this *ability to choose* as the last of the human freedoms. "We who lived in concentration camps can remember the men who walked through the huts comforting others, giving away their last piece of bread. They may have been few in number, but they offer sufficient proof that everything can be taken from a man but one thing: the last of the human freedoms—to choose one's attitude in any given set of circumstances, to choose one's own way" (p. 86).

Coaches work with clients to help them become more aware of the thinking, language, and stories that they use to construct their perspectives and experience. Clients can then begin to explore more helpful alternatives and responses, which typically opens up far more options and possibilities for them. As clients become more aware of how their current thinking is limiting them and realize that they have far more choice in their responses than they were previously aware of, self-responsibility and an increased sense of personal agency often ensue.

A third notion fundamental to the coaching approach is the focus on the client's strengths and values versus focusing on shortcomings and weaknesses (Cooperrider & Whitney, 1999; Cooperrider, Whitney, & Stavros, 2003; Seligman, 2002). In applying coaching to issues of life balance, the coaching perspective would be to assist clients to identify the extent to which their lifestyle is congruent with their strengths and values. The coaching focus would include assisting them to understand their strengths and values and what is truly important to them and then incorporate these more into their life. Recent theoretical and empirical research on human flourishing informs this approach (Aspinall & Staudinger, 2003; Emmons, 2003; Frederickson, 2003; Keys & Haidt, 2003; Ryan & Deci, 2001; Seligman, 2002; Snyder & Lopez, 2002). This research, among others, provides more detailed accounts of human strengths, resilience, the importance of values, and the role of meaning for well-being.

Of particular note is the model of authentic happiness put forward by Martin Seligman (2002). Seligman proposes that happiness (or subjective well-being) is a function of three different elements and thus integrates different perspectives on happiness and well-being. The first component of happiness is the *pleasant life*, which depends on minimizing negative emotions and maximizing positive emotions. "Feeling good" in this sense, though, makes only a small contribution to overall happiness. The second component of happiness is *engagement*, which is generated when individuals find opportunities to use their strengths. The third component is *meaning*, which involves individuals using their strengths in services of a cause that is greater than their own self.

ADLERIAN APPROACH TO COACHING

All professional coaching aims to partner with the client to produce fulfilling results in their personal and or professional lives. Within this framework, there are minor variations in philosophy and approach. One is the Adlerian approach. This approach to coaching incorporates some of the basic tenets of the work of Alfred Adler, in particular, the concept that humans are motivated primarily by two desires: (1) to fulfill their own potential and (2) to make a meaningful contribution to the community (Dreikurs, 1953).

In the Adlerian approach to professional coaching, nine guiding principles provide coaches with direction as they engage in the coaching process with the client (Sinclair & Russell, 2002). These principles reflect one of the fundamental ideas addressed in coaching, and one that all humans face: We find fulfillment and hence balance through reconciling the paradox between expressing our unique selves while at the same time living in relationship with others and the world. The nine principles are organized into three groups (Sinclair, 2002). Each group reflects three areas of human development that contribute to successful resolution of this paradox: (1) principles that capture the nature of the human core self as being unique, creative, and meaning making; (2) principles that reflect each human's capacity to grow and develop through using their full range of capacities, reflection and inquiry, and exercising choice; and (3) principles that guide us in relating to others and the world (Sinclair, 2002). The nine principles are:

Principles Anchoring Us in Our Essential Selves

The first set of principles aims to anchor us in our unique, best self.

1. Every human being is creative and self-creating.
2. Every human being is by nature meaning seeking and meaning making.
3. Every human being has unique strengths and gifts with which to create a meaningful life.

Principles Supporting Development of Our Potential

The next set of principles focuses on developing our potential to its fullest.

4. Reflection and inquiry are essential for enhanced awareness, which in turn is a key in the quest for greater excellence and meaning in working and living.
5. A human being is an integrated whole consisting of many different aspects—mind, body, spirit, thinking, feeling, imagination, and so forth. Effective and meaningful working and living require congruence and synergy among these different elements.
6. As human beings, we have both the freedom and the responsibility to choose.

Principles for Entering Into Meaningful and Productive Relationships With Others and the World

The third set of principles guides us in relating to others and the world around us.

7. Our subjective view of reality—our beliefs, assumptions, mental models, and stories about ourselves, others, and the world in which we operate—influences our choices and actions.
8. As human beings, we are embedded in a multifaceted life, and we form part of many different systems of relationships.
9. The guiding principles outlined above serve to provide the grounding for intentional action leading to the creation of meaningful results. (Sinclair, 2002, pp. 2.4–2.5)

HOW PROFESSIONAL COACHING WORKS

As previously indicated, improving life balance involves making lasting lifestyle changes. For most, change can be daunting to take on alone, as it often requires getting rid of old habits that have taken years to develop and are deeply engrained and replacing them with new, unfamiliar, and at times initially uncomfortable habits. Working through the coaching process assists clients to go beyond identifying desired new habits to offering them an ally and the support they need to actually make the change occur in their lives. The coach provides much more than active listening and a sounding board for the client. Coaching's success is based on the careful orchestration of several tools and contexts designed to prompt client awareness, reflection, and behavior change. This relationship is unlike any other.

As described later in this chapter, the coaching profession appears to be at an emerging-discipline phase of its growth. Research and models specifically defining and describing the coaching processes are limited. The ICF outlines 11 core coaching competencies that are grouped into four main skill categories: (1) setting the foundation, (2) cocreating the relationship, (3) communicating effectively, and (4) facilitating learning and results. The ICF (2008) indicates that the skills in each area are "critical for any competent coach to demonstrate." Skills and approaches observed or demonstrated during a coaching session likely are derived from, or mirror, the ICF competencies. For more details regarding the coaching core competencies, visit www.coachfederation.org.

The co-active coaching model by Whitworth et al. (2007) is one current model that has many similarities to the concepts covered in the ICF competencies. The model uses the term *co-active* to refer to "the fundamental nature of a coaching relationship in which the coach and client are active collaborators" (p. 3) in meeting the clients' goals. The model includes five contexts that a coach brings to the coaching relationship that are continuously at work. The constant presence of these contexts, with the client in the center, make coaching unique.

1. *Listening at a deeper level.* This type of listening goes beyond the superficial level of what is being said and takes in information from all the senses throughout the exchange with the client. "It is the listening for the meaning behind the story, for the underlying process, for the theme that will deepen the learning. The coach is listening for the appearance of the client's vision, values, purpose" (Whitworth et al., 2007, pp. 10–11). Active listening on the part of the coach is crucial for supporting the client and mirroring to the client what is being said and what is going unsaid. Often a coach may notice that a client is avoiding a situation or forward movement or is stuck in a difficult situation, or he or she may notice where the client's true passion and values are and then offer it as feedback to the client. For example, a client may indicate that he wants to start his own business yet offers several excuses as to why he can't. During the coaching session, it becomes apparent that the real issue needing to be addressed is the client's fear of failure, not his excuses about why a business is not possible.

2. *Intuition.* Coaches strive to synthesize information from clients and from impressions about what they are saying. This includes the coach listening to his or her own gut responses and offering them to the client. Intuition may be triggered by a "visual image or an unexplained shift in emotion or energy" (Whitworth et al., 2007, p. 54). For example, the coach may say "I have a feeling that what is really bothering you is _____," "I am wondering if _____," or "I have a hunch that there is something more than what you are saying about _____." Once offered, the coach invites the client to reflect and accept, reject, or expand on the coach's impression. According to Whitworth et al. (2007), the value of coaches expressing their intuition in the coaching process lies in moving clients forward and furthering the client's understanding of their situation, not in whether the intuitive reaction is accurate.

3. *Curiosity.* Coaches operate from the premise that "clients are capable and resourceful and have the answers" (Whitworth et al., 2007, pp. 11–12); they come from a place of curiosity or openness toward what is occurring for the client. In the spirit of being curious, a coach asks powerful questions to create reflection and learning. Powerful questions are "really strong, provocative questions that send them [the client] into uncharted territory" (p. 77). Powerful questions can set the stage for the client to see situations from other points of view, to expand possibilities, and to initiate forward movement for finding their own answers. A coach may ask, "What is _____ about for you?" or "How is _____ working for you?" or "Where do we go from here?" Examples of powerful questions are limitless, and sometimes it is the simplest or, as Whitworth et al. indicate, the "dumb" question that best provokes the clients to become aware of his or her core truths or beliefs (p. 79).

4. *Forward and deepen.* Forwarding action and deepening learning are where coaches assist clients to stretch themselves to perform at a higher level. In this way, clients gain "resourcefulness, expanded possibilities, and stronger muscles for change" (Whitworth et al., 2007, p. 12). Some key strategies used by coaches to assist clients to forward action and deepen their learning include the following:

> ▣ *Establish goals.* Goals are established with the coach supporting the clients to imagine the future that clients want to invent and to set an overall intention of attaining that future. The coach encourages the client to open his or her perspective or expand his or her beliefs to the range of possibilities available. Intentions are then broken down into small steps or short-term behavioral goals that are meaningful and challenging yet realistic and manageable. For example, a client wanting to return to college may feel overwhelmed with where and how to begin. By breaking the overall intention of returning to college into smaller steps, such as researching potential career options, discussing related financial needs with a spouse, and investigating possible schools, and then taking one step at a time, the client is no longer paralyzed by the daunting task ahead and is able to move forward.

> ▣ *Develop challenges.* Challenges, requests, or experiments may be created in line with the client's goals. For example, a client struggling to begin a job search may be challenged to complete his résumé by the next coaching session, or a client wishing to create more time for herself may be asked to experiment with saying "no" to requests from friends and family demanding her time and noting the responses that occur.

> ▣ *Create accountability.* Accountabilities, commitments, or agreements are set between the coach and the client to forward the action on goals. These include agreeing on what steps the client will take, by when, and how progress will be communicated. It is the accountability part of coaching that is crucial to its success. This is an important step in the process, because when clients know that they will be reporting back to someone, it increases the likelihood of following through and takes them a step closer to meeting their goal.

> ▣ *Take an action–reflection–learning approach.* Coaching takes an action–reflection–learning approach. Once a client has tried to adopt a new behavior or make change, in a subsequent coaching session, the coach prompts him or her to reflect on what was learned. Areas of questioning include what worked, what didn't, what got in the way, and what needs to be done differently.

> ▣ *Use additional strategies.* Other strategies include requesting clients to put a physical or symbolic structure in place to remind them of the area or goal they are focusing on and, overall, heighten awareness. A structure may be as simple as hanging a note on the bathroom mirror with a goal or question written on it, tracking how many times a particular behavior occurs, such as agreeing to things one doesn't want to do, or burning a candle at bedtime as a reminder to reflect on one thing that went well during the day.

5. *Self-management.* For the coaching process to be successful, coaches must self-manage by setting aside their personal judgments and advice to allow clients to find their own answers. "The coach needs to be 'over there' with the client, immersed in the client's situation and struggle, not 'over here,' dealing with his or her judgments and thoughts" (Whitworth et al., 2007, p. 13). The values of the coach and the client may be very different, yet it is the role of the coach to accept what is being said as the client's reality and hold the client's agenda. Skills that a coach may use here include creating a clearing to bring the client's attention to the coaching session, "bottom-lining" to get to the essence of the client's message, asking permission to give candid feedback, and championing by providing acknowledgement of strengths.

PROFESSIONAL COACHING PROCESS

There are various ways coaching can take place: on the telephone, face-to-face, electronically, or a hybrid of these (Chapman, Lesch, & Pappas Baun, 2007; Grant & Zackon, 2004). Over-the-phone coaching is currently the most popular method (Grant & Zackon, 2004), as it is less expensive and can be more convenient than face-to-face sessions, not to mention it allows coaching to take place from great distances. Face-to-face coaching sessions are the second most commonly used and are thought to be more effective due to the more personal nature of meeting in person. Electronic coaching, such as using e-mail, is the least commonly used method, although many coaches use some electronic communication with clients (Grant & Zackon, 2004). Coaches may also use a mix of these modalities, depending on the needs of the client and the coach's availability. As technology develops, there is also mention in the coaching literature of the development of "computer-based coaching" in which the "coach is the computer program and the participant is communicating only through the computer" (Chapman et al., 2007, p. 2). This type of coaching may actually use "artificial intelligence, self-learning systems, and query engine logic in its operation" (p. 2). Although this type of coaching may allow participants convenient access, some of them may not be comfortable communicating directly with a computer. Motivation may also be decreased because participants know there is not another human being directly holding them accountable.

Some coaches specialize in working with teams, such as work groups, families, or other partnerships, to enhance performance as well as transition through changes (Whitworth et. al, 2007). These forms of coaching have an added layer of complexity in managing the individuals as well as the dynamics of the group and the interdependence of its members.

Another emerging area for coaching lies in coaching a group of individuals who have similar needs. Klippel (2006) uses the example of writers working with a coach in a group teleconference to write a book. Other examples might include coaching individuals with a particular diagnosis or disability or coaching in an area of common interest such as relationships or career transition. Although evidence-based research is lacking at this time, group coaching may be more cost-effective than one-on-one coaching and offer participants a sense of community or peer support as well as networking opportunities (Whitworth et al. as cited in Klippel, 2006).

Coaching sessions typically range in length from 30 to 60 minutes, with sessions occurring on average three times per month (Grant & Zackon, 2004). It is also common for coaching clients to have homework to complete between sessions (Klippel, 2006). Whitworth et al. (2007) describe homework inquiries as a type of powerful question that is asked at the end of a coaching session, "meant to give clients time for continued reflection and exploration" (p. 80). An example may be as simple as requesting the client to consider the question "What do I want?" or "What is getting in the way?" as they go about their week. Clients may also be asked to do homework in the form of journaling, experimenting with new behaviors, or looking at situations in a different way. The typical duration of the coaching relationship is 3 to 6 months, with many lasting 6 to 12 months (Grant & Zackon, 2004). This may be negotiated at the beginning of the coaching relationship, depending on the individual client.

PROFESSION OF COACHING: AN EMERGING DISCIPLINE

The concept of coaching is not new; however, the emergence of coaching as a profession is new. Coaching as a professional role can be traced back to examples of coaching relationships noted in the Bible (Chapman et al., 2007) and in the workplace, date back as far as 1937 in the periodical *Factory Management and Maintenance* (as cited in Stober & Grant, 2006) with a focus on coaching within organizations. In the 1960s and 1970s, coaching further developed out of the human potential movement. During this time, individuals were looking to expand their "perspectives, beliefs, and behaviors" to achieve self-actualization (Sorensen, 2005, p. 11). In the mid-1980s, Thomas Leonard, a financial planner, coined the term *life coaching* based on his belief that he was spending more time dealing with his clients' life issues than their actual finances (as cited in Klippel, 2006). Overall, the origins of coaching are grounded in organizational behavior and the potentiation of human performance in the workplace.

Despite this long history, in the academic and professional sense, coaching is still considered an emerging discipline. Although there have been thousands of references to coaching in the popular literature, there have been few in the academic literature (Grant & Cavanagh, 2004). Grant and Cavanagh's (2004) extensive review of academic literature on coaching indicates that "the coaching industry is far from meeting the basic requirements of a true profession" (p. 3). This is in part due to the challenges inherent in measuring and documenting its effectiveness. In some of the popular press, people have made "sensational claims about its [coaching's] ability to create the perfect life for clients" (Cavanagh et al., 2005, p. 6), inviting criticism as to its credibility. Grant, who coined the term *evidence-based coaching* (Stober & Grant, 2006, p. 4), says, "An evidence-based approach to coaching can make the difference between the often over-hyped coaching that tends to be adapted from personal development and motivational programs and professional coaching that draws on solid theory and research" (Cavanagh et al., 2005, p. 7). On the basis of this, it is most appropriate to say that coaching is an emerging profession with a history of citations in the literature dating back to the 1960s (Grant & Cavanagh, 2004).

Coaching Clients

In recent years, there has been an explosion of interest in the application of coaching in a wide variety of fields for achieving behavior change, optimal performance, health, and fulfillment. Research is slowly emerging that shows coaching is highly effective with various populations, including people with heart disease (Vale, Jelinek, Best, & Santamaria, 2002), people with HIV/AIDS (Garfinkel & Blumenthal, 2001), people with addictions (Shafer, Kiebzak, & Dwoskin, 2003), spinal cord injuries (Brachtesende, 2005), diabetes (Joseph, Griffin, Hall, & Sullivan, 2001; Kelly, Crowe, & Shearer, 2005), obstetrics (Hadikin, 2001), older adults (Holland, Greenberg, Tidwell, & Newcomer, 2003; Lynch, Morse, Mendelson, & Robins, 2003), health promotion (Irwin & Morrow, 2003), families in crisis (McGoldrick & Carter, 2001), workers who are stressed and underproductive (Yen, Edington, McDonald, Hirschland, & Edington, 2001), women who are mildly depressed (Pechinik, 2003), and executives (Kampa-Kokesch & Anderson, 2001).

Although many of the previous examples refer to applications of coaching within the health care context, it appears to be used more extensively by the private sector and the general public at this time. Non-health care uses of coaching include assisting people such as high-potential employees who have developmental needs; people going through transitions such as job search or change, retirement, divorce, or adjustment to disability; those experiencing a feeling of discontentment or that something is missing in their lives; or people having difficulty balancing roles and responsibilities.

According to Grant and Cavanaugh (2004) in a 2003 study using data collected from ICF members, coaching engagements tend to fall into three main categories: (1) executive coaching, (2) workplace coaching, and (3) life coaching. *Executive coaching* addresses areas such as improving strategic planning, team building, and leadership development. Generally, the client is someone who has managerial responsibilities. *Workplace coaching* is often used with nonexecutives in the workplace and emphasizes skill enhancement and transfer of training. There is minimal focus on personal or professional issues. *Life coaching* is holistic and is focused more on personal issues and life goals than those of the workplace (Cavanagh et al, 2005). It is in this latter context that issues of life balance will more likely be immediately raised. It is significant to mention, however, that life–balance concerns are often raised by clients in any of the coaching areas.

It is important to note that, "while often therapeutic, coaching is not a substitute for appropriate medical or psychological therapy" (Grant & Cavanagh, 2004, p. 11). Coaches are trained to be on the alert for clients who are in need of therapy and refer them as necessary. This is also reflected and supported in the ICF code of ethics. It is the responsibility of the coach to refer clients to other professionals when deemed appropriate (ICF, 2007b).

Reflecting again on Grant and Cavanagh's (2004) research, coach respondents indicated that they typically work with adults between the ages of 18 and 64. Of these clients, 73.9% are women. Coaches indicated that their clients were typically managers, executives, entrepreneurs, owners of small businesses, and professionals in private practice.

Many coaching practitioners coach in a particular niche area. Some examples include financial coach, writing coach, career coach, retirement coach, small business owner coach, women in transition coach, and artist coach (Klippel, 2006; Yousey, 2001). This allows the field to accommodate many types of clients and the various needs for change they may be seeking.

In addition to individuals, organizations use coaching. Coaching has become an "expected intervention component of any serious [worksite] wellness program initiative" (Chapman et al., 2007, p. 1). The types of health and wellness coaching provided for employees might include disease-management coaching, financial-planning coaching, and physical-training coaching. Educational institutions are also using professional life coaching. Principals and superintendents in some schools in high-poverty areas are being trained to become coaches in an effort to increase student achievement and enhance learning experiences for staff (Killion, 2002).

Training and Regulation of Professional Coaching

Currently coaching is not a regulated profession, meaning there are no licensing standards or professional review boards (Grant, 2003). Professional-coach training programs vary in format from workshops and seminars to programs lasting 2 years, with parts being in person, over the phone, or on-line. Required hours and experiences are variable. Training costs can range from the cost of a workshop to the cost of a university graduate degree. Like many professions, there are an abundance of continuing-education opportunities in a variety of formats available to practitioners.

Although there are many organizations that indicate they credential coaching programs or provide coaching training, it seems that the International Coach Federation is the most recognized worldwide. The ICF was founded in 1995 (ICF, 2007c) with the intention of being the "voice for the coaching profession" (ICF, 2007d). The ICF describes itself as the "largest worldwide resource for business and personal coaches, and the source for those who are seeking a coach" (ICF, 2007d). Currently, the organization has over 11,000 members in over 80 countries. The ICF is a nonprofit organization whose mission is to "build, support and preserve the integrity of the coaching profession" (ICF, 2007d). ICF developed and promotes the coaching profession's code of professional standards and coaching core competencies as well as the first "universally accepted accreditation process" with standardized credentialing (ICF, 2007d). The ICF accredited coach training programs (ACTP) must include the following: a minimum of 125 hours of coach-specific training, 100 direct client coaching hours of which 75 hours were paying clients, a minimum of 6 observed coaching sessions with an experienced coach, and a comprehensive final exam that evaluates a student's coaching competency. Certified graduates of an ACTP may apply for an ICF credential (ICF, 2007e).

The ICF offers credentialing at three levels: associate certified coach, professional certified coach, and master certified coach (ICF, 2007f). Each designation has specifically outlined requirements largely met through hours of experience. The master certified coach level has the most advanced requirements (2,500 hours of direct client coaching hours). Applicants to each level of certification must show evidence of training at an ACTP or accredited coach-specific training hours (ACSTH), documented hours with mentors, logged coaching experiences, coach references, and successful completion of an examination.

Although the ICF has a credentialing program in place, uncredentialed practitioners and training programs do not need to follow the standards that the ICF has set. Some coaching schools indicate that they are "aligned with" the ICF's core competencies and training requirements but do not necessarily meet ICF accreditation standards. According to research conducted in 2003 (Grant & Zackon, 2004), coaches in the marketplace have varying ranges of training. Results showed that 57.3% of coaches who responded claimed to hold a coaching credential, while only 19% held an ICF credential. Also of interest, 28.3% of respondents shared that they had not graduated from any coaching program, and approximately 10% of respondents had never been enrolled in a coach training program. It is highly possible that these statistics may be changing with growing public awareness and the maturity of the coaching profession. Nevertheless, there is a diverse range of training in the coaching field. Consumers currently need to satisfy themselves of a prospective coach's training, credentials, and background. Lacking a definite system for regulating training and practice is one of the criticisms about coaching and a hurdle for it to overcome to be viewed as an evidence-based profession. By having accredited training and credentialing standards that are grounded in rigorous research and articulated best practice standards, coaching is establishing credibility and professional recognition and demonstrating evidence of its effectiveness.

Profile of Professional Coaches

In 2006, ICF commissioned PricewaterhouseCoopers to undertake a global survey of coaches. In all, 5,415 coaches from 73 countries responded. Results indicated that the majority of those who responded hold an advanced degree such as a master's degree or a PhD. Over two-thirds of respondents were women. The biggest grouping in terms of age was 46 to 55 years. Consistent with the newness of the profession, the majority of respondents had been coaching for less than 10 years (ICF & PricewaterhouseCoopers, 2008).

Looking at the ICF member data from 2003, 99.9% of coaches came from a previous professional career, with 85.9% indicating they had some form of postsecondary education. Of those who responded to the survey, 40.8% indicated they had previously worked as consultants, 30.2% as executives, 30.8% as managers, 15.7% as teachers, and 13.8% as sales people. Also noteworthy is that out of this sample, 18.8% indicated backgrounds in the helping professions, such as social work, psychology, or counseling (Grant & Zackon, 2004, p. 6).

Finding a Professional Coach

ICF recommends a number of questions to ask when considering hiring a coach (ICF, 2007g). These include inquiring about the coach's background, such as type of training, credentials and years of experience, philosophy about coaching, logistics, and process of coaching. It may also be beneficial to ask the coach to share examples of success stories they have had working with individuals. Depending on your area of focus, it may be beneficial to consider searching for a coach who has a specialty or niche area of practice.

Of significant importance when looking for a professional coach is finding someone you feel you can be yourself with. This includes being able to speak freely while being honest about your thoughts and feelings. Ultimately, being comfortable having a professional relationship with the person coaching you is of utmost necessity for the coaching relationship to be a success.

Many coaches will offer a free introductory coaching session. This can be an effective method of determining your fit with a particular coach, as well as a way to learn more about the coaching process and if it is right for you.

CONCLUSION

There is an abundance of evidence to indicate that coaching is, at a minimum, here to stay or, even more likely, has the potential to be a major driving force in the future. The fact that the ICF alone has doubled its membership in the past 5 years (Ferrette, 2007) speaks to people's interest in making life changes and the effectiveness of coaches in assisting individuals in making these changes. The promising future for professional coaching is also evident in the focus of our health care systems. In efforts to cut costs, systems are shifting from the traditional medical model of fixing or treating illnesses toward a more proactive stance with a focus on prevention and wellness. In response to this shift, professional coaching is becoming more widely accepted as a vehicle for assisting people to make behavioral changes more quickly and in an individualized manner, whether to maintain and achieve good health or prevent illness.

Described as "a dynamic and vibrant emerging discipline with a distinct flavour and methodologies of its own" (Grant and Zackon, 2004, p. 13), professional coaching, by its very nature, can have a profound impact on life balance. The benefits of coaching are limitless. The process of coaching enables individuals to produce extraordinary results in their lives that they may not have been able to achieve on their own. With the support of a coach, clients are able to determine what it is they truly value in their lives and make choices that align with those defined values. Through this process of deeper learning, understanding, and taking action, individuals take steps toward bringing their ideal life balance to fruition. Coaching has the potential to precipitate transformation in individuals at a variety of levels; "Evidence-based professional coaching has the very real potential to become a powerful methodology for individual, organizational, social, and systemic change" (Stober and Grant, 2006, p. 6).

Erich Fromm said, "Man's main task in life is to give birth to himself, to become what he potentially is" (BrainyQuote, n.d.). The concept of life balance, although not universally defined, indicates that it is about living in a way in which one's true potential is recognized, utilized, and maximized. Life balance is reflected in what we do, the lifestyle we create, and the feelings surrounding it. Life balance is a process that occurs over time, is ongoing, and should be our life's work. It requires making intentional lifestyle choices and embracing change. Given the challenges inherent in achieving life balance, professional coaching, with its focus on supporting individuals as they realize their potential, appears to be a powerful resource for those desiring a more balanced life.

REFERENCES

Aspinall, L. G., & Staudinger, U. M. (Eds.). (2003). *A psychology of human strengths: Fundamental questions and future directions for a positive psychology.* Washington, DC: American Psychological Association.

Brachtesende, A. (2005). Life goals don't have to end with injuries. *OT Practice, 10*(9), 7–8.

BrainyQuote. (n.d). *Erich Fromm quotes.* Retrieved on January 7, 2008, from http://www.brainyquote.com/quotes/authors/e/erich_fromm.html

Cavanagh, M., Grant, A., & Kemp, T. (2005). *Evidence-based coaching: Theory, research, and practice from the behavioural sciences,* (Vol. 1). Bowen Hills, Queensland, Australia: Australian Academic Press.

Chapman, L., Lesch, N., & Pappas Baun, M. (2007). The role of health and wellness coaching in worksite health promotion. *American Journal of Health Promotion 21,* 1–10.

Cooperrider, D. L., & Whitney, D. (1999). *Appreciative inquiry.* San Francisco: Berrett-Koehler Communications.

Cooperrider, D. L., Whitney, D., & Stavros, J. M. (2003). *Appreciative inquiry handbook.* San Francisco: Berrett-Koehler Publishers.

DePoy, E., & Gitlin, L. (2005). *Introduction to research: Understanding and applying multiple strategies* (3rd ed.). St. Louis: Elsevier Mosby.

Dreikurs, R. (1953). *Fundamentals of Adlerian Psychology.* Chicago: Alfred Adler Institute.

Emmons, R. A. (2003). Personal goals, life meaning, and virtue: Wellsprings of a positive life. In C. L. M. Keys & J. Haidt, J. (Eds.), *Flourishing: Positive psychology and the life well-lived* (pp. 105–128). Washington, DC: American Psychological Association.

Ferrette, C. (2007) *Life coaches help answer: What's next?* Retrieved October 18, 2007, from http://www.thejournalnews. com/apps/pbcs.dll/article?AID=2007710010355

Frankl, V. (1984). *Man's search for meaning.* New York: Washington Square Press.

Frederickson, B. (2003). The value of positive emotions [Electronic version]. *American Scientist, 91,* 330–335.

Garfinkel, M., & Blumenthal, E. (2001). Co-active coaching and HIV. *AIDS Alert, 16,* 105–108.

Glasser, W. (2000). *Choice theory: The new reality therapy.* New York: HarperCollins.

Grant, A., & Cavanagh, M. (2004). Toward a profession of coaching: Sixty-five years of progress and challenges for the future. *International Journal of Evidence Based Coaching and Mentoring, 2,* 1–16.

Grant, A., & Zackon, R. (2004). Executive, workplace and life coaching: Findings from a large-scale survey of International Coach Federation Members. *International Journal of Evidence Based Coaching and Mentoring, 2*(2), 1–15.

Grant, P. (2003). Coaches for the game of life. *More, 6*(6), 70–73.

Hadikin, R. (2001). Co-active coaching: An introduction. *Practicing Midwife, 4*(7), 36–37.

Holland, S. K., Greenberg, J., Tidwell, L., & Newcomer, R. (2003). Preventing Disability through community-based health coaching. *Journal of the American Geriatrics Society, 51,* 265–269.

Hollis, J. (2001). *Creating a life: Finding your individual path.* Toronto: Inner City Books.

International Coach Federation. (2007a). *What is coaching?* Retrieved October 7, 2007, from http://www.coachfederation.org/ICF/For+Coaching+Clients/What+is+a+Coach/

International Coach Federation. (2007b). *The ICF code of ethics.* Retrieved October 7, 2007, from http://www.coachfederation.org/ICF/For+Current+Members/Ethical+Guidelines/Code+of+Ethics/

International Coach Federation. (2007c). *Background information and membership facts.* Retrieved October 7, 2007, from http://www.coachfederation.org/NR/rdonlyres/257CE43D-C730-4556-9D4B-F8B53061AA56/6927/sept_07Page01.pdf

International Coach Federation. (2007d). *The International Coach Federation.* Retrieved October 7, 2007, from http://www.coachfederation.org/ICF/For+Coaching+Clients/What+is+ICF/

International Coach Federation. (2007e). *Coach training programs.* Retrieved October 7, 2007, from http://www.coachfederation.org/ICF/For+Current+Members/Coach+Training/For+Prospective+Students/

International Coach Federation. (2007f). *Become credentialed.* Retrieved October 7, 2007, from http://www.coachfederation.org/ICF/For+Current+Members/Credentialing/Become+Credentialed/

International Coach Federation. (2007g). *A guide to choosing a professional coach.* Retrieved October 7, 2007, from http://www.coachfederation.org/NR/rdonlyres/257CE43D-C730-4556-9D4B-F8B53061AA56/6235/coach.pdf

International Coach Federation. (2008). *Coaching core competencies.* Retrieved April 7, 2008, from http://www.coachfederation.org/ICF/For+Current+Members/Credentialing/Why+a+Credential/Competencies/

International Coach Federation, & PricewaterhouseCoopers. (2008). *International Coach Federation global coaching study executive summary revised February 2008.* Retrieved April, 7, 2008, from http://www.coachfederation.org/NR/rdonlyres/257CE43D-C730-4556-9D4B-F8B53061AA56/7778/ExecutiveSummaryFinalversion20.pdf

Irwin, J. D., & Morrow, D. (2003, November). *The co-active coaching method as a theoretical grounded strategy for "doing" health promotion.* Proceedings of the First International Coach Federation Research Symposium. Denver.

Joseph, D., Griffin, M., Hall, R., & Sullivan, E. (2001). Peer coaching: An intervention for individuals struggling with diabetes. *Diabetes Educator, 27,* 703–710.

Kampa-Kokesch, S., & Anderson, M. Z. (2001). Executive coaching: A comprehensive review of the literature. *Consulting Psychology Journal, 53,* 205–229.

Kegan, R. (1982). *The evolving self: Problem and process in human development.* Cambridge, MA: Harvard University Press.

Kegan, R. (1994). *In over our heads: The mental demands of modern life.* Cambridge, MA: Harvard University Press.

Kelly, J., Crowe, P., & Shearer, M. (2005). The Good Life Club project: Telephone coaching for chronic disease self-management. *Australian Family Physician, 34,* 31–34.

Keys, C. L. M., & Haidt, J. (Eds.). (2003). *Flourishing: Positive psychology and the life well-lived.* Washington, DC: American Psychological Association.

Killion, J. (2002). Soaring with their own life coach: Participants concentrate on 12 strategies for success in all areas of life. *Journal of Staff Development, 23*(2), 19–22.

Klippel, L. (2006). A horse of a different color: Mental health, occupational therapy, and coaching. *Mental Health Special Interest Section Quarterly, 29*(1), 1–4.

Lynch, T. R., Morse, J. Q., Mendelson, T., & Robins, C. J. (2003). Dialectical behaviour therapy for depressed older adults. *American Journal of Geriatric Psychiatry, 11,* 33–45.

May, R. (1953). *Man's search for himself.* New York: Dell.

May, R. (1975). *The courage to create.* New York: Norton.

May, R. (1983). *The discovery of being: Writings in existential psychology.* New York: Norton.

McGoldrick, B., & Carter, B. (2001). Advances in coaching: Family therapy with one person. *Journal of Marital and Family Therapy, 27,* 281–300.

Mezirow, J. (2000). *Learning as transformation: Critical perspectives on a theory in progress.* San Francisco: Jossey-Bass.

Pechinik, J. (2003). *Treatment of mild depression in female employees: A program design.* Dissertation Abstracts International, 64 (12-B), 428. U.S.: L Univ. Microfilms International.

Ryan, R. M., & Deci, E. L. (2001). *On happiness and human potential: A review of research on hedonic and eudaimonic well-being. Annual Review of Psychology.* Retrieved February 3, 2004, from http://www.findarticles.com/cf_0/m1175/3_33/62215085/p1/article.jhtml

Seligman, M. E. P. (2002). *Authentic happiness: Using the new positive psychology to realize your potential for lasting fulfillment.* New York: The Free Press.

Shafer, K. C., Kiebzak, L., & Dwoskin, J. (2003). Coaching: A new role for addictions. Journal of Social Work Practice in Addictions 3, *105–112.*

Sinclair, M. (2002) *Moving toward artful coaching—Approach and philosophy overview.* Toronto: Adler School of Professional Coaching

Sinclair, M., & Russell, D. (2002). *Foundations of professional coaching [Binder].* Toronto: Adler School of Professional Coaching.

Snyder, C. R. & Lopez, S. J. (Eds.). (2002). *Handbook of positive psychology.* Oxford: Oxford University Press.

Sorensen, J. (2005). Coaching: Another emerging practice area. *Advance, 21*(16), 11.

Stober, D., & Grant, A. (2006). *Evidence based coaching handbook: Putting best practices to work for your clients.* Hoboken, NJ: John Wiley & Sons.

Thurman, R. (2005). *The jewel of Tibet: The enlightenment engine of Tibetan Buddhism.* New York: Free Press.

Vale, M. J., Jelinek, M. V., Best, J. D., & Santamaria, J. D. (2002). Coaching patients with coronary heart disease to achieve the target cholesterol: A method to bridge the gap between evidence-based medicine and the "real world"—randomized controlled trial. *Journal of Clinical Epidemiology, 55,* 245–252.

Vaillant, G. (2002). *Aging well.* Boston: Little, Brown.

Whitworth, L., Kimsey-House, K., Kimsey- House, H., & Sandahl, P. (2007). *Co-active coaching: New skills for coaching people toward success in work and life.* Mountain View, CA: Davies-Black.

Yen, L., Edington, M. P., McDonald, T., Hirschland, D., & Edington, D. (2001). Changes in health risks among the participants in United Auto Workers-General Motors LifeSteps Health Promotion Program. *American Journal of Health Promotion, 16,* 7–15.

Yousey, J. R. (2001). Life coaching: A one on one approach to changing lives. *OT Practice, 16*(1), 11–14.

SECTION V

Future Research on Life Balance

CHAPTER 17

Research Directions for Advancing the Study of Life Balance and Health

CATHERINE BACKMAN AND DANA ANABY

INTRODUCTION

Life balance can be viewed in a number of ways, and the complexity of the construct has been illuminated by the different perspectives on balance described in the preceding chapters. The various authors offered historical, theoretical, empirical, and practical considerations in their particular perspective or line of inquiry. Some of these ideas had been presented by the authors at the International Life Balance Conference held in Kingston, Ontario, in 2007. To bring the conference to a close, the final discussion focused on generating a research agenda to advance the study of life balance, health, and well-being. Participants were asked to consider if life balance is a legitimate construct and if so, to identify gaps in knowledge and propose directions for ongoing scholarly activity (Figure 17-1). These responses influenced the development of the present chapter, the purpose of which is to articulate potential research directions for the study of life balance and health, drawing on the preceding chapters for examples of research questions.

The research agenda presented here is a first draft. Although the topics are drawn from the book as a whole, they are not the result of a consensus or priority exercise. They are simply suggestions potentially worthy of systematic inquiry. A preliminary organizational scheme is presented in Table 17-1. In this scheme, research topics are loosely categorized as either theoretical or applied research. Theoretical topics are those that contribute to conceptual clarity as well as the development of conceptual models that explore relationships among the various factors contributing to life balance and potentially explain how life balance influences health. The applied research category offers topics for empirical study, such as developing valid tools for measuring life balance, methodological approaches congruent with theoretical assumptions, and observational and intervention studies aimed at testing theoretical relationships and approaches to enhancing life balance.

The lack of conceptual clarity was a substantial source of discussion and debate at the conference. Whether life balance is distinct from other constructs or a renaming of old ideas generated lively discussion. This discussion was aimed at determining whether or not life balance could be defined succinctly and distinctly in a manner that satisfied the attendees.

K. Matuska & C. Christiansen (Eds.)
Life balance: Multidisciplinary theories and research (pp 257–268)
© 2009 SLACK Incorporated and AOTA Press

LIFE BALANCE (LB) AS A PATTERN OF ACTIVITY

✦ LB refers to the orchestration of daily activities.

✦ LB considers roles, activities, and time.

LIFE BALANCE AS CONGRUENCE OR DISCREPANCY BETWEEN WHAT IS AND WHAT IS DESIRED

✦ *Congruence* may be a more appropriate term than *balance*.

✦ The foundation of LB is congruence with personal values—what's important.

✦ Life congruence = demands and expectations balanced with what one wants to do.

✦ LB = the match or discrepancy between desired reality and actual reality.

✦ LB = the match between actual and ideal arrangement of energy, time, resources, and skills in carrying out life roles.

✦ LB = the match between what people do and what they want to do or value.

✦ Achieving LB may require adjusting both desires and expectations.

LIFE BALANCE AS TIME USE

✦ LB has to do with the way we partition time.

✦ LB = the actual use of time relative to what is important to the person.

LIFE BALANCE IS INFORMED BY THEORY.

LIFE BALANCE IS INDIVIDUALLY DEFINED BASED ON WHAT IS IMPORTANT AND MEANINGFUL.

LIFE BALANCE REQUIRES MULTIPLE DEFINITIONS DEPENDING ON THE LEVEL AT WHICH IT IS EXAMINED.

✦ LB occurs at individual, corporate, societal, and other levels.

✦ Behaviors at each level influence perceived LB at every other level.

✦ People lacking control, at least at the individual level, cannot achieve congruence between desired and actual state of affairs.

LIFE BALANCE REQUIRES MEASURABLE OUTCOMES.

✦ Measuring discrepancy between what is and what is desired may be a start.

LIFE BALANCE IS DIFFERENT FROM

✦ Quality of life

✦ Stress.

Figure 17-1. Defining Life Balance: Issues raised by participants at the International Life Balance Conference, 2007.

DEFINING LIFE BALANCE

The discussion suggested that reaching consensus on a definition is likely not possible. However, we do not view this as problematic, because we propose that a single definition of *life balance* is not necessary to advance the research agenda. A defining characteristic of the construct is its subjectivity. Consider, for example, Marks and MacDermid's single-item measure "Nowadays I seem to enjoy every part of my life equally well," wherein the individual is invited to decide what is relevant rather than having the researcher decide this (Marks & MacDermid, 1996). Some elements of life balance may be relevant to one person or group but not to another; relevance may

Table 17-1

RESEARCH AGENDA

GENERAL GOALS	RESEARCH ISSUES OR QUESTIONS	READ MORE IN CHAPTER
THEORETICAL AND PHILOSOPHICAL TOPICS		
Conceptual Clarity	Is life balance a universal construct?	Chapter 3
	Is a balanced life a better life?	Chapter 11
	Is life balance distinct from other concepts (e.g., psychological well-being)? Is there a definition of life balance that resolves the circularity problem (in which the predictor and the outcome are conceptualized in the same way)?	Chapter 6
	Is imbalance necessarily to be avoided, or can it have benefits?	Chapter 6
	Why is the life in balance better than a life not so? In what manner, precisely, is life in balance better? What is being balanced in the balanced life?	Chapter 2
	Is there a stable distribution of time, a time balance, which is just appropriate to maintain society?	Chapter 8
	How much time is too much? Can one desire too much of a good thing?	Chapter 14
	How do different populations experience (im)balance in everyday life?	Chapter 10
Theoretical Relationships	How does life balance affect happiness? How does life balance relate to personal stress?	Chapter 8
	If people live up to their potential, will they consider themselves more balanced and happier?	Chapter 16
	What characteristics of everyday activity (occupations) contribute to life balance? How do control, meaning, manageability, and occupational balance interact to impact health?	Chapter 9
	Is the absence of work–life balance the most important factor explaining stress? (Other factors, such as satisfaction with work, level of control, involvement, and recognition, may be more important).	Chapter 2
	Does engaging in activities deemed passionate, to which one is highly committed, increase energy and balance? Test the scarcity theory—To what degree does limited time and energy fit with how people experience their everyday lives?	Chapter 5
	Test the value congruence theory—To what degree does making choices congruent with both values and environmental demands impact well being?	Chapter 12

Table 17-1 continued

General Goals	Research Issues or Questions	Read More in Chapter
Applied Research Topics		
Measurement	How can the presence of a state of balance within a person's life be quantified?	
	Are balance and imbalance opposite extremes of a single dimension, or are they differing dimensions? (Could a person be both balanced and unbalanced at the same time?)	Chapter 6
	Create and validate appropriate measures of life balance (e.g., discrepant time use profile)	
	How does time use differ among people who are balanced or imbalanced?	Chapter 8
	How is balance assessed when a person cannot understand the abstract concept, regulate emotions, or adapt to stress? If balance is a perceived, subjective phenomenon and a person has impaired cognition, how do they perceive balance?	Chapter 15
	Is imbalance reflected by the discrepancy between what a person has and wants? Is this gap related to well-being? What discrepancy methods/approaches could better explain well-being?	Chapter 7
Patterns of Engaging in Activity	What are the costs and benefits of students working part-time?	Chapter 14
	Chart lifestyle mixes to assess balance and happiness.	Chapter 4
	How do (specify a target population) experience and perceive balance within their daily occupations?	Chapter 9
	What are the consequences (negative and positive) of structured time?	Chapter 13
	How do people frame their lives and achieve life balance in the presence of limited roles and functional and adaptive limitations (e.g., disturbed affect following brain injury)	Chapter 15
	What kinds of activity patterns enable people to meet basic and important needs? What makes an activity meaningful, and how does this impact perceived balance?	Chapter 11
	Does retirement lead to lack of need fulfillment, life purpose, and identity?	Chapter
Prevalence of (Im)balance	Are the most hurried children stressed? What proportion of children are hurried?	Chapter 13

Table 17-1 continued

GENERAL GOALS	RESEARCH ISSUES OR QUESTIONS	READ MORE IN CHAPTER
Impact of Social Location	What factors promote balance at micro-, meso-, and macro-levels?	Chapter 9
	How do social spaces enable or constrain balance?	Chapter 8
	Examine the cultural alternatives to locating balance (e.g., "joyful community" where participants fully commit and engage in all activities.)	Chapter 5
	Is life balance relevant in an environment where, structurally and practically, productivity, caregiving, obligation, and relatedness happen in a culturally meaningful, naturalistic, and meshed way?	Chapter 3
	Study balance at the level of a social unit (e.g., family. How do resources vs. values drive family lifestyles?)	Chapter 13
Preventing Illness	What factors prevent imbalance? Does preventing imbalance prevent ill health?	Chapter 9
	Are there certain internal factors or personal characteristics that increase the risk for burnout?	Chapter 11
	To what extent does life coaching contribute to balance and prevention of imbalance/ill health?	Chapter 16

also change over time or in response to various circumstances. Instead of a consensus definition, we propose that there are elements to consider in articulating a definition to be used to guide each specific study or avenue of scholarly inquiry. A coherent terminology for these elements (yet to be fully developed) may serve as a starting point for researchers to create a definition of life balance appropriate to the study purpose. Such an operational or working definition assists in the design and conduct of research and in communicating the findings.

A rigorous study is typically influenced by one or more theoretical approaches. The theoretical definition serves as the basis for an operational definition to guide a systematic study plan. Moreover, as has been illustrated in this book, there are a number of closely related concepts that will figure more or less prominently in any definition of life balance, depending on the guiding theory. Subjective well-being and happiness are two examples that may be viewed as overlapping, related to, or distinct from life balance. Examining the theoretical relationships among all these concepts is one avenue for further research. Such studies will contribute to an enhanced understanding of life balance as well as articulate more precise definitions.

What elements should be considered when operationalizing life balance? Life balance seems to apply nearly universally, albeit in differing ways. Various aspects of life balance are important to children, working and nonworking adults, and people of various ages and cultures and with differing abilities living various settings. Life balance seems applicable across the life span and across ability continua, but different aspects may be of greater or lesser importance in the context of one's life. That which constitutes life balance for a middle-class working mother in suburban North America may be quite different from that of a mother whose family is homeless in the inner city. And both may experience life balance differently than a mother (and her family) displaced from their village due to war or conflict in countries experiencing political unrest. Many notions of life balance favor the privileged in stable societies, where the basic needs for surviving and thriving are accessible, but a theory-driven definition of life balance should acknowledge layers of complexity and contain elements applicable to myriad settings and circumstances. This multidimensional framework should have the following characteristics:

- *Subjective.* The concept of life balance is internally determined and reflects the person's point of view. People experience balance (Backman, in press; Jonsson & Persson, 2006); it cannot be objectively observed (although there may be observable behaviors indicating more or less life balance). Contextual factors may influence the extent to which a subjective view is perceived as an individual, self-oriented view versus a collective view (see, for example, Whiteford's [2009] discussion of Grandmothers Against Poverty and AIDS in Chapter 3).

- *Individual.* Definitions of life balance should be able to reflect the values, roles, and activities of greatest importance to the person (or group) participating in the research or using the research findings. Life balance will vary from one person and group to another, and that's okay. Definitions that allow for individual interpretation will incorporate multiple dimensions and move away from dichotomous categories such as work–life balance, work–family balance, and work–leisure balance. These dichotomies miss the complexity of patterns in daily activity and role occupancy.

- *Dynamic.* Life balance fluctuates and changes over time (Håkansson, Dahlin-Ivanoff, & Sonn, 2006), be it within a year, a life span, or in response to specific events (Marks, 2009). Cummins (2009) proposes subjective well-being as an indicator of balance, noting that it is relatively stable due to homeostasis. Therefore, subjective well-being ratings that fall outside an anticipated range indicate substantive fluctuations in life balance (or homeostatic failure).

- *Contextual.* Life balance is influenced by the environment, including time, space, and societal expectations. Pentland and McColl (2009) describe how environmental demands and expectations may create tension when responding to them is not in accordance with one's values, strengths, and sense of meaning—a condition contrary to life balance viewed from the perspective of emotional state. Giving consideration to contextual factors requires that choices be congruent with one's values and responsive to the environment: Excluding neither individual integrity nor environmental demands and expectations leads to well-being (Pentland & McColl, 2009).

◻ *Theoretically consistent.* As previously noted, variations in definitions of life balance, or even the label itself, reflect differences in theory. To effectively communicate research findings, the underlying theory should be made explicit, and its terminology carried throughout the definition of the construct and design of subsequent research or inquiry. For example, in this text we have read about *lifestyle balance* (Matuska & Christiansen, 2009), *occupational integrity* (Pentland & McColl, 2009), *role balance* (Marks, 2009), and *occupational balance* (Erlandsson & Håkansson, 2009)—each construct defined in a way that is consistent with a specific theoretical position, yet each still offering a perspective on life balance in general.

◻ *Related to "bigger" outcomes.* Life balance is hypothesized to be an indicator of health and well-being. A working definition should describe the anticipated link between life balance and these or other outcomes. Is it a metaphor for subjective well-being? And if so, under what circumstances?

Matuska and Christiansen (Chapter 11) define a *balanced lifestyle* as "a satisfying pattern of daily occupations that is healthful, meaningful, and sustainable to an individual within the context of his or her current life circumstances" (p. 150 in this volume). This generally incorporates most of the elements outlined above, although we may make different inferences about what contributes to each element, such as assuming the dynamic nature of balance is recognized by the phrase "current life circumstances." Regardless, this notion of a pattern of occupation or activity is emerging as one way of conceptualizing balance and has the potential to recognize many layers in the construct. Time use is one such layer, illustrated by the way people actually spend their time, their satisfaction with time use, and whether or not there is a gap between the actual versus the ideal use of time (Cummins, Chapter 7; Harvey & Singleton, Chapter 8; Sheldon, Chapter 6). Other layers incorporated in activity patterns consider the number, duration, intensity, and complexity of activities (Erlandsson & Håkansson, Chapter 9; Harvey & Singleton, Chapter 8; Hofferth, Kinney, & Dunn, Chapter 13; Marks, Chapter 5; Matuska & Christiansen, Chapter 11; Veenhoven, Chapter 4), offering several targets for quantifying factors representing the rhythm or pattern of activities characterizing life balance.

It is further assumed that the qualities or characteristics of the activities themselves influence perceived balance. These characteristics include (1) meeting psychological needs (Christiansen & Matuska, Chapter 11); (2) having congruence with personal values (Pentland & McColl, Chapter 12); (3) demonstrating competence (Westhorp, 2003); (4) providing different affective experiences such as relaxation or excitement (Jonsson & Persson, 2006; Persson & Jonsson, Chapter 10); and (5) having a positive and facilitating impact on each activity within the person's (or group's) cluster of current activities, not a negative and interfering impact (Christiansen, 1996; Riediger & Freund, 2004). Therefore, those measuring life balance need to consider not just the observable pattern of activities (as in time use) but also the nature and quality of the activities (as in judging congruence with personal or societal values).

For example, from the perspective of daily rhythms, a "workaholic" might be perceived as being imbalanced—this is an outsider's (or etic) view. However, from the perspective of quality and congruence, this same person may feel optimal life balance because the challenge, meaning, and satisfaction gained from the work not only contributes to a sense of well-being but also feeds it and produces more energy (Marks, Chapter 5). This is the insider's (or emic) view. Both outside and inside (etic and emic) perspectives may be important in developing better measures of life balance.

MEASURING LIFE BALANCE

Measuring life balance has been a challenge, in part due to the lack of conceptual clarity. Once a theoretical approach and operational definition are specified to explore a research hypothesis, it is necessary to select a measure congruent with that definition. Is life balance a one-dimensional or two-dimensional concept? Are balance and imbalance opposing anchors on a single continuum, or are they independent dimensions that can coexist? The answer influences the measurement strategy: As a one-dimensional concept, both balance (e.g., positive or high scores) and imbalance (e.g., negative or low scores) are measured on one scale. As a two-dimensional concept, each factor is measured separately: one scale for balance (positive aspect) and one scale for imbalance (negative aspect). The two-dimensional measurement strategy would answer questions like the one posed by Marks (2009): Is it possible to experience balance and imbalance at the same time? For example, a person might feel that their daily pattern fits with their interests and values (balanced life) but does not fit the environmental expectation (unbalanced). There are empirical ways to test this claim, such as confirmatory factor analysis (where we expect a two-factor solution) or evaluating how each of the two dimensions are independently associated with well-being, assuming well-being is even the outcome of life balance! In our own research, there is evidence that negative indicators of life balance are inversely associated with well-being, while positive indicators are not, supporting the two-dimensional view (Anaby, Jarus, & Backman, 2009).

Creating and validating measures of life balance is an avenue that requires exploration. The extent to which a measure is congruent with the selected theoretical and operational definitions is just the beginning. Measures are required that can discriminate among groups (on the basis of age, ability, and so on), and might also be evaluated for applicability to differing life views. That, however, brings us full circle to selecting a measure compatible with the theoretical definition—and that definition is likely to be quite different when based upon the life view arising from Eastern versus Western philosophies, for example.

ORGANIZING A RESEARCH AGENDA ON LIFE BALANCES

In this chapter, we have attempted to synthesize much of the discussion on life balance that occured at the international conference into a draft research agenda. This was challenging, because the chapters presented in this book offered myriad ideas worthy of further exploration and generated numerous additional research questions we could consider. In sifting through these ideas, it was not feasible to itemize all emerging questions, but a selection was presented in Table 17-1. Beyond the theoretical studies and measurement studies that are necessary, we believe there is a need to look for new information (as Sheldon points out in Chapter 6). Cross-sectional and longitudinal studies may explore the personal, social, and cultural factors associated with life balance and, in turn, its association with health and illness. Very little is known about the dynamic nature of life balance—for example, how it changes across the life span, and the impact of critical life events such as immigration; transition to new life roles (e.g., parent, spouse); losses arising from divorce, death, or disability; or milestones (e.g., graduation, new employment, special achievements). Intervention studies will help identify which, if any, strategies and behaviors improve life balance, and for whom.

Figure 17-1 presents a structure for organizing hypotheses for further study, based on our theoretical upbringing in occupational science and occupational therapy. However, the occupational-balance curve depicted here assumes that balance is a one-dimensional concept. Given the earlier discussion, this curve might be visualized as a double rainbow—with balance on one curve and imbalance on a second curve—to test both one- and two-dimensional perspectives. Another way of comparing balance and imbalance is through use of a classic quadrant (2 x 2 matrix; see Figure 17-2).

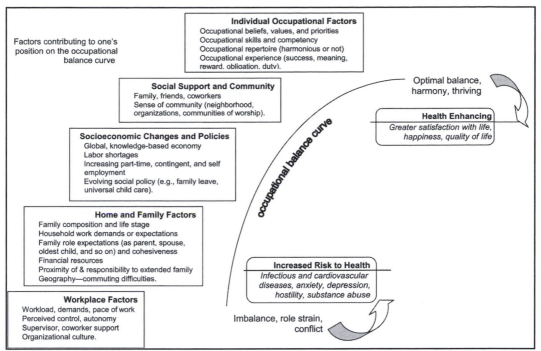

Figure 17-1. Studying life balance; a framework for organizing research questions and hypotheses. (Reprinted with permission from Backman, C. (in press). Occupational balance and well-being. In C.H. Christiansen and E.A. Townsend (Eds.) *Introduction to occupation: The art and science of everyday living.* Prentice-Hall.)

Figure 17-2. Preliminary organizational scheme.

low balance high imbalance	high balance high imbalance
low balance low imbalance	high balance low imbalance

balance (horizontal axis)

imbalance (vertical axis)

CONCLUSION

We view life balance as a concept that defies a single, universal definition. As a construct for further study, it requires careful consideration of specific elements when operationalized for research purposes. We propose that definitions of life balance should be subjective, individual, dynamic, contextual, theoretically consistent, and related to bigger outcomes, such as health and well-being.

We hypothesize that life balance and imbalance can coexist and that the former is enhanced and the latter reduced when everyday activities and life roles are congruent with values and priorities, sufficiently stimulating or challenging, and free from conflict (Backman, in press). Do we believe that life balance is a legitimate construct, worthy of research? Yes.

REFERENCES

Anaby, D., Jarus, T., & Backman, C. L. (2009). *Measuring occupational balance and its relationship to well-being.* Manuscript submitted for publication.

Backman, C. (in press). Occupational balance and well-being. In C. H Christiansen & E. A. Townsend (Eds.), *Introduction to occupation: The art and science of everyday living* (2nd ed.). Upper Saddle River, NJ: Prentice-Hall.

Christiansen, C. H. (1996). Three perspectives on balance in occupation. In R. Zemke & F. Clark (Eds.), *Occupational science: The evolving discipline.* (pp. 431–451). Philadelphia: F. A. Davis.

Christiansen, C. H., & Matuska, K. M. (2006). Lifestyle balance: A review of concepts and research. *Journal of Occupational Science, 13,* 49–61.

Cummins, R. A. (2009). Measuring life balance through discrepancy theories and subjective well-being. In K. Matuska, C. Christiansen, & H. J. Polatajko (Eds.), *Life balance: Multidisciplinary theories and research* (pp. TK). Bethesda, MD/Thorofare, NJ: AOTA Press/SLACK Incorporated.

Erlandsson, L.-K., & Håkansson, C. (2009). Aspects of daily occupations the promote life balance among women in Sweden. In K. Matuska & C. Christiansen (Eds.), *Life balance: Multidisciplinary theories and research* (pp. 83–103). Bethesda, MD/Thorofare, NJ: AOTA Press/SLACK Incorporated.

Håkansson, C., Dahlin-Ivanoff, S., & Sonn, U. (2006). Achieving balance in everyday life. *Journal of Occupational Science, 13,* 74–82.

Harvey, A. S., & Singleton, J. (2009). Time use and balance. In K. Matuska & C. Christiansen (Eds.), *Life balance: Multidisciplinary theories and research* (pp. 127-142). Bethesda, MD/Thorofare, NJ: AOTA Press/SLACK Incorporated.

Hofferth, S. L., Kinney, D. A., & Dunn, J. S. (2009). The "hurried" child: Myth versus reality. In K. Matuska & C. Christiansen (Eds.), *Life balance: Multidisciplinary theories and research* (pp. 201–223). Bethesda, MD/Thorofare, NJ: AOTA Press/SLACK Incorporated.

Jonsson, H., & Persson, D. (2006). Towards an experiential model of occupational balance: An alternative perspective on flow theory analysis. *Journal of Occupational Science, 13,* 63–73.

Marks, S. R. (2009). Multiple roles and life balance: An intellectual journey. In K. Matuska & C. Christiansen (Eds.), *Life balance: Multidisciplinary theories and research* (pp. 49–66). Bethesda, MD/Thorofare, NJ: AOTA Press/SLACK Incorporated.

Marks, S. R., & MacDermid, S. M. (1996). Multiple roles and the self: A theory of role balance. *Journal of Marriage and the Family, 58,* 417–432.

Matuska, K., & Christiansen, C. (2009). A model of lifestyle balance and imbalance. In K. Matuska & C. Christiansen (Eds.), *Life balance: Multidisciplinary theories and research* (pp. 163-179). Bethesda, MD/Thorofare, NJ: AOTA Press/SLACK Incorporated.

Pentland, W., & McColl, M.A. (2009). Another perspective on life balance: Living in integrity with values. In K. Matuska, C. Christiansen, H. J. Polatajko, & Jane Davis (Eds.), *Life balance: Multidisciplinary theories and research* (pp. TK). Bethesda, MD/Thorofare, NJ: AOTA Press/SLACK Incorporated.

Persson, D., & Jonsson, H. (2009). The importance of experiential challenges in a balanced life: Micro- and macro-perspectives. In K. Matuska, C. Christiansen, & H. J. Polatajko (Eds.), *Life balance: Multidisciplinary theories and research* (pp. TK). Bethesda, MD/Thorofare, NJ: AOTA Press/SLACK Incorporated.

Riediger, M., & Freund, A. M. (2004). Interference and facilitation among personal goals: Differential associations with subjective well-being and persistent goal pursuit. *Personality and Social Psychology Bulletin, 30,* 1511–1523.

Sheldon, K. M. (2009). Defining and validating measures of life balance: Suggestions, a new measure, and some preliminary results. In K. Matuska, C. Christiansen, & H. J. Polatajko (Eds.), *Life balance: Multidisciplinary theories and research* (pp. TK). Bethesda, MD/Thorofare, NJ: AOTA Press/SLACK Incorporated.

Veenhoven, R. (2009). Optimal lifestyle mix: An inductive approach. In K. Matuska, C. Christiansen, & H. J. Polatajko (Eds.), *Life balance: Multidisciplinary theories and research* (pp. TK). Bethesda, MD/Thorofare, NJ: AOTA Press/SLACK Incorporated.

Westhorp, P. (2003). Exploring balance as a concept in occupational science. *Journal of Occupational Science, 10,* 99–106.

Whiteford, G. E. (2009). Problematizing life balance: Difference, diversity, and disadvantage. K. Matuska, C. Christiansen, & H. J. Polatjko (Eds.), *Life balance: Multidisciplinary theories and research* (pp. TK). Bethesda, MD/Thorofare, NJ: AOTA Press/SLACK Incorporated.

Zuzanek, J. (2009). Time-use imbalance: Developmental and emotional costs. In K. Matuska, C. Christiansen, & H. J. Polatajko (Eds.), *Life balance: Multidisciplinary theories and research* (pp. TK). Bethesda, MD/Thorofare, NJ: AOTA Press/SLACK Incorporated.

Index

Note: Page numbers in italics indicate figures and tables.